PROGRESS IN BRAIN RESEARCH

VOLUME 185

HUMAN SLEEP AND COGNITION
PART I: BASIC RESEARCH

PROGRESS IN BRAIN RESEARCH

VOLUME 185

HUMAN SLEEP AND COGNITION
PART I: BASIC RESEARCH

EDITED BY

GERARD A. KERKHOF

Department of Psychology,
University of Amsterdam
Amsterdam
The Netherlands

HANS P.A. VAN DONGEN

Sleep and Performance Research Center
Washington State University Spokane
Spokane, WA
USA

ELSEVIER

AMSTERDAM – BOSTON – HEIDELBERG – LONDON – NEW YORK – OXFORD
PARIS – SAN DIEGO – SAN FRANCISCO – SINGAPORE – SYDNEY – TOKYO

Elsevier
Radarweg 29, PO Box 211, 1000 AE Amsterdam, The Netherlands
Linacre House, Jordan Hill, Oxford OX2 8DP, UK
360 Park Avenue South, New York, NY 10010-1710

First edition 2010

Library of Congress Cataloging-in-Publication Data
A catalog record for this book is available from the Library of Congress

British Library Cataloguing in Publication Data
A catalogue record for this book is available from the British Library

ISBN: 978-0-444-53702-7
ISSN: 0079-6123

Printed and bound in Great Britain

10 11 12 13 10 9 8 7 6 5 4 3 2 1

List of Contributors

P. Achermann, Institute of Pharmacology and Toxicology, University of Zürich; Zürich Center for Integrative Human Physiology, University of Zürich, Zürich, Switzerland
E. Altena, Department Sleep and Cognition, Netherlands Institute for Neuroscience, an Institute of the Royal Netherlands Academy of Arts and Sciences, Amsterdam, The Netherlands
S. Banks, Centre for Sleep Research, University of South Australia, Adelaide, SA, Australia
T.E. Bjorness, Department of Psychiatry, University of Texas Southwestern, Dallas, TX, USA
S. Fulda, Max Planck Institute for Psychiatry, Munich, Germany
A. Geiger, Child Development Center, University Children's Hospital Zürich; Zürich Center for Integrative Human Physiology, University of Zürich, Zürich, Switzerland
J.M. Hinson, Department of Psychology, Washington State University, Pullman, WA, USA
O.G. Jenni, Child Development Center, University Children's Hospital Zürich; Zürich Center for Integrative Human Physiology, University of Zürich, Zürich, Switzerland
B. Kemp, Sleep Centre, Medical Centre Haaglanden, The Hague; Department of Neurology, Leiden University Medical Centre, Leiden, The Netherlands
W.D.S. Killgore, Neuroimaging Center, McLean Hospital, Harvard Medical School, Belmont, MA, USA
L. Lack, School of Psychology, Flinders University, Adelaide, SA, Australia
N. Lovato, School of Psychology, Flinders University, Adelaide, SA, Australia
G.R. Poe, Departments of Anesthesiology and Molecular and Integrative Physiology, University of Michigan, Ann Arbor, MI, USA
J.R. Ramautar, Department Sleep and Cognition, Netherlands Institute for Neuroscience, an Institute of the Royal Netherlands Academy of Arts and Sciences, Amsterdam, The Netherlands
A.C. Reynolds, Centre for Sleep Research, University of South Australia, Adelaide, SA, Australia
H. Schulz, Department of Educational Science and Psychology, Free University Berlin, Berlin, Germany
Y.D. Van Der Werf, Department Sleep and Cognition, Netherlands Institute for Neuroscience, an Institute of the Royal Netherlands Academy of Arts and Sciences, Department of Anatomy and Neurosciences, VU University Medical Center, Amsterdam, The Netherlands
E.J.W. Van Someren, Department Sleep and Cognition, Netherlands Institute for Neuroscience, an Institute of the Royal Netherlands Academy of Arts and Sciences, Amsterdam; Sleep Center Leiden, Departments of Neurology and Radiology, Leiden Institute for Brain and Cognition, Leiden University Medical Center, Leiden; Department of Integrative Neurophysiology, Faculty of Earth and Life Sciences, VU University Amsterdam, Amsterdam, The Netherlands
M.P. Walker, Sleep and Neuroimaging Laboratory, Department of Psychology, Helen Wills Neuroscience Institute, University of California, Berkeley, CA, USA
C.M. Walsh, Neuroscience Interdepartmental Program, University of Michigan, Ann Arbor, MI, USA
J. Waterhouse, Research Institute for Sport and Exercise Sciences, Liverpool John Moores University, Liverpool, UK
P. Whitney, Department of Psychology, Washington State University, Pullman, WA, USA

To Emmy and Judith

Preface

It is increasingly recognized that there is a critical, bi-directional relationship between sleep and cognition. The literature in this area, encompassing rich and multi-dimensional research foci, is dotted with important discoveries – but surprisingly scattered. For example, dozens of recent papers in about as many different scientific journals are hotly debating what happens in the human brain during sleep and sleep deprivation and how this affects cognitive performance. For psychologists, sleep researchers, neuroscientists, clinicians and others working in a range of disciplines where sleep and cognition are highly relevant, it is difficult to get a good overview of the basic principles, latest discoveries and outstanding challenges. Perhaps because of the inter-disciplinary nature of the science of sleep and cognition, it is not a clearly defined sub-discipline in any established academic field, and as yet not well integrated.

Human Sleep and Cognition (Parts 1 and 2) aims to bring together and make accessible cutting-edge research on the topic in the basic, clinical and applied sciences, in order to review current knowledge and understanding, provide a starting point for researchers and practitioners entering the field, and build a platform for further research and discovery. Volume 1 deals with the basic aspects, primarily based on human data but also including some relevant animal research. The volume is organized into the following three sections: ‘Basic aspects of sleep and cognition’, ‘Sleep manipulation and impact on cognition’ and ‘Developmental aspects of sleep and cognition’.

In Part 1: Basic Research, Poe, Walsh and Bjorness describe brain mechanisms underlying cognitive processes and the impact of sleep on these processes, in particular learning and memory (Poe et al., 2010). Walker (2010) reviews the role of sleep in the regulation of cognitive and emotional brain processes, with intriguing implications for mood disorders. Whitney and Hinson (2010) emphasize that the interpretation of measures of overall task performance without consideration of the distinct cognitive processes involved can yield misleading conclusions. In a discussion of methodological issues for studies of sleep and cognition, Fulda and Schulz (2010) draw examples from investigations of treatment effects in sleep-disordered patients. Focusing on the technology of recording sleep, Kemp (2010) highlights methodological pitfalls and offers novel approaches for quantifying sleep processes. Reynolds and Banks (2010) juxtapose the effects of sleep deprivation, sleep restriction and sleep disruption on cognitive functioning. Killgore (2010) discusses whether sleep deprivation affects cognitive capabilities globally through degraded alertness, or whether it impairs specific components of cognition more than others. Waterhouse (2010) explains the effects of circadian rhythm and time awake on cognitive performance, in particular in relation to time zone transitions and shift work. Lovato and Lack (2010) compare the benefits of short versus long naps as a means to restore alertness, with a brief discussion of the detrimental effect of sleep inertia immediately after awakening. In the context of developmental changes, Geiger, Achermann and Jenni look for associations between sleep, intellectual ability and cognitive processing, arguing that general traits should be differentiated from state-dependent fluctuations (Geiger et al., 2010). And, upon reviewing the age- and insomnia-related changes in cognition and brain, Altena, Ramautar, Van Der Werf and Van Someren contend that age-related cognitive decline may be partially due to degraded sleep quality (Altena et al., 2010).

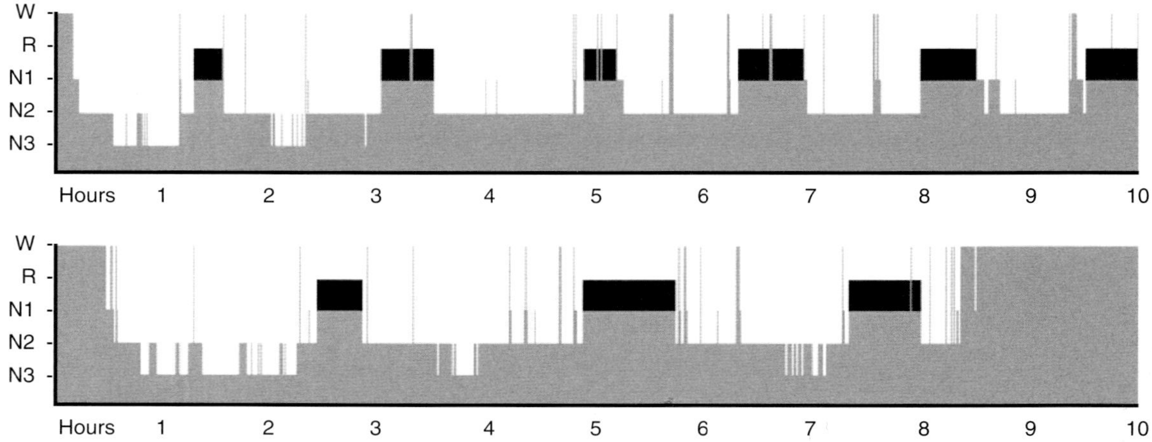

Fig. 1. Illustration of stereotypical and variant sleep structures in healthy young adults. Human sleep is conventionally characterized by means of polysomnography, which involves the recording of small electrical signals from the brain (electroencephalogram; EEG), eyes (electro-oculogram; EOG) and muscles (electromyogram; EMG), in addition to other physiological signals such as breathing and heart rate. Visual scoring criteria have been established (Iber et al., 2007; Rechtschaffen and Kales, 1968) to classify polysomnographically recorded sleep on the basis of the EEG, EOG and EMG – which change dynamically as sleep time progresses – into distinct sleep stages, specifically, rapid eye movement (REM) sleep and different levels of non-REM sleep. Top: Example hypnogram of a stereotypical nocturnal baseline pattern of sleep stages recorded during 10 h nocturnal time-in-bed (TIB) from 22:00 until 08:00. The hypnogram shows six sleep cycles of about 100 min duration on average, each consisting of an episode of non-REM (stages N1–N3) sleep followed by an episode of REM sleep (stage R; black bars). Notice that slow wave sleep (deep sleep) stage N3 is present only in the first few sleep cycles, whereas stages N2 and N1 (light sleep) are more prevalent during later sleep cycles. REM sleep is also expressed more towards the end of the nocturnal sleep period. There are occasional sleep stage transitions and brief intermittent awakenings (W), but overall, sleep is highly consolidated. Bottom: Example hypnogram of a variant nocturnal baseline pattern of sleep stages, in another subject recorded during 10 h TIB from 22:00 until 08:00. The subject exhibited no behavioural, psychological or clinical abnormalities, no recognized sleep-wake or circadian disorder, and no history of restricted or unusual sleep. Nevertheless, the sleep structure in this subject deviates significantly from the stereotype, with longer sleep cycle duration, more stage N3 sleep and earlier final awakening. Such inter-individual variations in sleep structure are considerably trait-like, but their functional relevance is unknown. Sleep was recorded here with Nihon Kohden equipment, and sleep stages were scored visually based on the criteria set forth by the American Academy of Sleep Medicine (Iber et al., 2007).

Intensive research over the past few decades has elucidated many psychophysiological, neuroanatomical and biomolecular aspects of sleep, but the function(s) of sleep and its various stages (see Fig. 1) remain to be uncovered. In the process of further unravelling sleep, researchers benefit substantially from input from the cognitive sciences. For example, inconsistent results regarding the effects of sleep deprivation on cognitive task performance are being clarified through a detailed understanding of the cognitive processes involved in performing the task at hand. For the cognitive sciences, there is also much to learn from studies of sleep and sleep loss. A good example is the improved understanding of memory processes resulting from research on the role of sleep in learning and memory. As such, studies of sleep in the context of cognition, and vice versa, are fruitful for progress in both areas. This is true across development and aging, as well as in pathological conditions including sleep disorders and neurological disease. Additionally, there are clear advantages to studying sleep and cognition in applied settings, not the least of which is concerned with improvements in safety that can be achieved by managing sleep, fatigue and cognitive impairment in 24-h operational environments.

The chapters in *Human Sleep and Cognition,* Part 1: Basic Research, provide an in-depth overview of the state-of-the-art of basic research on sleep and cognition, and a solid and fascinating foundation for the clinical and applied chapters of Part 2: Clinical and Applied Research.

Gerard A. Kerkhof
Hans P.A. Van Dongen

References

Altena, E., Ramautar, J. R., Van Der Werf, Y. D., & Van Someren, E. J. W. (2010). Do sleep complaints contribute to age-related cognitive decline? In: Kerkhof, G. A., Van Dongen, H. P. A. (Eds.), *Human sleep and cognition. Part 1: Basic research. Progress in Brain Research. Vol. 185*, Elsevier, Amsterdam.

Fulda, S., & Schulz, H. (2010). How treatment affects cognitive deficits in patients with sleep disorders: Methodological issues and results. In: Kerkhof, G. A., Van Dongen, H. P. A. (Eds.), *Human sleep and cognition. Part 1: Basic research. Progress in Brain Research. Vol. 185*, Elsevier, Amsterdam.

Geiger, A., Achermann, P., & Jenni, O. G. (2010). Sleep, intelligence and cognition in a developmental context: Differentiation between traits and state-dependent aspects. In: Kerkhof, G. A., Van Dongen, H. P. A. (Eds.), *Human sleep and cognition. Part 1: Basic research. Progress in Brain Research. Vol. 185*, Elsevier, Amsterdam.

Iber, C., Ancoli-Israel, S., Chesson Jr., A. L., & Quan, S. F. (2007). *The AASM manual for the scoring of sleep and associated events. Rules, terminology and technical specifications.* American Academy of Sleep Medicine, Westchester.

Kemp, B. (2010). Measurement of sleep. In: Kerkhof, G. A., Van Dongen, H. P. A. (Eds.), *Human sleep and cognition. Part 1: Basic research. Progress in Brain Research. Vol. 185*, Elsevier, Amsterdam.

Killgore, W. D. S. (2010). Effects of sleep deprivation on cognition. In: Kerkhof, G. A., Van Dongen, H. P. A. (Eds.), *Human sleep and cognition. Part 1: Basic research. Progress in Brain Research. Vol. 185*, Elsevier, Amsterdam.

Lovato, N., & Lack, L. (2010). The effects of napping on cognitive functioning. In: Kerkhof, G. A., Van Dongen, H. P. A. (Eds.), *Human sleep and cognition. Part 1: Basic research. Progress in Brain Research. Vol. 185*, Elsevier, Amsterdam.

Poe, G. R., Walsh, C. M., & Bjorness, T. E. (2010). Cognitive neuroscience of sleep. In: Kerkhof, G. A., Van Dongen, H. P. A. (Eds.), *Human sleep and cognition. Part 1: Basic research. Progress in Brain Research. Vol. 185*, Elsevier, Amsterdam.

Rechtschaffen, A., & Kales, A. (1968). *A manual of standardized terminology, techniques, and scoring system for sleep stages of human subjects.* UCLA Brain Information Service, Los Angeles.

Reynolds, A. C., & Banks, S. (2010). Sleep deprivation, chronic sleep restriction and sleep disruption. In: Kerkhof, G. A., Van Dongen, H. P. A. (Eds.), *Human sleep and cognition. Part 1: Basic research. Progress in Brain Research. Vol. 185*, Elsevier, Amsterdam.

Walker, M. P. (2010). Sleep, memory and emotion. In: Kerkhof, G. A., Van Dongen, H. P. A. (Eds.), *Human sleep and cognition. Part 1: Basic research. Progress in Brain Research. Vol. 185*, Elsevier, Amsterdam.

Waterhouse, J. (2010). Circadian rhythms and cognition. In: Kerkhof, G. A., Van Dongen, H. P. A. (Eds.), *Human sleep and cognition. Part 1: Basic research. Progress in Brain Research. Vol. 185*, Elsevier, Amsterdam.

Whitney, P., & Hinson, J. M. (2010). Measurement of cognition in studies of sleep deprivation. In: Kerkhof, G. A., Van Dongen, H. P. A. (Eds.), *Human sleep and cognition. Part 1: Basic research. Progress in Brain Research. Vol. 185*, Elsevier, Amsterdam.

Contents

Section III. Developmental aspects of sleep and cognition

G. A. Kerkhof and H. P. A. Van Dongen (Eds.)
Progress in Brain Research, Vol. 185
ISSN: 0079-6123

CHAPTER 1

Cognitive neuroscience of sleep

Gina R. Poe[†,*], Christine M. Walsh[‡] and Theresa E. Bjorness[§]

[†]*Departments of Anesthesiology and Molecular and Integrative Physiology, University of Michigan, Ann Arbor, MI, USA*
[‡]*Neuroscience Interdepartmental Program, University of Michigan, Ann Arbor, MI, USA*
[§]*Department of Psychiatry, University of Texas Southwestern, Dallas, TX, USA*

Abstract: Mechanism is at the heart of understanding, and this chapter addresses underlying brain mechanisms and pathways of cognition and the impact of sleep on these processes, especially those serving learning and memory. This chapter reviews the current understanding of the relationship between sleep/waking states and cognition from the perspective afforded by basic neurophysiological investigations. The extensive overlap between sleep mechanisms and the neurophysiology of learning and memory processes provide a foundation for theories of a functional link between the sleep and learning systems. Each of the sleep states, with its attendant alterations in neurophysiology, is associated with facilitation of important functional learning and memory processes. For rapid eye movement (REM) sleep, salient features such as PGO waves, theta synchrony, increased acetylcholine, reduced levels of monoamines and, within the neuron, increased transcription of plasticity-related genes, cumulatively allow for freely occurring bidirectional plasticity, long-term potentiation (LTP) and its reversal, depotentiation. Thus, REM sleep provides a novel neural environment in which the synaptic remodelling essential to learning and cognition can occur, at least within the hippocampal complex. During non-REM sleep Stage 2 spindles, the cessation and subsequent strong bursting of noradrenergic cells and coincident reactivation of hippocampal and cortical targets would also increase synaptic plasticity, allowing targeted bidirectional plasticity in the neocortex as well. In delta non-REM sleep, orderly neuronal reactivation events in phase with slow wave delta activity, together with high protein synthesis levels, would facilitate the events that convert early LTP to long-lasting LTP. Conversely, delta sleep does not activate immediate early genes associated with *de novo* LTP. This non-REM sleep-unique genetic environment combined with low acetylcholine levels may serve to reduce the strength of cortical circuits that activate in the ~50% of delta-coincident reactivation events that do not appear in their waking firing sequence. The chapter reviews the results of manipulation studies, typically total sleep or REM sleep deprivation, that serve to underscore the functional significance of the phenomenological associations. Finally, the implications of sleep neurophysiology

[*] Corresponding author.
Tel.: (+) 734-763-2128; Fax: (+) 734-764-9332.
E-mail: ginapoe@umich.edu

DOI:10.1016/B978-0-444-53702-7.00001-4

for learning and memory will be considered from a larger perspective in which the association of specific sleep states with both potentiation or depotentiation is integrated into mechanistic models of cognition.

Keywords: Bidirectional plasticity; long-term potentiation (LTP); depotentiation; spindles; theta; slow waves; acetylcholine (ACh); norepinephrine (NE); serotonin (5HT); memory consolidation; Spike Timing Dependent Plasticity (STDP)

In the last 20 years, evidence linking sleep traits and cognitive processes underlying learning and memory has developed in several research domains. Other chapters in this volume describe aspects of the relationship between sleep and cognition gleaned from behavioural paradigms and/or neuroimaging data in humans to elucidate the functional anatomy underlying sleep and cognition. The focus of this chapter is the physiological knowledge gained from research, conducted almost exclusively in animals, that has provided an outline of the underlying mechanisms whereby sleep affects learning and memory. Two broad areas will be covered: (1) physiological traits of rapid eye movement (REM) sleep, non-rapid eye movement sleep (non-REM) sleep and the Stage 2 transition to REM state that affect the substrate of learning and memory, synaptic plasticity; and (2) revelations from sleep deprivation studies that demonstrate a functional role for sleep in the normal expression of learning and memory. The chapter concludes with a summary of unresolved controversies and future directions.

Cognitive processes involve neural oscillations and synchronization among brain regions that are active during attention, perception, working memory, short- and long-term memory acquisition, retention and recall, imagination and thought (Axmacher et al., 2006; Crick and Koch, 1998; Llinas and Ribary, 1993). Dynamic cognitive networks that become engaged in a thought or task work through temporary bands of activity that synchronize multiple brain areas into a functional unit. For example, Jones and Wilson (2005) showed that the hippocampus and prefrontal cortex oscillate together when rats perform a spatial memory task requiring both areas. Just as periods of synchronization occur while performing cognitive tasks during waking (e.g. Brown and McCormack, 2006), periods of synchronization also appear in all other states in various frequencies and extent of brain areas involved. Cheng et al. (2008) propose that sleep states themselves are a less useful categorization schema in which to examine what occurs offline for cognition. Instead, predominant electroencephalographic (EEG) frequencies, which often coincide with particular sleep states, should be examined to uncover the role of sleep for cognition. Specific sleep traits, including dominant frequencies, neurochemical milieu and neuronal activation patterns, can be dissociated from their normal state under relatively normal conditions. Here we examine the role of each state with particular emphasis on their traits, and the role of each trait for cognition with particular regard to learning and memory.

Spontaneous physiological processes during natural sleep to support cognition

REM sleep

Two books that nicely explain the role of REM sleep for memory were published 22 years apart (Winson, 1985; Walter, 2007). Walter reviews most of the literature and consensus findings in 'REM Illumination: Memory Consolidation', providing a framework to understand current ongoing research. Theoretical perspectives in 'Brain and Psyche: the Biology of the Unconscious' by Jonathan Winson in 1985 presented many of the concepts of REM sleep involvement in memory consolidation that are now found in most publications concerning REM sleep and learning. Winson and Pavlides (Pavlides and Winson, 1989; Pavlides et al., 1988) were the first to record hippocampal unit activity during activity and subsequent sleep, revealing startlingly non-random activity patterns during sleep. Their findings stimulated many others to measure the physiological processes at work supporting cognition during sleep on a cellular level, as discussed further below.

Not long after Pavlides and Winson joined the handful of those actively engaged in sleep and memory research (e.g. Hennvin, Guerrin, LeConte and Smith), two studies were published back to back in *Science* that highlighted the sleep and learning field for a broader scientific audience. The first (Karni et al., 1994), later replicated and expanded in 2002 (Mednick et al., 2002), showed that REM sleep effects on memory consolidation were circuit-specific. A visual perceptual learning task that causes focal synaptic changes to occur in the visual cortex needed REM sleep for strong, lasting improvements. The REM sleep–associated synaptic gains were specific to the circuits trained and did not generally transfer to all other visual processing fields. This elegant study kindled new excitement in the puzzle of REM sleep and memory and revitalized the sleep and memory field in general. The other landmark paper (Wilson and McNaughton, 1994) was met with equal enthusiasm, and amplified the Pavlides and Winson (1988, 1989) finding of orderly hippocampal reactivation during sleep; it will be discussed in greater detail under non-REM sleep, below.

Learning increases REM sleep

Spontaneous increases in REM sleep follow training and precede large increases in performance during learning (Bramham et al., 1994; Fishbein et al., 1974; Hennevin et al., 1974; Lucero, 1970; Portell-Cortes et al., 1989; Smith and Rose, 1996; Smith and Wong, 1991; Smith et al., 1980) associated with acquiring the task (Datta, 2000; Hennevin et al., 1995). REM sleep increases in humans just after intensive learning trials as well (De Koninck et al., 1989; Mandai et al., 1989; Smith, 1995; Smith and Lapp, 1991). Learning can either prolong and/or intensify REM sleep (Dujardin et al., 1990; Guerrien et al., 1989; Mandai et al., 1989; Smith et al., 1980). While it is not the case that smarter animals have more REM sleep (Siegel, 2001), studies of increased REM sleep during times of learning have never been made across species. It appears from the majority of studies that the total time in REM sleep is not as important as the REM sleep augmentation that is accomplished during times of high learning demands.

PGO waves increase with learning

Waves of excitation originating from the brainstem, called ponto-geniculo-occipital (PGO) waves, or P-waves in the rat, occur only during REM sleep and the transition to REM sleep (TR) (Jouvet, 1962). PGO waves are coincident with REMs and middle ear muscle activity as well as occasional myoclonic jerks of postural musculature (Lai and Siegel, 1991). Both auditory and somatosensory stimuli influence PGO wave activity [for review, see Callaway et al. (1987)]. The dorsal part of the nucleus subcoeruleus of the pons in the rat is the most effective area for inducing PGO waves and probably initiates their propagation through the medial reticular formation (MRF) to the forebrain. This area projects to the hippocampus and amygdala, among other structures (Datta et al., 1998). During intensive learning, PGO waves increase in intensity and density during REM sleep and TR, and their increase is directly correlated with task retention (Datta, 2000). PGO waves are hypothesized by Datta et al. (2004) to be a potent regulator of synaptic plasticity in both the hippocampus and the amygdala, as they comprise large, synchronous excitatory waves of glutamate that terminate directly on forebrain targets.

Hippocampus for associative learning and memory consolidation

The rapid encoding structure of the hippocampus is where the building block for memory encoding, long-term potentiation (LTP), was discovered (Bliss and Lomo, 1973). Memory consolidation is the transfer of this hippocampal plasticity to more permanent long-term storage sites distributed throughout the neocortex. LTP requires postsynaptic membrane depolarization coincident with presynaptic action potentials to allow the intracellular cascade of molecular events that effect long-term increases in synaptic strength. LTP is easily induced during wakefulness and REM sleep in the hippocampus (Bramham and Srebro, 1989).

REM sleep neuronal reactivation

Pavlides and Winson (1989) were the first to show increased firing of hippocampal neurons in REM sleep that had been active in prior waking. Many others have repeated and enhanced that work. Hippocampal pyramidal cells can act as place field encoders, or place cells, firing rapidly in a particular area of the environment as the animal navigates through, then falling silent elsewhere. Studies have shown that place cells that have overlapping fields in an environment and therefore fire in an ordered, overlapping fashion show increased co-activation during 'offline' hippocampal large irregular activity (LIA), which occurs during non-REM sleep and quiet waking (QW) (Wilson and McNaughton, 1994). Very structured replay of the waking track running sequences were also seen during REM sleep (Louie and Wilson, 2001). Our study (Poe et al., 2000) showed that spontaneous reactivation of hippocampal neurons during REM sleep occurs in a theta-specific pattern concordant with the induction of both LTP and with its reversal, depotentiation, during the REM sleep state.

Theta phase specificity

Place cells fire in a specific relationship to the ongoing EEG theta (5–10 Hz) rhythm activity during active waking. Most spikes occur at the peaks (corresponding to the maximum depolarization of the cell membrane) of theta, as the cell discharges through the place field (Buzsaki et al., 1983; Fox et al., 1986). Pavlides et al. (1988) found that stimulation on the positive phase of the hippocampal theta rhythm induced LTP; stimulation at the opposite phase, the theta trough, induced a decrease in synaptic efficacy (depotentiation). Huerta and Lisman (1995) found that LTP and depotentiation could be induced at the theta peak and trough, respectively, with a burst of only four 200 Hz stimuli lasting 20 ms and applied to the Schaeffer collaterals. Others have shown this result in the intact animal (Hyman et al., 2003; Orr et al., 2001). These experiments showed that LTP could be induced with physiologically feasible stimuli, if timed to the naturally occurring theta activity.

Acetylcholine (ACh) inputs allow the hippocampus to display theta activity during active waking and REM sleep. Givens (1996) found a stimulus-evoked resetting of the dentate theta rhythm during working memory tasks in rats. ACh is important to the induction of LTP in the intact animal and to learning in the hippocampus (Givens, 1996; Hasselmo and Bower, 1993; Mizumori et al., 1990; Rashidy-Pour et al., 1996; Winson, 1978). Similarly, disruptions of hippocampal theta impair learning [see Vertes and Kocsis (1997)]. Hasselmo and Bower (1993) suggest and Détári et al. (1999) showed that cholinergic activity may be modulated by ongoing memory or cognitive demands in the system.

Hippocampal measures of ACh release during REM sleep exceed those measured during waking, although they are probably equal to levels present during active waking behaviours (Marrosu et al., 1995). Stimulation of the MRF, the same area that propagates PGO waves during waking startle and REM sleep, induces theta rhythm activity in the hippocampus (Vertes, 1982). The evidence suggests that the timing of incoming stimuli relative to the cell's membrane polarity, which normally oscillates with theta, influences the induction of LTP and depotentiation; dampened theta amplitudes are less conducive to learning. When the reticular formation is stimulated in REM sleep, increasing hippocampal theta, rats improve significantly on memory retention tasks over those given the same stimulation in slow wave sleep (e.g. Hennevin et al., 1989). Reticular stimulation can reverse the mnemonic impairments imposed by REM sleep deprivation (Hars and Hennevin, 1983). Reticular neurons exert their influence on hippocampal theta through projections to the supramammillary nucleus, which in turn projects to the septal nuclei that provide timed cholinergic and GABAergic inputs to CA1 pyramidal cells and interneurons (Vertes and Kocsis, 1997).

We found that neurons active in novel places discharge at the peaks of local theta oscillations in both waking and REM sleep (Poe et al., 2000). Such peak theta phase firing is consistent with establishing LTP in support of memory formation. Once the place becomes familiar to the animal, neurons that were active in these places *reverse phase* at which they fire with respect to local theta oscillations during REM sleep. That is, although place cells fired at theta peaks in REM sleep when the environment was novel, they fired at theta troughs in REM sleep once the environment is familiar. Cells active only in familiar areas of the environment in waking fire at theta troughs in REM sleep. Although the mechanism of such reversed phase firing during REM sleep is unclear, such phase-reversed firing during theta is consistent with patterns that induce the depotentiation of previously potentiated synapses.

The importance of depotentiation

Depotentiation is important to theories of learning and memory that incorporate a temporary associative memory structure such as the hippocampus. The hippocampus is a temporary storage facility for memory; hippocampal synapses are more limited in number as compared to the entire neocortical mantle, where long-term memories are probably stored in a parallel, distributed fashion. Thus, if the hippocampus serves to form associative memories and temporarily store them until they are consolidated to the neocortex, it is logical that the hippocampal network of weighted synapses involved with consolidated memories should be recycled for future differential weighting of associative memories in other functional assemblies. Depotentiation may serve that synaptic recycling function in the CA1 region of the hippocampus where there is no adult neurogenesis.

A growing literature suggests that depotentiation is also critical to cognitive function (Braunewell and Manahan-Vaughan, 2001; Manahan-Vaughan and Braunewell, 1999; Nakao et al., 2002). Depotentiation seems to be associated with the addition of new stimuli to a contextual frame (Kemp and Manahan-Vaughan, 2004). Biphasic changes in synaptic strength could separate the acquisition of different types of information. Novel spatial exploration induces depotentiation of previously induced but irrelevant LTP (Xu et al., 1998). After two exposures to an environment with the same objects always located in the same spatial locations, depotentiation was expressed after a third exposure merely by changing the configuration of the objects. The re-association of objects within a particular spatial context triggers depotentiation, probably due to the necessity of rewiring the memory network to accommodate the new change in formation for efficient storage.

Requirements of depotentiation met in REM sleep: NE and 5HT absence

Depotentiation may be more reliably induced in the absence of norepinephrine (NE), which pushes the net effect of all activity towards LTP. NE, working at both beta and alpha1 receptors, blocks depotentiation in the hippocampus and enhances LTP (Katsuki et al., 1997; Thomas et al., 1996; Yang et al., 2002). Either stimulation of the noradrenergic cells of the locus coeruleus (LC), or direct intracerebroventricular application of NE enhances and prolongs LTP (Almaguer-Melian et al., 2005).

REM sleep is a time when noradrenergic inputs are suppressed (Aston-Jones and Bloom, 1981; Nitz and Siegel, 1997). Noradrenergic neurons are tonically active in all states except REM sleep (Aston-Jones and Bloom, 1981), and in brief periods before each spindle wave during non-REM sleep. Therefore, we hypothesize that REM sleep and possibly the TR are the only times when theta trough activity in the CA1 region has the opportunity to depotentiate synapses from spontaneous neural activity in the intact animal.

Serotonin (5HT) is present in the hippocampus in all states but is vastly diminished in REM sleep (Park et al., 1999), when dorsal raphe serotonergic neurons are inactive (McGinty and Harper, 1976). We hypothesize that the absence of 5HT in the hippocampus during REM sleep allows that state to serve a depotentiation function supporting the reworking of networks for maximally efficient cognitive function.

Both depotentiation and habituation to an environment were inhibited by 5HT agonist application (Kemp and Manahan-Vaughan, 2004). 5HT agonist application also improved acquisition but impaired memory consolidation (Meneses and Hong, 1997). The pre-training stimulation of serotonergic type 4 (5-HT_4) receptors enhanced the acquisition of a conditioned response, while post-training activation of postsynaptic 5-HT_4 receptors impaired the consolidation of learning. Thus, it may be that 5-HT_4 receptor activation is beneficial for certain types of information acquisition that depend on LTP and detrimental for other types that depend on depotentiation. The available studies show that, through the 5-HT_4 receptor, 5HT depresses depotentiation and impairs memory consolidation.

These two neurotransmitter systems, noradrenaline and 5HT, influence synaptic excitability and plasticity and fall uniquely silent during REM sleep (Aston-Jones and Bloom, 1981; McGinty and Harper, 1976), allowing the hippocampus to both strengthen and refine the memories it encodes. Thus, the neurochemical environment of REM sleep and specific reactivation patterns relative to the theta rhythm are consistent with a unique opportunity to depotentiate, or weaken, those synapses encoding memories already consolidated to structures outside the hippocampus. Such depotentiation would be especially important during intensive learning periods such as during development and for integrating old knowledge with changing novel information.

More evidence for synaptic plasticity in REM sleep: gene studies

It could also be true that neural reactivation in any stage of sleep or wakefulness serves no purpose for learning and memory. This is unlikely to be the case, especially in REM sleep when ACh levels are high, theta is present in the hippocampus, the forebrain is activated by PGO waves and LTP is readily induced as mentioned above (Bramham and Srebro, 1989). Furthermore, Ribeiro et al. (1999, 2002) have shown that *zif*-268, an immediate early gene involved in LTP, is upregulated in the hippocampus and associated neocortical structures during REM sleep following waking learning and LTP. Further, the zif-268 activation occurs in the hippocampus and entorhinal cortex in the first REM sleep period after learning, then in primary and secondary associated structures in ensuing REM sleep periods, as though consolidation of the memory from the hippocampus to the neocortex were being accomplished in one sleep session.

Multiple cellular tests of LTP and depotentiation are now available in the freely behaving animal. Thus, the question of whether reactivation results in synaptic plasticity and learning will be directly addressed in future research.

Non-REM sleep

Learning amplifies slow waves (Huber et al., 2004; Wamsley et al., 2010). Slow waves, shown in a rat recording in Fig. 1, allow a reactivation of neurons that were involved in learning or encoding during theta states on a much accelerated ($\sim 300\times$),

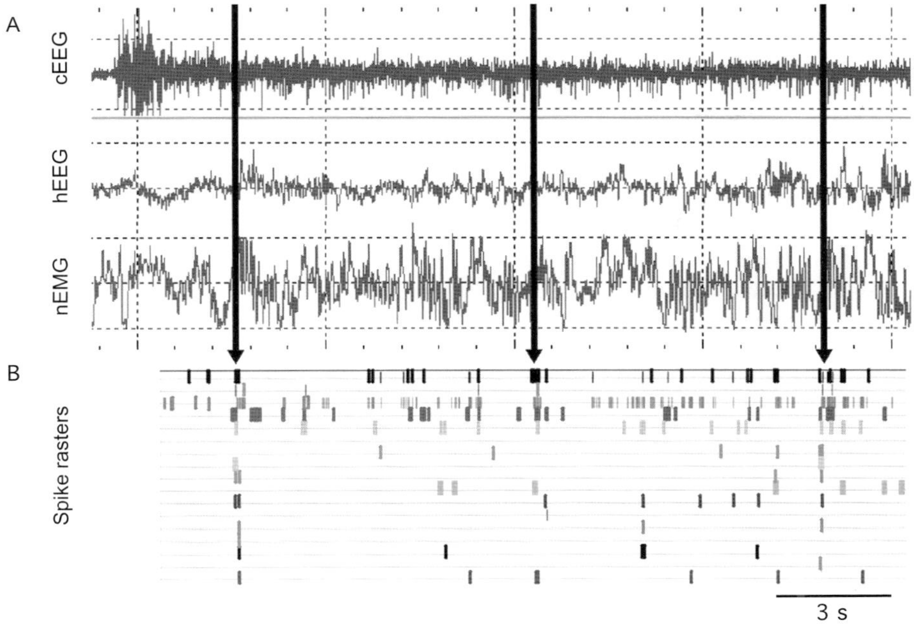

Fig. 1. Electroencephalographic (EEG) and electromyographic (EMG) signals across 20 s of recording time. (A) Vertical grid spacing is 200 μV. Cortical EEG was taken as the differential signal from screw electrodes placed over the frontal cortices. Hippocampal EEG (hEEG) was recorded from a tetrode (4 individual 12 μm nichrome recording wires twisted together such that the distance between wires is ~15 μm) placed at the hilus and referenced to a tetrode placed in the corpus callosum. These data were taken from a rat implanted with a tetrode assembly (12 tetrodes) recorded from a resting pot after a maze run during a period of wakefulness (high variable EMG) without voluntary movement, allowing slow waves rather than theta to appear in the hEEG trace. Slow waves appear in the hippocampus both during non-REM sleep and during quiet wakefulness. (B) Times of action potentials from 17 simultaneously recorded hippocampal neurons (1 spike raster row for each cell) show bursts of coincident reactivation at the depolarized peaks of the hippocampal slow waves (arrows) during this period of quiet wakefulness. (For interpretation of the references to colour in this figure legend, the reader is referred to the web version of this book.)

condensed time scale (Kudrimoti et al., 1999; Pavlides and Winson, 1989; Wilson and McNaughton, 1994).

Part B of Fig. 1 shows an example of multiple single units recorded in our laboratory during hippocampal slow waves. Many laboratories have documented a rise in slow wave activity during slow wave sleep associated with increased waking task requirements demanded from the same area of neocortex (Borbely and Achermann, 2005; Borbely et al., 1981; Esser et al., 2007; Ferrara et al., 2008; Franken et al., 1991; Krueger and Obal, 1993; Riedner et al., 2007; Vyazovskiy et al., 2000, 2007). Such reactivation events occur during these delta or sharp waves (e.g. Kudrimoti et al., 1999; Ribeiro and Nicolelis, 2004; Wilson and McNaughton, 1994), which we will henceforth call slow waves.

Non-REM sleep reactivation for memory interleaving and consolidation

The function of such coordinated offline reactivation has been proposed to be for memory consolidation. A host of multiple single unit publications hypothesize that slow wave-dependent activity would serve to strengthen memory circuits even though most of them have shown that cross correlations strong at the start of slow wave activity are weakened within 10–20 min of such activity (Kudrimoti et al., 1999; Wilson and McNaughton, 1994). LTP requires postsynaptic membrane depolarization coincident with presynaptic action potentials to allow the intracellular cascade of molecular events that effect long-term increases in synaptic strength. The conditions of LTP may be well satisfied during hippocampal slow wave oscillations and reactivations (Tsukamoto-Yasui et al., 2007). Cells are synchronously depolarized, allowing the opening of voltage-gated Ca^{2+} channels and the unblocking of NMDA channels associated with plasticity changes. Interconnected neurons that synchronously fire together allow spike timing-dependent plasticity (STDP) (Bi and Poo, 1998) to occur at their synapses.

Neurochemistry not right for LTP in non-REM sleep

However, direct evidence of a synaptic plasticity function of spontaneous offline hippocampal reactivation, whether during waking or sleep, is lacking. Synchronous firing may not be enough. ACh, so influential for synaptic plasticity as mentioned in the REM sleep section above, is at a minimum in the forebrain during non-REM sleep. In fact, ACh is not present in the slow wave-producing hemisphere during unihemispheric sleep (Lapierre et al., 2007). The addition of ACh eliminates slow waves (Lapierre et al., 2007; Vanderwolf and Stewart, 1986).

Genes not available for LTP in non-REM sleep

Further complicating the hypothesis that reactivation during non-REM sleep serves synaptic plasticity is the problem that no one has successfully induced LTP in vivo in the absence of ACh, during slow wave sleep (Bramham and Srebro, 1989; Leonard et al., 1987). More evidence against slow wave reactivation as the state to enhance LTP includes the finding that calcium-dependent gene expression related to synaptic plasticity is absent during non-REM sleep (Pompeiano et al., 1994; Ribeiro et al., 1999, 2002). Indeed, there is a rise in depotentiation-related genes and drop in LTP-related genes during sleep (Basheer et al., 1997; Cirelli and Tononi, 2000a, 2000b; Pompeiano et al., 1994, 1995, 1997).

Non-REM sleep reduces synaptic strength?

The best two pieces of physiological evidence to date that slow wave-dependent processing affects synaptic weights are (1) a rise in the amplitude of slow waves after extended waking experience that becomes attenuated again after a period of slow wave activity ensues (Hanlon et al., 2009; Steriade, 2004; Vyazovskiy et al., 2000), and (2) the decline in evoked potentials across sleep (Esser et al., 2006). These results support a role of slow wave processing in reducing the strength of synapses, rather than increasing them, which runs counter to most hypotheses of the role of slow wave processing for learning and memory.

Mechanisms for non-REM sleep downscaling

One mechanism whereby slow wave coincident reactivation could lead to synaptic downscaling or depotentiation rather than LTP is the finding that slow waves activate voltage-gated Ca^{2+} channels to allow in a little calcium, and that small amount of intracellular Ca^{2+} is not augmented by simultaneous pre- and postsynaptic depolarization in the $\sim$50% of slow waves that do not include ordered replay (Foster and Wilson, 2006; Karlsson and Frank, 2009). A disorderly replay would cause heterosynaptic depotentiation, caused by the asynchronous activation of post- then presynaptic elements according to the rules of STDP. If postsynaptic activity is also not amplified by muscarinic ACh receptor activation during non-REM sleep, then the intracellular cascade and absent strong activation of beta adrenergic receptors is set up to produce long-term depression

(LTD) instead of LTP. Small rises in intracellular Ca^{2+} set into motion a cascade of events that lead to LTD or depotentiation, rather than LTP [for review, see Blitzer et al. (2005)].

Synaptic stabilization and embossing

Instead of *de novo* synaptic strengthening, non-REM sleep may be a time for the secondary and tertiary changes required to convert short-term potentiation (early LTP, lasting minutes to a few hours) into long-lasting LTP (late LTP, measured for months). Protein synthesis, which is required for long-term LTP (late-LTP) (Frey et al., 1988; Krug et al., 1984; Otani et al., 1989), is extensively increased during the non-REM sleep (Ramm and Smith, 1990). Without protein synthesis, early LTP, which is protein synthesis-independent, would not turn into late-LTP and would only last for 4–6 h (Abraham, 2003; Abraham and Bear, 1996; Frey et al., 1988; Krug et al., 1984; Reymann and Frey, 2007), which is, perhaps not by mere coincidence, the same critical window for sleep-dependent consolidation of novel learning (see 'Sleep deprivation: physiological ramifications' section, below). Thus, non-REM sleep reactivation may serve to stabilize synapses by completing the necessary protein synthesis for those synapses that underwent sufficient LTP during prior wakefulness to induce such protein synthesis.

At the same time, non-REM sleep could serve to downscale synapses that were only weakly potentiated. If a neuron is used in an established cognitive circuit during wakefulness, then its synapses may be enhanced and 'tagged' (see below), but may not be sufficiently strengthened. Familiar circuit activation would lack the extra reverberatory firing that novelty imparts or the push towards LTP that neuromodulators such as cortisol and noradrenaline, induced by novelty, would give. Such weak synaptic enhancement of established circuits without modification during wakeful cognition would create a synaptic tag (exact mechanisms still unknown, Frey and Frey, 2008; Frey and Morris, 1997, 1998) that would degrade over a few hours if not stabilized by plasticity-related proteins. Strong stimuli at another synapse (circuit reformation) would, however, set into motion the production of such plasticity-related protein synthesis.

We propose that the approximate length of time that a tagged synapse has to be boosted or degraded probably depends on how near the synapse is to the cell soma and thus how much interference it receives through backpropagation (Golding et al., 2001) as well as how active the cell is in other circuits. The closer to the soma and the more active the cell is in other cognitive tasks, the more likely the early LTP will be degraded through heterosynaptic depotentiation mechanisms. This process may explain proactive interference. The length of time that a tagged synapse has to survive before being degraded or enhanced probably also defines the timing of the sleep-critical window (Smith, 1985). Further, the strength of the waking experience may dictate whether only non-REM sleep-related protein synthesis is needed in that window, or also *de novo* synaptic strengthening that can be induced by REM sleep reactivation. Non-REM sleep-related synaptic interference could downscale weakly potentiated synapses whose 'tag' was not picked up. Protein synthesis in non-REM sleep could stabilize strongly strengthened synapses and their weakly tagged neighbors. But, it is probably only during REM sleep that synaptic remodelling (*de novo* LTP and targeted depotentiation) occurs, thereby embossing the memory system, downscaling some synapses and strengthening others, for all the reasons outlined in the 'REM sleep' section, above.

If downscaling of reactivated familiar memories occurs during non-REM sleep (noise elimination), then the hypothesis that REM sleep is for forgetting purported by Francis Crick and Graemi Mitchison (1983) would also apply to the state of non-REM sleep.

A very notable exception to the idea that non-REM sleep allows the strongly potentiated synapses (and strong paired with weak) to be stabilized while weak synapses are allowed to fade is the activity and neurochemical environment surrounding the occurrence of sleep spindles, which also occur during non-REM sleep, but normally during the ascending Stage 2 of non-REM sleep, also known as intermediate sleep or the TR.

TR/Stage 2 sleep spindles

Rats trained on a spatial maze showed enhanced correlated firing between the hippocampus and medial prefrontal cortical areas during a working spatial memory task compared with a non-spatial task (Jones and Wilson, 2005), but Romcy-Pereira and Pavlides (2004) found that transmission between the medial prefrontal cortex and the hippocampus is strongest during a non-REM sleep. Siapas and Wilson (1998) and Siapas et al. (2005) showed that strong synchronization between the hippocampus and prefrontal cortex occurred during a state characterized by the simultaneous appearance of cortical sleep spindles (during non-REM sleep) and hippocampal theta (characterizing REM sleep) in the normal learning rat. We have observed such dissociated states in learning rats (Emrick et al., 2008).

One of the fascinating characteristics of sleep spindles is that they are generated by the thalamic reticular nucleus, and do not occur in the presence of NE. In fact, LC neurons fall silent in the second preceding each spindle (Aston-Jones and Bloom, 1981), allowing the reticular neurons to hyperpolarize until they emit Ca^{2+} spikes in the spindle frequency and coordinate the cortical projection neurons to cause cortical cells to oscillate together in a characteristic spindle (11–16 Hz) fashion (Lee and McCormick, 1996). 5HT and ACh in the thalamus also prevent spindling. Thus, spindles occur in a neurochemical environment similar to that of REM sleep, but perhaps in the absence of ACh and only in brief (1–3 s) bursts during non-REM sleep.

In several studies, there is a very good correlation between spindle occurrences during sleep and waking learning (Molle et al., 2006). And in the highly plastic visual cortex of the kitten, synaptic changes after monocular deprivation are well correlated with spindle density (Frank et al., 2001). Datta et al. (Datta, 2000; Datta et al., 2004; Mavanji and Datta, 2003) found that the TR state showed the highest increase (>300%) after intensive two-way active avoidance training in those animals that retained the task best between the training and the testing period.

If neuronal activity between the hippocampal output CA1/subiculum region and prefrontal cortex are coordinated during spindles or theta/spindle complexes, while NE is absent and 5HT levels are low, then the hippocampus could cause the same kind of targeted bidirectional synaptic reorganization in the prefrontal cortex during non-REM sleep that it may cause within itself during REM sleep. Further, the strong reactivation of the LC that initiates the termination of each spindle (Aston-Jones and Bloom, 1981) could allow the *de novo* synaptic strengthening that the circuit could need for memory consolidation. Such coordination between the hippocampus and prefrontal cortex may not occur during REM sleep, as it has been observed that the two areas do not fire together during REM sleep.

Waking 'offline' processing

The hippocampus also exhibits slow wave activity during 'offline' waking, here called quiet waking. A paper by Foster and Wilson (2006) showed that reactivation sequences occurring in the hippocampus during waking slow waves are backward in firing order compared to waking experience. STDP principles would dictate that reversed reactivation sequences may actually reverse the LTP gains on the maze run. The CA1 cells we record receive their major inputs from the CA3 region of the hippocampus, which is extensively recurrently connected. If postsynaptic target neurons fire *before* the presynaptic inputs arrive, as would be the case with backwards reactivation, then LTD or depotentiation should result. Such a result would be consistent with the observation that increased periods of wakefulness from the time of training to testing, without intervening sleep, serve to interfere with memory performance.

Waking reactivation may serve an opposing plasticity function to waking learning and sleep reactivation, consistent with behavioural data of reduced performance across post-training wakefulness (Jenkins and Dallenbach, 1924; Wamsley et al., 2010). This unravelling of memory during prolonged wakefulness may be why the traits of sleep are so important for memory preservation and consolidation. The theoretical need for reactivation to occur offline is to interleave the new information in with the old in the absence of sensory interference (Dave and Margoliash, 2000; Jenkins and Dallenbach, 1924; McClelland et al., 1995; Melton and Irwin, 1940; Winson, 1990). In songbirds learning their song, Derégnaucourt et al. (2005) found that across waking experience the song becomes more complex and error filled, but the song simplifies with the preservation of correct learned elements across sleep. Both song and speech learning literature indicates a 40–50% decrease in dendritic spines in zebra finches and mynah birds, respectively (Rausch and Scheich, 1982; Wallhausserfranke et al., 1995). It would make sense that such pruning of unneeded synaptic elements would occur during a sleep state where depotentiation and synaptic pruning were allowed.

Dissociated states

The traits mentioned for each state listed above are largely dissociable from that state, even under normal conditions. Thus, it may be less useful to ask what state serves what cognitive function, than what set of traits is necessary for each stage of preparing the brain for maximal waking effectiveness. Intermediate sleep is much increased under certain psychiatric conditions; whereas in normal persons transitions are scored at less than 10%; under psychiatric illness it can comprise up to 40% of total sleep time (Akindele et al., 1970; Nielsen, 2000). Features of REM sleep can appear in other states, a phenomenon Nielsen called 'covert REM' (Nielsen, 2000). Persons suffering under depression have altered brain neurochemistry. It could be that the noradrenergic and serotonergic environment and hippocampal patterned reactivation necessary for memory consolidation could occur, under certain conditions (e.g. prolonged sleep restriction and psychiatric illness), during the normally short state of intermediate sleep at the transition from non-REM sleep to REM sleep (Lairy et al., 1967; Mahowald and Schenck, 1992). Data from Subimal Datta's laboratory show drastic increases in transitions to REM sleep during intensive learning (Datta, 2000; Datta et al., 2004; Mavanji and Datta, 2003). However, very little overall time in any state with the right traits present may be necessary to accomplish LTP or depotentiation. Single bursts of theta frequency stimuli can cause LTP and depotentiation (Huerta and Lisman, 1995), so plasticity effects could be obtained in only a few seconds of replay in the proper phase of the ongoing EEG.

Sleep deprivation: physiological ramifications

Controversies and consensus

Our understanding of how sleep is important to cognition has been greatly aided by many informative sleep loss studies looking at what changes between those deprived of all or various stages of sleep and paired controls. There have been some mixed results in the sleep deprivation and learning field, however. An important early review by McGrath and Cohen (1978) gave logical methodological reasons for the discrepancies, but still, given the relative dearth of knowledge in both the sleep and the learning fields, interest in the crossover between them waned for more than a decade. Some generalities that can be pulled from the data are as follows.

For rats, tasks requiring little change in the animal's behavioural repertoire are REM sleep independent, according to Seligman (1970). When training intensity is high, the need for REM sleep for memory consolidation is more immediate (Smith, 1995); if REM sleep is prevented in the first few hours after training, memory for the task will be impaired even if total time spent in REM sleep is not diminished over the sleep period (Smith and Butler, 1982; Smith and Rose, 1996). Animals allowed to enter REM sleep in the first few hours after training perform normally the next day, even when deprived of REM sleep in a later time window of the sleep cycle. Thus, the idea of critical REM windows for memory consolidation was introduced (Smith, 1985; Smith and Butler, 1982).

There may also be critical windows for non-REM sleep-dependent reactivation. The critical window for the conversion of early LTP to late LTP that varies with the strength of LTP as well as other factors (discussed above) could be the physiological basis for these critical sleep windows.

LTP effects of sleep deprivation

More recent studies have delved into the cellular consequences of sleep deprivation. REM sleep deprivation inhibits LTP induction and maintenance (Campbell et al., 2002; Davis et al., 2003; Marks and Wayner, 2005; McDermott et al., 2003; Romcy-Pereira and Pavlides, 2004). Even basic cellular excitability metrics are depressed after the platform over water method of REM sleep deprivation (McDermott et al., 2003).

Hippocampal neurogenesis

Hairston et al. (2005) found that even only 6 h of gentle REM sleep restriction impaired place learning and abolished the learning-dependent rise in hippocampal dentate gyrus neurogenesis. Two years earlier Guzman-Marin et al. (2003) found that total sleep deprivation for 96 h on an intermittently powered treadmill reduced neurogenesis in the dentate by 40% and specifically those cells with neuronal cell markers by over 50% (Guzman-Marin et al., 2005). Because adult neurogenesis is involved in learning and memory (Gould et al., 1999), it is likely that such sleep deprivation-induced reductions in neurogenesis would impact future learning. One unanswered question is how long such depression in neurogenesis lasts after recovery from sleep deprivation, and how long the behavioural effects of prior suppression of neurogenesis lasts.

Neurogenesis occurs in the dentate and CA3 regions of the hippocampus (Tonchev and Yamashima, 2006), the novelty encoding network. These are structures of the hippocampus that do not fire primarily at theta troughs in REM sleep (Buzsaki, personal communication) and, also unlike the CA1 region, they do not receive direct temporo-ammonic (TA) inputs from the entorhinal cortex layer III to their distal dendrites. Therefore, these two areas may not be able to depotentiate and refresh their synapses for novel encoding, but instead, once their synaptic structure is saturated, they must be replaced with new neurons with fresh dendritic trees. The inability to replenish saturated dendritic trees with new neurons may be the origins of the sense of brain saturation and of feeling cognitively impaired after periods of sleep deprivation.

Other informative effects of sleep deprivation

Because other chapters in this book cover the human and imaging sleep and cognition data, including the effects of sleep deprivation, we will only list some of the other effects that could give clues as to the mechanisms of sleep impacting cognition here. Sean Drummond's laboratory has shown (Drummond et al., 2001) that sleep deprivation causes the subjects to recruit more brain areas in the performance of the same cognitive task. Matt Walker showed that hippocampal function is drastically reduced in an fMRI study after one overnight total sleep deprivation (Yoo et al., 2007). One of the arguments against the relationship between sleep and cognition is that people treated for depression with monoamine oxidase inhibitors (MAOIs) and other antidepressants obtain little to no REM sleep for long periods of time, yet have no obvious learning and memory deficits. However, learning and memory deficits have been documented for persons and animals on antidepressant medications (Burgos et al., 2005; Burt et al., 1995). Furthermore, while it is true that drugs like MAOIs significantly reduce REM sleep time, depending on the dose and individual, they often do not eliminate REM sleep altogether; on any given night the amount of REM sleep recorded from persons on MAOIs is from 0 to 75% of baseline (Akindele et al., 1970; Nicholson et al., 1989; Riemann et al., 2001). Learning needs may make homeostatic demands on the REM sleep generating mechanisms (e.g. the PGO wave generator and/or the theta generator) that either temporarily increase REM sleep levels in these people despite their medications, or cause the traits to dissociate into other states. Interestingly, reticular stimulation either electrically or with carbachol (an ACh agonist) induces a dissociation of PGO waves into non-REM sleep and can reverse the mnemonic impairments imposed by REM sleep deprivation (Datta and Siwek, 2002; Hars and Hennevin, 1983).

Some unsolved mysteries

The mysteries still outnumber the things known and hold pace with the unsolved questions in both the sleep and learning fields. The principles of *working memory* are only beginning to be understood among neuroscientists, and there are few studies describing the effects of sleep loss on working memory (Hagewoud et al., 2010; Smith et al., 1998). It is not yet known whether memory recall always requires *reconsolidation*, what is the cellular basis for reconsolidation, and whether there is a sleep function for reconsolidation. There are major implications of sleep-dependent reconsolidation for those suffering from sleep disturbance. For example, those with Alzheimer's disease have abnormal sleep and would thus, perhaps, *not* want to perform memory recall exercises if reconsolidation mechanisms are not in place; memories could be erased faster. Do *dreams* matter? If our brain is metaplastic during REM sleep, and we are dreaming, would the content of the dream, even if not consciously remembered, change our synaptic network structure and thus change our mind?

Future directions

This chapter presents phenomenological studies that outline mechanisms through which sleep could serve learning and memory and general synaptic circuit reorganization. A missing piece of the puzzle is direct evidence that the events occurring during sleep have lasting effects on brain circuitry. The best studies published thus far were done by Frank and colleagues (Aton et al., 2009; Frank et al., 2001), who showed that sleep deprivation following monocular deprivation did not allow the plasticity events that occurred during wakefulness to stabilize and be amplified. But there are many tests of synaptic plasticity in intact functional circuits that can and should be employed in the online sleeping and learning brain. Such tests will probably reveal a startling amount of neural plasticity over sleep and waking states.

Summary

This chapter describes neurophysiologic processes during sleep that impact cognition and those processes compromised by sleep loss. REM sleep traits such as PGO waves, theta synchrony, high ACh levels, the loss of NE and 5HT and the return of plasticity-related gene transcription allow for freely occurring bidirectional plasticity: LTP or its reversal, depotentiation. This bidirectional plasticity during REM sleep affords synaptic remodelling in support of learning and cognition in the hippocampal complex. Traits of non-REM Stage 2 sleep, especially spindles and the neurochemical milieu that promotes them, are also probably highly conducive to synaptic plasticity – perhaps allowing targeted bidirectional plasticity in the neocortex. Neuronal reactivation of waking sequences at peaks of slow wave delta activity during non-REM sleep, together with high protein synthesis levels, could serve to convert early LTP to late LTP, but not engender new plasticity. Reactivation events on delta waves are some–times disordered, even backward, which could depotentiate synaptic circuits by the principles of STDP, especially as delta sleep is characterized by low ACh levels and by the activation of genes supporting depotentiation. Such depotentiation events at delta peaks could serve to downscale synapses of certain circuits during non-REM sleep and perhaps quiet wakefulness. Finally, sleep deprivation studies revealed deficits in neuronal excitability and LTP mechanisms that would affect future learning as well as memory consolidation and possibly reconsolidation. The evidence set forth points to an overall function of embossing of synaptic circuits to add definition to and integrate memories, distinguishing them from the noise introduced to synaptic weights throughout wakefulness. The activity patterns, neurochemical and gene environments of sleep thus serve to clear noise and strengthen weakened networks of neural circuits for efficient subsequent cognitive processing demands.

Abbreviations

5HT	Serotonin
ACh	acetylcholine
EEG	electroencephalographic
LC	locus coeruleus
LIA	large irregular activity
LTD	long-term depression
LTP	long-term potentiation
MAOIs	monoamine oxidase inhibitors
MRF	medial reticular formation
NE	norepinephrine
non-REM sleep	non-rapid eye movement sleep
PGO waves	ponto-geniculo-occipital waves
QW	quiet waking
REM sleep	rapid eye movement sleep
STDP	spike timing-dependent plasticity
TA	temporo-ammonic
TR	transition to REM sleep

Acknowledgements

Research described herein in the Poe et al., studies were supported by MH60670, MH 76280 and the Department of Anesthesiology at the University of Michigan. Special thanks to Victoria Booth, Ph.D. and to Brett Riley for their contributions to the development of some of these concepts.

References

Abraham, W. C. (2003). How long will long-term potentiation last? *Philosophical Transactions of the Royal Society of London Series B: Biological Sciences*, *358*, 735–744.

Abraham, W. C., & Bear, M. F. (1996). Metaplasticity: The plasticity of synaptic plasticity. *Trends of Neuroscience*, *19*, 126–130.

Akindele, M. O., Evans, J. I., & Oswald, I. (1970). Mono-amine oxidase inhibitors, sleep and mood. *Electroencephalography and Clinical Neurophysiology*, *29*, 47–56.

Almaguer-Melian, W., Rojas-Reyes, Y., Alvare, A., Rosillo, J. C., Frey, J. U., & Bergado, J. A. (2005). Long-term potentiation in the dentate gyrus in freely moving rats is reinforced by intraventricular application of norepinephrine, but not oxotremorine. *Neurobiology of Learning and Memory*, *83*, 72–78.

Aston-Jones, G., & Bloom, F. E. (1981). Activity of norepinephrine-containing locus coeruleus neurons in behaving rats anticipates fluctuations in the sleep-waking cycle. *Journal of Neuroscience*, *1*, 876–886.

Aton, S. J., Seibt, J., Dumoulin, M., Jha, S. K., Steinmetz, N., & Coleman, T., et al. (2009). Mechanisms of sleep-dependent consolidation of cortical plasticity. *Neuron*, *61*, 454–466.

Axmacher, N., Mormann, F., Fernández, G., Elger, C., & Fell, J. (2006). Memory formation by neuronal synchronization. *Brain Research Reviews*, *52*, 170–182.

Basheer, R., Sherin, J. E., Saper, C. B., Morgan, J. I., Mccarley, R. W., & Shiromani, P. J. (1997). Effects of sleep on wake-induced c-fos expression. *Journal of Neuroscience*, *17*, 9746–9750.

Bi, G. Q., & Poo, M. M. (1998). Synaptic modifications in cultured hippocampal neurons: Dependence on spike timing, synaptic strength, and postsynaptic cell type. *Journal of Neuroscience*, *18*, 10464–10472.

Bliss, T. V., & Lomo, T. (1973). Long-lasting potentiation of synaptic transmission in the dentate area of the anaesthetized rabbit following stimulation of the perforant path. *Journal of Physiology*, *232*, 331–356.

Blitzer, R. D., Iyengar, R., & Landau, E. M. (2005). Postsynaptic signaling networks: Cellular cogwheels underlying long-term plasticity. *Biological Psychiatry*, *57*, 113–119.

Borbely, A. A., & Achermann, P. (2005). Sleep homeostasis and models of sleep regulation. In: Kryger, M. H., Roth, T., Dement, W. C. (Eds.), *Principles and practice of sleep medicine.* Elsevier Saunders, Philadelphia.

Borbely, A. A., Baumann, F., Brandeis, D., Strauch, I., & Lehmann, D. (1981). Sleep deprivation: Effect on sleep stages and EEG power density in man. *Electroencephalography and Clinical Neurophysiology*, *51*, 483–495.

Bramham, C. R., Maho, C., & Laroche, S. (1994). Suppression of long-term potentiation induction during alert wakefulness but not during 'enhanced' REM sleep after avoidance learning. *Neuroscience*, *59*, 501–509.

Bramham, C. R., & Srebro, B. (1989). Synaptic plasticity in the hippocampus is modulated by behavioral state. *Brain Research*, *493*, 74–86.

Braunewell, K. H., & Manahan-Vaughan, D. (2001). Long-term depression: A cellular basis for learning? *Review of Neuroscience*, *12*, 121–140.

Brown, G., & McCormack, T. (2006). The role of time in human memory and binding: A review of the evidence. *Binding in Human Memory: A Neurocognitive Approach* 251–290

Burgos, H., Mardones, L., Campos, M., Castillo, A., Fernandez, V., & Hernandez, A. (2005). Chronic treatment with clomipramine and desipramine induces deficit in long-term visuospatial memory of rats. *International Journal of Neuroscience*, *115*, 47–54.

Burt, D. B., Zembar, M. J., & Niederehe, G. (1995). Depression and memory impairment: A meta-analysis of the association, its pattern, and specificity. *Psychological Bulletin*, *117*, 285–305.

Buzsaki, G., Leung, L. W., & Vanderwolf, C. H. (1983). Cellular bases of hippocampal EEG in the behaving rat. *Brain Research*, *287*, 139–171.

Callaway, C. W., Lydic, R., Baghdoyan, H. A., & Hobson, J. A. (1987). Pontogeniculooccipital waves: Spontaneous visual system activity during rapid eye movement sleep. *Cellular and Molecular Neurobiology*, *2*, 105–149.

Campbell, I. G., Guinan, M. J., & Horowitz, J. M. (2002). Sleep deprivation impairs long-term potentiation in rat hippocampal slices. *Journal of Neurophysiology*, *88*, 1073–1076.

Cheng, R., Williams, C., & Meck, W. (2008). Oscillatory bands, neuronal synchrony and hippocampal function: Implications of the effects of prenatal choline supplementation for sleep-dependent memory consolidation. *Brain Research*, *1237*, 176–194.

Cirelli, C., & Tononi, G. (2000a). Differential expression of plasticity-related genes in waking and sleep and their regulation by the noradrenergic system. *Journal of Neuroscience*, *20*, 9187–9194.

Cirelli, C., & Tononi, G. (2000b). Gene expression in the brain across the sleep-waking cycle. *Brain Research*, *885*, 303–321.

Crick, F., & Koch, C. (1998). Consciousness and neuroscience. *Cerebral Cortex*, *8*, 97–107.

Crick, F., & Mitchison, G. (1983). The function of dream sleep. *Nature*, *304*, 111–114.

Datta, S. (2000). Avoidance task training potentiates phasic pontine-wave density in the rat: A mechanism for sleep-dependent plasticity. *Journal of Neuroscience*, *20*, 8607–8613.

Datta, S., & Siwek, D. F. (2002). Single cell activity patterns of pedunculopontine tegmentum neurons across the sleep-wake cycle in the freely moving rats. *Journal of Neuroscience Research*, *70*, 611–621.

Datta, S., Mavanji, V., Ulloor, J., & Patterson, E. H. (2004). Activation of phasic pontine-wave generator prevents rapid eye movement sleep deprivation-induced learning impairment in the rat: A mechanism for sleep-dependent plasticity. *Journal of Neuroscience*, *24*, 1416–1427.

Datta, S., Siwek, D. F., Patterson, E. H., & Cipolloni, P. B. (1998). Localization of pontine PGO wave generation sites and their anatomical projections in the rat. *Synapse*, *30*, 409–423.

Dave, A. S., & Margoliash, D. (2000). Song replay during sleep and computational rules for sensorimotor vocal learning. *Science*, *290*, 812–816.

Davis, C. J., Harding, J. W., & Wright, J. W. (2003). REM sleep deprivation-induced deficits in the latency-to-peak induction and maintenance of long-term potentiation within the CA1 region of the hippocampus. *Brain Research*, *973*, 293–297.

De Koninck, J., Lorrain, D., Christ, G., Proulx, G., & Coulombe, D. (1989). Intensive language learning and increases in rapid eye movement sleep: Evidence of a performance factor. *International Journal of Psychophysiology*, *8*, 43–47.

Derégnaucourt, S., Mitra, P. P., Fehér, O., Pytte, C., & Tchernichovski, O. (2005). How sleep affects the developmental learning of bird song. *Nature*, *433*, 710–716.

Détári, L., Rasmusson, D. D., & Semba, K. (1999). The role of basal forebrain neurons in tonic and phasic activation of the cerebral cortex. *Progress in Neurobiology*, *58*(3); 249–277.

Drummond, S. P., Gillin, J. C., & Brown, G. G. (2001). Increased cerebral response during a divided attention task following sleep deprivation. *Journal of Sleep Research*, *10*, 85–92.

Dujardin, K., Guerrien, A., & Leconte, P. (1990). Sleep, brain activation and cognition. *Physiology & Behavior*, *47*, 1271–1278.

Emrick, J., Riley, B., Cropp, E., Zheng, C., Booth, V. & Poe, G. (2008) Cortical and hippocampal EEG show different simultaneous sleep states after learning. *Society for Neuroscience Abstract.* Washington, D.C.: Society for Neuroscience.

Esser, S. K., Hill, S. L., & Tononi, G. (2007). Sleep homeostasis and cortical synchronization: I. Modeling the effects of synaptic strength on sleep slow waves. *Sleep*, *30*, 1617–1630.

Esser, S. K., Huber, R., Massimini, M., Peterson, M. J., Ferrarelli, F., & Tononi, G. (2006). A direct demonstration of cortical LTP in humans: A combined TMS/EEG study. *Brain Research Bulletin*, *69*, 86–94.

Ferrara, M., Iaria, G., Tempesta, D., Curcio, G., Moroni, F., & Marzano, C., et al. (2008). Sleep to find your way: The role of sleep in the consolidation of memory for navigation in humans. *Hippocampus*, *18*, 844–851.

Fishbein, W., Kastaniotis, C., & Chattman, D. (1974). Paradoxical sleep: Prolonged augmentation following learning. *Brain Research*, *79*, 61–75.

Foster, D. J., & Wilson, M. A. (2006). Reverse replay of behavioural sequences in hippocampal place cells during the awake state. *Nature*, *440*, 680–683.

Fox, S. E., Wolfson, S., & Ranck Jr., J. B. (1986). Hippocampal theta rhythm and the firing of neurons in walking and urethane anesthetized rats. *Experimental Brain Research*, *62*, 495–508.

Frank, M. G., Issa, N. P., & Stryker, M. P. (2001). Sleep enhances plasticity in the developing visual cortex. *Neuron*, *30*, 275–287.

Franken, P., Dijk, D. J., Tobler, I., & Borbely, A. A. (1991). Sleep deprivation in rats: Effects on EEG power spectra, vigilance states, and cortical temperature. *American Journal of Physiology*, *261*, R198–R208.

Frey, S., & Frey, J. U. (2008). 'Synaptic tagging' and 'cross-tagging' and related associative reinforcement processes of functional plasticity as the cellular basis for memory formation. *Progress in Brain Research*, *169*, 117–143.

Frey, U., & Morris, R. G. (1997). Synaptic tagging and long-term potentiation. *Nature*, *385*(6616); 533–536.

Frey, U., & Morris, R. G. (1998). Synaptic tagging: implications for late maintenance of hippocampal long-term potentiation. *Trends in Neuroscience*, *21*(5); 181–188.

Frey, U., Krug, M., Reymann, K. G., & Matthies, H. (1988). Anisomycin, an inhibitor of protein synthesis, blocks late phases of LTP phenomena in the hippocampal CA1 region in vitro. *Brain Research*, *452*, 57–65.

Givens, B. (1996). Stimulus-evoked resetting of the dentate theta rhythm: Relation to working memory. *Neuroreport*, *8*, 159–163.

Golding, N. L., Kath, W. L., & Spruston, N. (2001). Dichotomy of action-potential backpropagation in CA1 pyramidal neuron dendrites. *Journal of Neurophysiology*, *86*, 2998–3010.

Gould, E., Tanapat, P., Hastings, N. B., & Shors, T. J. (1999). Neurogenesis in adulthood: A possible role in learning. *Trends in Cognitive Sciences*, *3*, 186–192.

Guerrien, A., Dujardin, K., Mandai, O., Sockeel, P., & Leconte, P. (1989). Enhancement of memory by auditory stimulation during postlearning REM sleep in humans. *Physiology & Behavior*, *45*, 947–950.

Guzman-Marin, R., Suntsova, N., Methippara, M., Greiffenstein, R., Szymusiak, R., & Mcginty, D. (2005). Sleep deprivation suppresses neurogenesis in the adult hippocampus of rats. *European Journal of Neuroscience*, *22*, 2111–2116.

Guzman-Marin, R., Suntsova, N., Stewart, D. R., Gong, H., Szymusiak, R., & Mcginty, D. (2003). Sleep deprivation reduces proliferation of cells in the dentate gyrus of the hippocampus in rats. *Journal of Physiology*, *549*, 563–571.

Hagewoud, R., Havekes, R., Novati, A., Keijser, J. N., Van Der Zee, E. A., & Meerlo, P. (2010). Sleep deprivation impairs spatial working memory and reduces hippocampal AMPA receptor phosphorylation. *Journal of Sleep Research*, *19*, 280–288.

Hairston, I. S., Little, M. T., Scanlon, M. D., Barakat, M. T., Palmer, T. D., & Sapolsky, R. M., et al. (2005). Sleep restriction suppresses neurogenesis induced by hippocampus-dependent learning. *Journal of Neurophysiology*, *94*, 4224–4233.

Hanlon, E. C., Faraguna, U., Vyazovskiy, V. V., Tononi, G., & Cirelli, C. (2009). Effects of skilled training on sleep slow wave activity and cortical gene expression in the rat. *Sleep*, *32*, 719–729.

Hars, B., & Hennevin, E. (1983). Reminder abolishes impairment of learning induced by paradoxical sleep retardation. *Physiology & Behavior*, *30*, 831–836.

Hasselmo, M. E., & Bower, J. M. (1993). Acetylcholine and memory. *Trends in Neurosciences*, *16*, 218–222.

Hennevin, E., Hars, B., & Bloch, V. (1989). Improvement of learning by mesencephalic reticular stimulation during post-learning paradoxical sleep. *Behavioral and Neural Biology*, *51*, 291–306.

Hennevin, E., Hars, B., Maho, C., & Bloch, V. (1995). Processing of learned information in paradoxical sleep: Relevance for memory. *Behavioral Brain Research*, *69*, 125–135.

Hennevin, E., Leconte, P., & Bloch, V. (1974). Paradoxical sleep increase triggered by learning, extinction and relearning of a response based on a positive reinforcement. *Brain Research*, *70*, 43–54.

Huber, R., Ghilardi, M. F., Massimini, M., & Tononi, G. (2004). Local sleep and learning. *Nature*, *430*, 78–81.

Huerta, P. T., & Lisman, J. E. (1995). Bidirectional synaptic plasticity induced by a single burst during cholinergic theta oscillation in CA1 in vitro. *Neuron*, *15*, 1053–1063.

Hyman, J. M., Wyble, B. P., Goyal, V., Rossi, C. A., & Hasselmo, M. E. (2003). Stimulation in hippocampal region CA1 in behaving rats yields long-term potentiation when delivered to the peak of theta and long-term depression when delivered to the trough. *Journal of Neuroscience*, *23*, 11725–11731.

Jenkins, J. G., & Dallenbach, K. M. (1924). Obliviscence during sleep and waking. *The American Journal of Psychology*, *35*, 605–612.

Jones, M., & Wilson, M. (2005). Theta rhythms coordinate hippocampal-prefrontal interactions in a spatial memory task. *PLoS Biology*, *3*, 2187.

Jouvet, M. (1962). Recherches sur les structures nerveuses et les mechanismes responsables des différentes phases du sommeil physiologique. *Archives Italiennes de Biologie*, *100*, 125–206.

Karlsson, M. P., & Frank, L. M. (2009). Awake replay of remote experiences in the hippocampus. *Nature Neuroscience*, *12*, 913–918.

Karni, A., Tanne, D., Rubenstein, B. S., Askenasy, J. J. M., & Sagi, D. (1994). Dependence on REM sleep of overnight improvement of a perceptual skill. *Science*, *265*, 679–682.

Katsuki, H., Izumi, Y., & Zorumski, C. F. (1997). Noradrenergic regulation of synaptic plasticity in the hippocampal CA1 region. *Journal of Neurophysiology*, *77*, 3013–3020.

Kemp, A., & Manahan-Vaughan, D. (2004). Hippocampal long-term depression and long-term potentiation encode different aspects of novelty acquisition. *Proceedings of the National Academy of Sciences of the United States of America*, *101*, 8192–8197.

Krueger, J. M., & Obal, F. (1993). A neuronal group theory of sleep function. *Journal of Sleep Research*, *2*, 63–69.

Krug, M., Lossner, B., & Ott, T. (1984). Anisomycin blocks the late phase of long-term potentiation in the dentate gyrus of freely moving rats. *Brain Research Bulletin*, *13*, 39–42.

Kudrimoti, H. S., Barnes, C. A., & McNaughton, B. L. (1999). Reactivation of hippocampal cell assemblies: Effects of behavioral state, experience, and EEG dynamics. *Journal of Neuroscience*, *19*, 4090–4101.

Lai, Y. Y., & Siegel, J. M. (1991). Pontomedullary glutamate receptors mediating locomotion and muscle tone suppression. *Journal of Neuroscience*, *11*, 2931–2937.

Lairy, G. C., Goldsteinas, L., & Guennoc, A. (1967). Disturbances of sleep in patients with confusional and demential syndromes. *Electroencephalography and Clinical Neurophysiology*, *23*, 286.

Lapierre, J. L., Kosenko, P. O., Lyamin, O. I., Kodama, T., Mukhametov, L. M., & Siegel, J. M. (2007). Cortical acetylcholine release is lateralized during asymmetrical slow-wave sleep in northern fur seals. *Journal of Neuroscience*, *27*, 11999–12006.

Lee, K. H., & McCormick, D. A. (1996). Abolition of spindle oscillations by serotonin and norepinephrine in the ferret lateral geniculate and perigeniculate nuclei in vitro. *Neuron*, *17*, 309–321.

Leonard, B. J., McNaughton, B. L., & Barnes, C. A. (1987). Suppression of hippocampal synaptic plasticity during slow-wave sleep. *Brain Research*, *425*, 174–177.

Llinas, R., & Ribary, U. (1993). Coherent 40-Hz oscillation characterizes dream state in humans. *Proceedings of the National Academy of Sciences of the United States of America*, *90*, 2078–2081.

Louie, K., & Wilson, M. A. (2001). Temporally structured replay of awake hippocampal ensemble activity during rapid eye movement sleep. *Neuron*, *29*, 145–156.

Lucero, M. A. (1970). Lengthening of REM sleep duration consecutive to learning in the rat. *Brain Research*, *20*, 319–322.

Mahowald, M. W., & Schenck, C. H. (1992). Dissociated states of wakefulness and sleep. *Neurology*, *42*, 44–51 discussion 52.

Manahan-Vaughan, D., & Braunewell, K. H. (1999). Novelty acquisition is associated with induction of hippocampal long-term depression. *Proceedings of the National Academy of Sciences of the United States of America*, *96*, 8739–8744.

Mandai, O., Guerrien, A., Sockeel, P., Dujardin, K., & Leconte, P. (1989). REM sleep modifications following a Morse code learning session in humans. *Physiology & Behavior*, *46*, 639–642.

Marks, C. A., & Wayner, M. J. (2005). Effects of sleep disruption on rat dentate granule cell LTP in vivo. *Brain Research Bulletin*, *66*, 114–119.

Marrosu, F., Portas, C., Mascia, M. S., Casu, M. A., Fa, M., & Giagheddu, M., et al. (1995). Microdialysis measurement of cortical and hippocampal acetylcholine release during sleep-wake cycle in freely moving cats. *Brain Research*, *671*, 329–332.

Mavanji, V., & Datta, S. (2003). Activation of the phasic pontine-wave generator enhances improvement of learning performance: A mechanism for sleep-dependent plasticity. *European Journal of Neuroscience*, *17*, 359–370.

McClelland, J. L., McNaughton, B. L., & O'Reilly, R. C. (1995). Why there are complementary learning systems in the hippocampus and neocortex: Insights from the successes and failures of connectionist models of learning and memory. *Psychology Review*, *102*, 419–457.

McDermott, C. M., Lahoste, G. J., Chen, C., Musto, A., Bazan, N. G., & Magee, J. C. (2003). Sleep deprivation causes behavioral, synaptic, and membrane excitability alterations in hippocampal neurons. *Journal of Neuroscience*, *23*, 9687–9695.

McGinty, D. J., & Harper, R. M. (1976). Dorsal raphe neurons: Depression of firing during sleep in cats. *Brain Research*, *101*, 569–575.

McGrath, M. J., & Cohen, D. B. (1978). REM sleep facilitation of adaptive waking behavior: A review of the literature. *Psychological Bulletin*, *85*, 24–57.

Mednick, S. C., Nakayama, K., Cantero, J. L., Atienza, M., Levin, A. A., & Pathak, N., et al. (2002). The restorative effect of naps on perceptual deterioration. *Nature Neuroscience*, *5*, 677–681.

Melton, A. W., & Irwin, J. M. (1940). The influence of degree of interpolated learning on retroactive inhibition and the overt transfer of specific responses. *American Journal of Psychology*, *53*, 175–203.

Meneses, A., & Hong, E. (1997). Effects of 5-HT4 receptor agonists and antagonists in learning. *Pharmacology Biochemistry and Behavior*, *56*, 347–351.

Mizumori, S. J., Perez, G. M., Alvarado, M. C., Barnes, C. A., & McNaughton, B. L. (1990). Reversible inactivation of the medial septum differentially affects two forms of learning in rats. *Brain Research*, *528*, 12–20.

Molle, M., Yeshenko, O., Marshall, L., Sara, S. J., & Born, J. (2006). Hippocampal sharp wave-ripples linked to slow oscillations in rat slow-wave sleep. *Journal of Neurophysiology*, *96*, 62–70.

Nakao, K., Ikegaya, Y., Yamada, M. K., Nishiyama, N., & Matsuki, N. (2002). Hippocampal long-term depression as an index of spatial working memory. *European Journal of Neuroscience*, *16*, 970–974.

Nicholson, A. N., Belyavin, A. J., & Pascoe, P. A. (1989). Modulation of rapid eye movement sleep in humans by drugs that modify monoaminergic and purinergic transmission. *Neuropsychopharmacology*, *2*, 131–143.

Nielsen, T. A. (2000). A review of mentation in REM and NREM sleep: 'Covert' REM sleep as a possible reconciliation of two opposing models. *Behavioral and Brain Sciences*, *23*, 851–866 discussion 904–1121.

Nitz, D., & Siegel, J. (1997). GABA release in the locus coeruleus as a function of sleep/wake state. *Neuroscience*, *78*(3); 795–801.

Orr, G., Rao, G., Houston, F. P., McNaughton, B. L., & Barnes, C. A. (2001). Hippocampal synaptic plasticity is modulated by theta rhythm in the fascia dentata of adult and aged freely behaving rats. *Hippocampus*, *11*, 647–654.

Otani, S., Marshall, C. J., Tate, W. P., Goddard, G. V., & Abraham, W. C. (1989). Maintenance of long-term potentiation in rat dentate gyrus requires protein synthesis but not messenger RNA synthesis immediately post-tetanization. *Neuroscience*, *28*, 519–526.

Park, S. P., Lopez-Rodriguez, F., Wilson, C. L., Maidment, N., Matsumoto, Y., & Engel Jr., J. (1999). In vivo microdialysis measures of extracellular serotonin in the rat hippocampus during sleep-wakefulness. *Brain Research*, *833*, 291–296.

Pavlides, C., Greenstein, Y. J., Grudman, M., & Winson, J. (1988). Long-term potentiation in the dentate gyrus is induced preferentially on the positive phase of theta-rhythm. *Brain Research*, *439*, 383–387.

Pavlides, C., & Winson, J. (1989). Influences of hippocampal place cell firing in the awake state on the activity of these cells during subsequent sleep episodes. *Journal of Neuroscience*, *9*, 2907–2918.

Poe, G. R., Nitz, D. A., McNaughton, B. L., & Barnes, C. A. (2000). Experience-dependent phase-reversal of hippocampal neuron firing during REM sleep. *Brain Research*, *855*, 176–180.

Pompeiano, M., Cirelli, C., Arrighi, P., & Tononi, G. (1995). c-Fos expression during wakefulness and sleep. *Neurophysiologie Clinique*, *25*, 329–341.

Pompeiano, M., Cirelli, C., Ronca-Testoni, S., & Tononi, G. (1997). NGFI-A expression in the rat brain after sleep deprivation. *Brain Research Molecular Brain Research*, *46*, 143–153.

Pompeiano, M., Cirelli, C., & Tononi, G. (1994). Immediate-early genes in spontaneous wakefulness and sleep: Expression of c-fos and NGFI-A mRNA and protein. *Journal of Sleep Research*, *3*, 80–96.

Portell-Cortes, I., Marti-Nicolovius, M., Segura-Torres, P., & Morgado-Bernal, I. (1989). Correlations between paradoxical sleep and shuttle-box conditioning in rats. *Behavioral Neuroscience*, *103*, 984–990.

Ramm, P., & Smith, C. T. (1990). Rates of cerebral protein synthesis are linked to slow wave sleep in the rat. *Physiology & Behavior*, *48*, 749–753.

Rashidy-Pour, A., Motamedi, F., Semnanian, S., Zarrindast, M. R., Fatollahi, Y., & Behzadi, G. (1996). Effects of reversible inactivation of the medial septal area on long-term potentiation and recurrent inhibition of hippocampal population spikes in rats. *Brain Research*, *734*, 43–48.

Rausch, G., & Scheich, H. (1982). Dendritic spine loss and enlargement during maturation of the speech control system in the mynah bird (*Gracula religiosa*). *Neuroscience Letters*, *29*, 129–133.

Reymann, K. G., & Frey, J. U. (2007). The late maintenance of hippocampal LTP: Requirements, phases, 'synaptic tagging', 'late-associativity' and implications. *Neuropharmacology*, *52*, 24–40.

Ribeiro, S., Goyal, V., Mello, C. V., & Pavlides, C. (1999). Brain gene expression during REM sleep depends on prior waking experience. *Learning & Memory*, *6*, 500–508.

Ribeiro, S., Mello, C. V., Velho, T., Gardner, T. J., Jarvis, E. D., & Pavlides, C. (2002). Induction of hippocampal long-term potentiation during waking leads to increased extrahippocampal zif-268 expression during ensuing rapid-eye-movement sleep. *Journal of Neuroscience*, *22*, 10914–10923.

Ribeiro, S., & Nicolelis, M. A. (2004). Reverberation, storage, and postsynaptic propagation of memories during sleep. *Learning & Memory*, *11*, 686–696.

Riedner, B. A., Vyazovskiy, V. V., Huber, R., Massimini, M., Esser, S., & Murphy, M., et al. (2007). Sleep homeostasis and cortical synchronization: III. A high-density EEG study of sleep slow waves in humans. *Sleep*, *30*, 1643–1657.

Riemann, D., Berger, M., & Voderholzer, U. (2001). Sleep and depression – results from psychobiological studies: An overview. *Biological Psychology*, *57*, 67–103.

Romcy-Pereira, R., & Pavlides, C. (2004). Distinct modulatory effects of sleep on the maintenance of hippocampal and medial prefrontal cortex LTP. *European Journal of Neuroscience*, *20*, 3453–3462.

Seligman, M. (1970). On the generality of the laws of learning. *Psychology Review*, *77*, 406–418.

Siapas, A. G., Lubenov, E. V., & Wilson, M. A. (2005). Prefrontal phase locking to hippocampal theta oscillations. *Neuron*, *46*, 141–151.

Siapas, A. G., & Wilson, M. A. (1998). Coordinated interactions between hippocampal ripples and cortical spindles during slow-wave sleep. *Neuron*, *21*, 1123–1128.

Siegel, J. M. (2001). The REM sleep-memory consolidation hypothesis. *Science*, *294*, 1058–1063.

Smith, C. (1985). Sleep states and learning: A review of the animal literature. *Neuroscience & Biobehavioral Reviews, 9*, 157–168.

Smith, C. (1995). Sleep states and memory processes. *Behavioural Brain Research, 69*, 137–145.

Smith, C., & Butler, S. (1982). Paradoxical sleep at selective times following training is necessary for learning. *Physiology & Behavior, 29*, 469–473.

Smith, C., & Lapp, L. (1991). Increases in number of REMS and REM density in humans following an intensive learning period. *Sleep, 14*, 325–330.

Smith, C., & Rose, G. M. (1996). Evidence for a paradoxical sleep window for place learning in the Morris water maze. *Physiology & Behavior, 59*, 93–97.

Smith, C., & Wong, P. T. (1991). Paradoxical sleep increases predict successful learning in a complex operant task. *Behavioral Neuroscience, 105*, 282–288.

Smith, C., Young, J., & Young, W. (1980). Prolonged increases in paradoxical sleep during and after avoidance- task acquisition. *Sleep, 3*, 67–81.

Smith, C. T., Conway, J. M., & Rose, G. M. (1998). Brief paradoxical sleep deprivation impairs reference, but not working, memory in the radial arm maze task. *Neurobiology of Learning & Memory, 69*, 211–217.

Steriade, M. (2004). Acetylcholine systems and rhythmic activities during the waking-sleep cycle. *Progress in Brain Research, Volume 145*, 179–196.

Thomas, M. J., Moody, T. D., Makhinson, M., & O'Dell, T. J. (1996). Activity dependent beta-adrenergic modulation of low frequency stimulation induced LTP in the hippocampal CA1 region. *Neuron, 17*, 475–482.

Tonchev, A. B., & Yamashima, T. (2006). Differential neurogenic potential of progenitor cells in dentate gyrus and CA1 sector of the postischemic adult monkey hippocampus. *Experimental Neurology, 198*, 101–113.

Tsukamoto-Yasui, M., Sasaki, T., Matsumoto, W., Hasegawa, A., Toyoda, T., & Usami, A., et al. (2007). Active hippocampal networks undergo spontaneous synaptic modification. *PLoS One, 2*, e1250.

Vanderwolf, C. H., & Stewart, D. J. (1986). Joint cholinergic-serotonergic control of neocortical and hippocampal electrical activity in relation to behavior: Effects of scopolamine, ditran, trifluoperazine and amphetamine. *Physiology & Behavior, 38*, 57–65.

Vertes, R. P. (1982). Brain stem generation of the hippocampal EEG. *Progress in Neurobiology, 19*, 159–186.

Vertes, R. P., & Kocsis, B. (1997). Brainstem-diencephalo-septohippocampal systems controlling the theta rhythm of the hippocampus. *Neuroscience, 81*, 893–926.

Vyazovskiy, V., Borbely, A. A., & Tobler, I. (2000). Unilateral vibrissae stimulation during waking induces interhemispheric EEG asymmetry during subsequent sleep in the rat. *Journal of Sleep Research, 9*, 367–371.

Vyazovskiy, V. V., Riedner, B. A., Cirelli, C., & Tononi, G. (2007). Sleep homeostasis and cortical synchronization: II. A local field potential study of sleep slow waves in the rat. *Sleep, 30*, 1631–1642.

Wallhausserfranke, E., Nixdorfbergweiler, B., & Devoogd, T. (1995). Song isolation is associated with maintaining high spine frequencies on zebra finch IMAN neurons. *Neurobiology of Learning and Memory, 64*, 25–35.

Walter, T. (2007). *REM illumination: Memory consolidation.* Lotus Magnus, LLC, Grove City, OH.

Wamsley, E. J., Tucker, M. A., Payne, J. D., & Stickgold, R. (2010). A brief nap is beneficial for human route-learning: The role of navigation experience and EEG spectral power. *Learning & Memory, 17*, 332–336.

Wilson, M. A., & McNaughton, B. L. (1994). Reactivation of hippocampal ensemble memories during sleep. *Science, 265*, 676–679.

Winson, J. (1978). Loss of hippocampal theta rhythm results in spatial memory deficit in the rat. *Science, 201*, 160–163.

Winson, J. (1985). *Brain and psyche: The biology of the unconscious.* Anchor Press/Doubleday, Garden City, NY.

Winson, J. (1990). The meaning of dreams. *Scientific American, 263*, 86–88 90–92, 94–96.

Xu, L., Anwyl, R., & Rowan, M. J. (1998). Spatial exploration induces a persistent reversal of long-term potentiation in rat hippocampus. *Nature, 394*, 891–894.

Yang, H. W., Lin, Y. W., Yen, C. D., & Min, M. Y. (2002). Change in bi-directional plasticity at CA1 synapses in hippocampal slices taken from 6-hydroxydopamine-treated rats: The role of endogenous norepinephrine. *European Journal of Neuroscience, 16*, 1117–1128.

Yoo, S. S., Hu, P. T., Gujar, N., Jolesz, F. A., & Walker, M. P. (2007). A deficit in the ability to form new human memories without sleep. *Nature Neuroscience, 10*, 385–392.

G. A. Kerkhof and H. P. A. Van Dongen (Eds.)
Progress in Brain Research, Vol. 185
ISSN: 0079-6123

CHAPTER 2

Measurement of sleep

Bob Kemp[†,‡,*]

[†]*Sleep Centre, Medical Centre Haaglanden, The Hague, The Netherlands*
[‡]*Department of Neurology, Leiden University Medical Centre, Leiden, The Netherlands*

Abstract: Rapid eye movement (REM) and non-REM sleep processes affect the electrical signals from brain, eyes and muscles. Recording these signals during sleep imposes special demands on electrodes, technicians and equipment. Both human and computerized signal analysis can then be applied to quantify the sleep processes. The most practical and state-of-the-art recording and analysis methods are discussed with emphasis on the most important details. Other analysis methods can be judged based on a few simple criteria.

Keywords: Sleep; EEG; recording; scoring; analysis

Introduction

Rapid eye movement (REM) and non-REM sleep states have well-known and immediate effects on brain activity, eye movements and submental-muscle tone. These effects are visible in the corresponding electroencephalogram (EEG), electrooculogram (EOG) and electromyogram (EMG) signals, respectively. It is therefore commonly accepted that these signals are the basis for recognizing the various states of sleep. This chapter discusses how to properly record those signals.

After recording, some kind of analysis must tell us what sleep states were underlying the observed signals. Two analysis methods are widely applied. The common method in sleep medicine (Iber et al., 2007) is the classification of sleep into a few discrete stages (Fig. 1, bottom trace), based on human (visual) recognition of sleep-related wave shapes in the EXG (EEG, EOG and EMG). Basic researchers, on the other hand, often use computerized amplitude (or its square, power) analysis (Fig. 1), usually based on bandpass filtering or Fourier analysis. Both methods have their merits and drawbacks and will be described briefly, while paying particular attention to some important but often neglected details.

[*] Corresponding author.
Tel.: (+) 31 71 5262188, 31 70 3302205; Fax: (+) 31 70 3882636.
E-mail: bk@hsr.nl

DOI:10.1016/B978-0-444-53702-7.00002-6

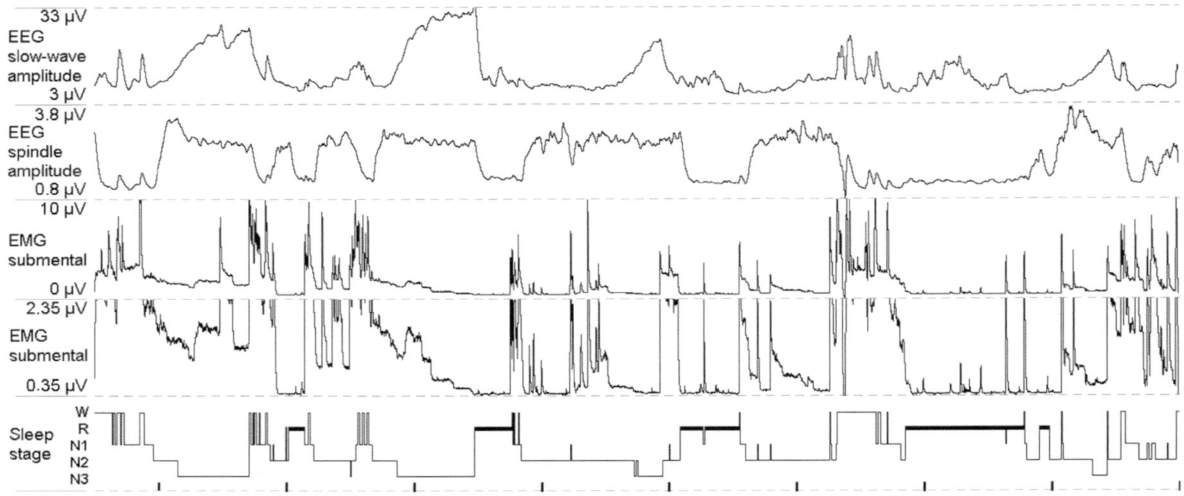

Fig. 1. Whole-night representation of sleep processes. Horizontal time axis: tick marks every hour. Starting at the top, amplitude plots of EEG slow waves (frequencies around 1 Hz), EEG sleep spindles (around 14 Hz), submental EMG (over 15 Hz) and the same EMG amplified five times. Bottom trace: hypnogram, that is visually detected sleep stages w(akefulness), R(EM sleep) and the non-REM sleep stages N1 (drowsiness), N2 (light sleep) and N3 (deep sleep). Note that slow waves increase from N1 to N2 and N3, spindles are active during N2 and N3, and EMG drops by only 0.2 μV at the transition from deep non-REM sleep (N3) to REM sleep.

Many new analysis methods are still being introduced. Only few resulted in new knowledge that could not have been obtained by amplitude analysis. Two of these methods will be described here: neuro-loop analysis and topographic mapping.

Recording EEG, EOG and EMG

Neurons, eyes and muscles maintain an electrical voltage and generate electrical current in the external body fluid. A tiny fraction of this current also flows along the skin. According to Ohm's law, this produces a tiny voltage (about 0.5–500 μV) between different locations on the skin. The voltage between any two locations can be measured by putting electrodes there. The effects of sleep on eye movements, muscle tone and neuronal activity are thus reflected by changes in that voltage. The voltages are small and easily disturbed by larger 'artefacts', that is unpredictable other voltages from neighbouring biological or technical sources. Therefore, optimizing the technical quality of EXG recording is crucial in measuring sleep. Errors and inaccuracies caused by suboptimal recording cannot be corrected later and will hamper any further analysis. Attention to the following details will largely improve recording quality.

The appropriate electrode locations are still subject of discussion. They depend on the orientation and location of the relevant signal and artefact sources. Although a standard grid of EEG electrode locations with corresponding electrode names has been widely accepted (Jasper, 1958), no sufficient data are available yet to select the ones that best reflect sleep. The same is true for EOG and EMG electrodes. As a consequence, the American Academy of Sleep Medicine (AASM) has recently suggested a variety of locations that can be used for visual sleep stage scoring

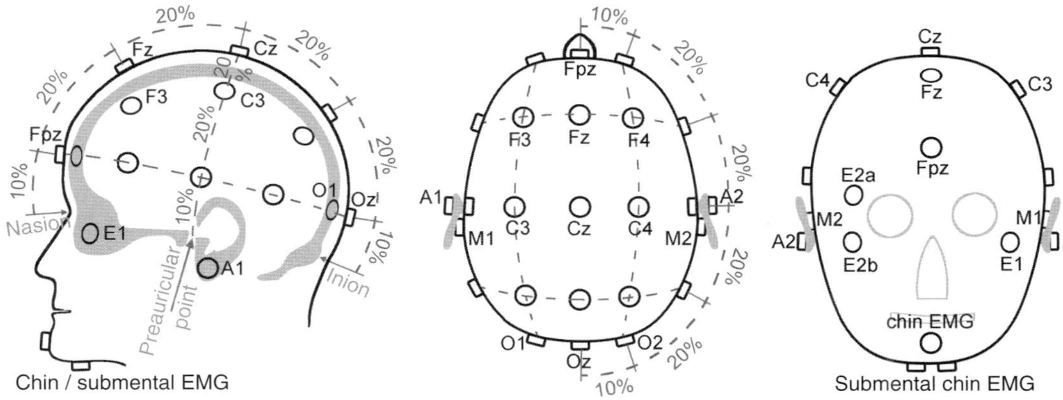

Fig. 2. Standardized electrode names and locations for sleep EXG: left view, top view and front view. Standard EEG electrodes that are not in any of the recommended sleep derivations are also shown, but without names. In sleep recordings, mastoid electrodes (M1 and M2) replace the earlobe electrodes (A1 and A2) that are commonly used in standard EEG.

(Iber et al., 2007, Fig. 2). Based on these locations, several optional electrode pairs were defined from which EXG can be derived. For instance, for measuring EEG slow waves one can choose to derive EEG from F4-M1, Fz-Cz, C4-M1 or Fpz-E1 pairs. Four options are also available for detecting eye movements: either Fpz or M2 must be paired with either E1 or E2. Some confusion may arise from the fact that two locations of E2 are specified: E2a and E2b in Fig. 2. Only the EMG recording was actually standardized: the electrode on the chin must be paired with one of the two submental ones (below the chin). The AASM derivations are widely applied but also subject of discussion (AASM FAQs, 2010). Other interesting ones are the fronto-central Fpz-Cz EEG because it is over the full slow-wave generating area (Happe et al., 2002) while being less sensitive to movement artefacts, the purely horizontally derived EOG because it is easier to interpret than the oblique AASM derivations and less affected by artefacts and large EEG waves such as K-complexes, and finally the purely submental EMG (derived from the two electrodes below the chin, see Fig. 2) because it is specific to REM sleep (Ferri et al., 2008; Jacobson et al., 1964; Rechtschaffen and Kales, 1968).

The type of electrode and its attachment to the skin are critical in any EXG recording, and even more so in sleep investigations because of their long duration. An electrode basically is a metal–salt contact between electrons flowing in the amplifier and ions flowing in the body. Any metal–salt contact acts like a battery with a voltage. In contrast to a real battery, the electrode voltage is not constant. Variations are caused by (amongst others) the random movement of the involved ions, their changing concentrations due to sweat or drying, temperature changes by bed linen or breathing and movements of the interface by body posture or neighbouring blood vessels. The effect of such factors is dramatic when the metal of the electrode (be it gold, silver, copper or tin) is in direct contact with the salts of the body: the two have nothing in common and cannot negotiate a stable equilibrium (battery) voltage. In that case, the electrode voltage is very vulnerable to the mentioned external factors, resulting in artefacts of several millivolts that completely hide EXG signals.

These artefacts can be strongly reduced by using a silver electrode covered by a silver chloride layer. This layer is electrically compatible with both the silver electrode and the chloride ions in the body.

Therefore, an equilibrium voltage settles that strongly dampens the mentioned external factors. Because the silver chloride layer wears off easily, electrodes that are a sintered mixture of silver and silver chloride powder perform even better in practice (Tallgren et al., 2005).

The contact to the body salts must be further improved by degreasing and abrading the skin and by applying a wet chloride-containing contact gel. The resulting low electrode-body resistance (typically less than 5 kΩ) effectively reduces artefacts induced by external electromagnetic fields. Another argument to minimize the resistance is that this reduces the spontaneous noise that is generated by the skin from about 20 to about 1 μV root mean square (rms) (Huigen et al., 2002). Only well-trained and highly experienced technicians know all the tricks for an optimal attachment of the electrode. They will (amongst others) optimally prepare the skin, apply the right amount of contact gel, firmly attach the right electrodes at the right place using collodion and other accessories, avoid drying out and check electrode resistance. They will pay particular attention to the submental EMG because only 0.2 μV (Fig. 1, trace 4) makes the difference between REM and non-REM sleep.

Cables connect the electrodes to a circuit of preamplifiers. Here, other artefacts due to mains interference, nylon clothing and amplifier noise may severely distort the small electrode voltages. Therefore, good EXG preamplifiers have some special characteristics. For safety reasons as well as to avoid signal distortion by external currents, the patient must not be grounded to the environment. Instead, an active-ground circuit using one or two extra electrodes connects the patient to the amplifier ground, while both stay electrically isolated from the environment. Cables should be as short and parallel as possible in order to avoid and cancel external electrical fields. Miniaturization also helps because smaller equipment picks up less of the external fields. The remaining mains interference is largely common at both electrodes and must be rejected by at least a factor of 100,000 (100 dB) from the measured voltage difference. Dedicated EXG amplifiers based on these criteria can record clean signals both in the hospital and at home under normal circumstances. Artefacts may still occur when close to electrical equipment or static charges, especially when cables or artefact source are moving. These artefacts can be removed almost completely by using cables with electrically guarded shields. Only in extreme research conditions with very small signals and very large external fields, a metal Faraday cage around the recording site may be required. Notch filters should be avoided at recording time because 50/60 Hz mains interference is a useful indication of deteriorating electrode quality and can be rejected off-line if necessary.

Some attention is still needed for hardware filtering and input noise because these are rather disappointing in some modern EXG amplifiers. In order to accurately record eye movements (Fig. 3), the time constant on the high-pass filter must be at least 5 s, which corresponds to a low cut-off frequency of at most 0.03 Hz. Several EXG amplifiers have a hardware filter that does not meet this specification and thus strongly attenuates and distorts the wave shapes. Because of the small EXG amplitudes, another concern is noise that is generated by the amplifier inputs and added to the EXG. It is often neglected that not only a noise voltage but also a noise current is generated. The current flows through the electrode-body resistances and therefore (by Ohms law) indirectly generates an extra input noise voltage proportional to the electrode-body resistance. Also sometimes forgotten is that one EXG signal contains noise from at least two amplifier inputs. An EXG from the lowest-noise recorder still contains about 0.3 μV rms amplifier noise at 1000 and 10,000 Ω electrode-body resistances, and 0.7 μV rms at 100,000 Ω. Ambulatory sleep recorders are commonly based on amplifier chips that consume less battery power but generate about the same noise as is coming from a well-prepared skin, that is 1 μV rms.

Although many EXG recorders still have an internal calibration signal, calibration by the user

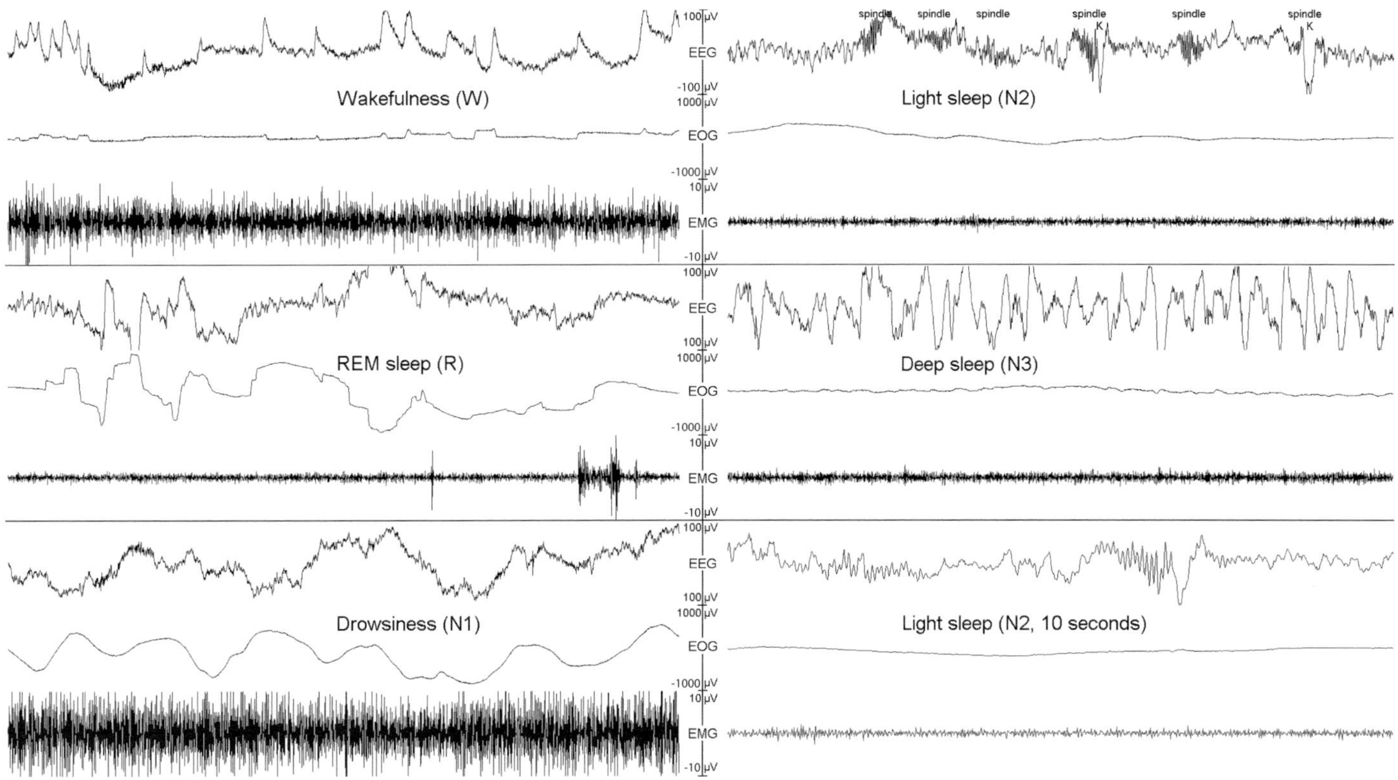

Fig. 3. The six sections are five 30-s epochs and one 10-s epoch, each showing Fpz-Cz EEG, horizontal EOG and submental EMG high-pass filtered at 0.1, 0.03 and 15 Hz, respectively. Note that the Fpz-Cz derivation also records vertical eye movements. Wakefulness (W) shows small mixed-frequency EEG, frequent eye movements and large EMG. REM sleep (REM) shows the same EEG but with sawtooth waves, rapid (saccadic) eye movements and a minimal EMG. Drowsiness (N1) shows a wake EEG and pendulating slow eye movements. Light sleep (N2) shows an EEG with sleep spindles and K-complexes, and no eye movements. Deep sleep (N3) shows many large slow waves in the EEG and no eye movements. The last section shows the 10-s centre of the light-sleep epoch, more clearly showing two 14 Hz sleep spindles.

has become obsolete. In contrast to the old systems with mechanical paper transport and ink-writers, modern recorders are fully solid state. Therefore, the inaccuracies in amplitude and time are orders of magnitude smaller than those caused by the variable location of electrodes and anatomy and by the limited frequency bandwidth that is recorded. Anyhow, built-in calibration signals may contain errors as well and often do not check the full signal path. Calibration is the responsibility of the manufacturer and should be performed using an independent and isolated external signal generator connected to the electrode inputs through a resistor network. This should be done at delivery and after any change of amplifiers or software.

Physiological calibration, on the other hand, can be very useful in each recording. For instance, a few standard eye movements will help detect misplaced or interchanged electrodes (see Fig. 2).

The amplified EXG must be entered into the computer for further analysis. An EXG is a continuous signal: it has no gaps in either time or amplitude and therefore represents an infinite amount of time and amplitude values. In contrast, a digital computer can only handle a limited number of discrete numbers. Therefore, the continuous EXG is digitized by an Analog-to-Digital Converter (ADC) as follows. At discrete times, for example every 4 ms, the ADC measures (samples) the EXG amplitude in microvolts and rounds this, for example by skipping all decimals after the first one. In this example, the sampling frequency of the ADC is thus 250 Hz and its amplitude resolution is 0.1 μV. The computer now has a representation of the signal at discrete times of 0.004, 0.008, 0.012 s, . . . and at discrete amplitudes of (both positive and negative) 0.0, 0.1, 0.2 μV . . . 37.3, 37.4, 37.5 μV, ...

The time resolution of 4 ms is quite sufficient for our wave shapes of interest. It is also sufficient for the representation of rhythmic activity up to 125 Hz, that is half the sampling frequency. However, the EXG also contains higher frequencies, for instance EMG coming from a nearby muscle. These frequencies would contribute to the sampled amplitudes and therefore be indistinguishable from frequencies below 125 Hz (a phenomenon called aliasing). Obviously, that would spoil the analysis of any specific frequency components such as slow waves or sleep spindles. Therefore, the excess frequencies are usually rejected by applying a low-pass filter before the ADC. However, frequency analysis is not the only method being used, and several non-linear analyses require a different type of low-pass filter and cut-off frequency (Kemp et al., 2000). Finally, in case of the submental EMG we are not interested in a sophisticated analysis but simply want to measure its amplitude. In that case, no low-pass filter should be applied at all because it would remove the largest part of the signal that we want to measure and thus dramatically reduce accuracy.

Generally speaking, the application of a low-pass filter strongly limits the analysis possibilities. The solution to this dilemma is to sample all EXGs at the highest possible frequency, for instance 2500 Hz while using a low-pass filter that rejects frequencies over 1250 Hz. Of course, we still want to reduce this sampling frequency to about 250 Hz in order to optimize storage capacity, computation time and review speed. But this reduction can now be done by software and thus accommodate the recorded signals and the required analyses. The 2500 Hz EEG and EOG signals can be subsampled to 250 Hz after applying a digital low-pass filter at 125 Hz, so the amplitude of frequencies up to 125 Hz can be analysed. Applying a different low-pass filter at 250 Hz allows the application of non-linear analysis. The 2500 Hz EMG amplitude can be computed (high-pass and notch filtering followed by rectifying or squaring) without applying a low-pass filter (because aliasing is not a confound here), and subsequently be averaged over 10 samples and thus also be reduced to 250 Hz. In general, higher sampling frequencies enable the application of more analysis methods.

The amplitudes of the ADC in this example are 0.1 μV apart. EXG signals cover an amplitude range of about ±1 mV, that is 20,000 of those amplitude values. Therefore, a 16-bit ADC is quite sufficient because it can handle $2^{16} = 65{,}536$ amplitude values, which corresponds to a range of ±3.7 mV. Apparently, signals of any ADC with more bits can be reduced to 16 bits without compromising range or accuracy, thus saving storage space and improving review speed. Even larger signals can easily be accommodated by 16 bits because ADC values may as well be 0.3 μV apart, thus increasing the 16-bit range to ±11 mV.

The recordings should preferably be saved into standard European data format files (EDF or EDF+, www.edfplus.info; Kemp and Olivan, 2003; Kemp et al., 1992). Such files can be sent to colleagues, subjected to independent review or analysis software, archived longer than a manufacturer's software is maintained and contribute to multi-centre studies. EDF+ is to be preferred over EDF because it is better defined and also saves annotations, events, manual scorings and computer analyses such as those in Fig. 1. Although EDF+ is of great benefit to the EEG and sleep field, commercial arguments still hold a few manufacturers back from supporting it. Therefore, customers may want to insist on EDF+ compatibility at least until the European normalization committee (CEN) has taken the intended steps to make EDF+ obligatory.

Human (visual) sleep staging

When compared to computer analysis, human specialists adapt better to unpredictable artefacts and individual characteristics in the EXG. Therefore, the most common sleep analysis procedure still is scoring of sleep stages by well-trained and experienced specialists. They page through the raw EXG signals, visually recognize specific sleep-related EXG characteristics, and decide what the most likely sleep stage is. Screen resolution is critical, in particular in the horizontal (time) direction. A good screen has at least 3000 horizontal pixels, which is still relatively expensive. Therefore, screen resolution is usually worse than desired and zooming is often necessary (Fig. 3, last section).

The scoring procedure for adults was standardized for the first time by a manual (Rechtschaffen and Kales, 1968) that describes the sleep-related EXG characteristics and how they define the six sleep stages. A recent update of the manual (Iber et al., 2007) only slightly modified this procedure. The manual defines wakefulness, REM sleep, the three non-REM stages N1 (drowsiness), N2 (light sleep) and N3 (deep sleep), and the corresponding EXG characteristics. Examples of the most important characteristics are presented in Fig. 3. A more comprehensive impression can be obtained by downloading some EDF sleep recordings (st7*.rec files) with corresponding sleep scorings (st7*.hyp files) from the sleep-EDF database at Physionet (www.physionet.org) and reviewing them using Polyman (www.edfplus.info) or EDFbrowser (www.teuniz.net). Note, however, that shape and amplitude of the EXG characteristics vary between individuals and also depend on age, gender, drugs, disorders, electrode location and so on. The manual has a separate section dedicated to child sleep.

Based on signal characteristics such as illustrated in Fig. 3, every 30-s epoch of the recording is classified into one sleep stage (Fig. 1, bottom trace). Scoring difficulties arise when sleep does not behave in accordance with the stage definitions and because of human limitations. For example, sleep spindles may occur in REM sleep (for instance due to the intake of temazepam) and spurious REMs may occur during non-REM sleep. In this case, the difficulty originates from the intrinsic assumption that REM and non-REM sleep processes cannot be active simultaneously. Another type of difficulty is illustrated by the scoring of drowsiness. The full AASM definition of stage N1 (Iber et al., 2007) mentions attenuation or slowing of the alpha rhythm and the presence of slow eye movements, 4–7 Hz EEG and vertex sharp waves. As is recognized by the manual, many subjects do not generate some or even any of these waves while they drowse like everybody else.

Therefore, not only does the definition introduce bias by individual variability of the EXG (see page 25 of the manual), it also requires humans to construct their own, subjective and patient specific, weighing of the various EXG characteristics. As a consequence, the overall disagreement (about 25%, depending on labs and patients) between two human sleep scorings of the same recording mainly involves stage N1 (Anderer et al., 2005). As a final example of scoring difficulties, distinguishing stage N2 from N3 requires measurement of all amplitudes and frequencies between 0.5 and 2 Hz in a 30-s epoch, a task that is impossible to do visually. Therefore, human specialists internalize their own, subjective, image of this difference.

In general, the disagreement between scorers can be reduced by ongoing training sessions that result in agreed consensus scorings. This is common practice in many sleep laboratories but does not solve the even larger differences between laboratories. Multi-laboratory training is already organized by networks of sleep centres in North America (www.aasmnet.org), Europe (www.thesiestagroup.com and www.esrs.eu), Australia and New Zealand (www.sleepaus.on.net). Training should also address important single-epoch scorings such as the detection of REM sleep onset, which has a large impact on the diagnosis and treatment of depressive disorders.

Computerized amplitude (or power) analysis

When compared to human scoring, computers can handle much larger amounts of data at much better accuracy. Therefore, computer analysis of the EXG signals is often used to quantify physiological sleep dynamics as well as the effects of drugs, pathology, sleep deprivation, daytime activities and so on.

Analysis of the submental EMG is rather simple and several solutions exist that do not differ essentially. Ours (Fig. 1) consists of a high-pass filter at 15 Hz (reducing artefacts from brain and electrodes), followed by a notch filter (rejecting any remaining 50/60 Hz mains interference), a rectifier, a sliding 1-s median filter (reducing ECG artefact) and a low-pass filter at 0.01 Hz. Polyman (www.edfplus.info) is equipped with these filters and can do this analysis while saving the result in an EDF file. EOG analysis is less relevant because distinguishing REM, wakefulness and non-REM sleep requires EMG and slow waves only, while eye movements vary strongly between and within subjects. Also, quantification of non-REM sleep depth requires only slow waves (including K-complexes that are in the same frequency band) and sleep spindles, while the other sleep-related EEG characteristics also vary strongly between and within subjects. Therefore, only the analysis of slow waves and sleep spindles will be discussed here.

The two have specific frequency bands roughly around 1 and 14 Hz, respectively. Different investigators prefer different bands, and the frequency band of sleep spindles also depends on the individual and on electrode location. Therefore, a common way to quantify slow waves and sleep spindles is to measure every frequency component separately. Such frequency analysis (also called power spectral analysis) is usually based on the Fourier algorithm. This algorithm samples a 1 Hz sine wave and a 1 Hz cosine wave along with the EEG. A 10 s epoch of EEG using the ADC mentioned above thus results in 2500 samples of the EEG as well as the sine wave and the cosine wave. In this epoch, each EEG sample is multiplied by the corresponding sine wave sample and all 2500 products are summed. Also, each EEG sample is multiplied by the corresponding cosine wave sample and all 2500 products are summed. If the EEG contains a 1 Hz component then either the cosine-sum or the sine-sum will be large, depending on the phase of the 1 Hz component. In fact, because $\sin^2(x) + \cos^2(x) = 1$, adding the sine-sum to the cosine-sum always reflects the power of the 1 Hz component, independent of its phase. The same procedure is repeated for all other frequencies, thus resulting in the power spectrum (Fig. 4). The frequency resolution is the inverse of the epoch

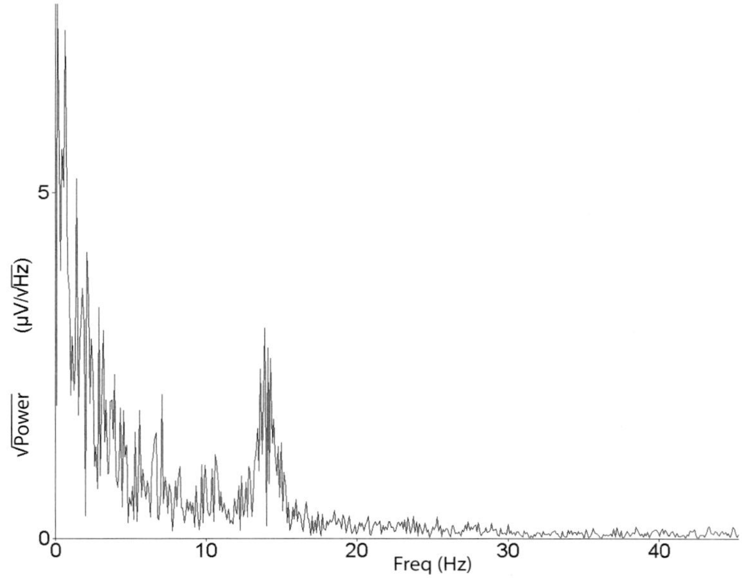

Fig. 4. Power spectrum of Fpz-Cz EEG during the 10 s of light sleep in the last section of Fig. 3. Horizontal axis: frequency. Vertical axis: amplitude, that is square root of power, at that frequency. Note the large estimator variability between adjacent frequencies.

duration (10 s). Thus, in this example the frequency resolution is 0.1 Hz. The thus computed power is the average squared amplitude and therefore reflects both amplitude and occurrence rate of each particular frequency in the EEG.

Sleep affects total slow-wave and spindle powers. These can be computed from the power spectrum by summing all relevant frequencies, for instance 0.5–2 and 12.5–16 Hz, respectively. Summation involves many frequency points (at 0.1 Hz apart) and thus averages out most of the estimator variance. The result is a slow-wave and spindle power estimate every 10 s. Better time resolution can be realized by using shorter epochs, however at the cost of more variance. Fourier analysis, although being a well-defined method, can be implemented with a variety of parameters such as epoch duration and epoch averaging, not to mention a few other commonly applied tricks such as epoch tapering and baseline correction. Plots of slow-wave and spindle amplitude (square root of power) based on Fourier analysis look similar to those in Fig. 1.

Slow waves and spindles also contain components outside the commonly specified frequency ranges. Therefore, the 0.1 Hz frequency selectivity of Fourier analysis is not required and may even have an adverse effect. Softening the edges of the frequency band, that is attenuating rather than blocking adjacent frequency components, essentially converts Fourier analysis into a relatively simple bandpass filter. Such a filter can be realized much more effectively by an algorithm that directly and momentarily converts the EEG into a signal that contains only the slow-wave or spindle component. Advantages are a much better time resolution and the user can see whether the chosen filter actually passes the relevant characteristics of the signal. After the filter, a rectifier (or squarer) converts all amplitudes to a positive value. Subsequent smoothing results in the average amplitude (or power). The bandpass filter and smoother can be implemented with a variety of filter algorithms and parameters. The slow-wave and spindle plots of Fig. 1 were obtained by resonance filters around 1 Hz (bandwidth 1.5 Hz) and 14 Hz (bandwidth 3.5 Hz), respectively, followed by rectification and two first-order low-pass filters at 0.003 Hz, applied to the Fpz-Cz EEG. One can easily reproduce these plots, and the EMG plot, because the recording is in the Physionet database while the filters are precisely specified (Kemp et al., 2000) and implemented in Polyman.

Figure 1 illustrates that the plots enable quantitative studies of slow-wave, spindle and submental-EMG processes. In this figure, we see, for instance, how the muscle tone can drop long before REM sleep starts and how sleep spindles decay while slow waves grow. Figure 5 was obtained in the same subject after administration of temazepam. This figure illustrates that temazepam causes sleep spindles to intrude in the first REM sleep episode. Apparently, processes that are usually attributed to non-REM sleep can be active during REM sleep. The same plots were also obtained from the Pz-Oz EEG (Fig. 5). These plots have smaller amplitudes (note their calibrations) but their shape is almost the same as that of the Fpz-Cz plots. Apparently, although slow waves and sleep spindles are bigger in Fpz-Cz, they show the same sleep-related trends in Pz-Oz. This implies some freedom in selecting derivations for automatic analysis, which can be used to reduce sensitivity to artefacts. For instance, the slow-wave plot obtained from Pz-Oz is less affected by eye movement artefacts.

As illustrated in Fig. 5, some trends may be caused by artefacts. Therefore, automatic analysis must be supervised by an expert who knows the raw data as well as the artefacts and understands how the algorithms handle these.

Neuro-loop analysis

Slow waves, alpha rhythm and sleep spindles are generated by neuronal loops. These loops propagate neuronal activity back to the original node.

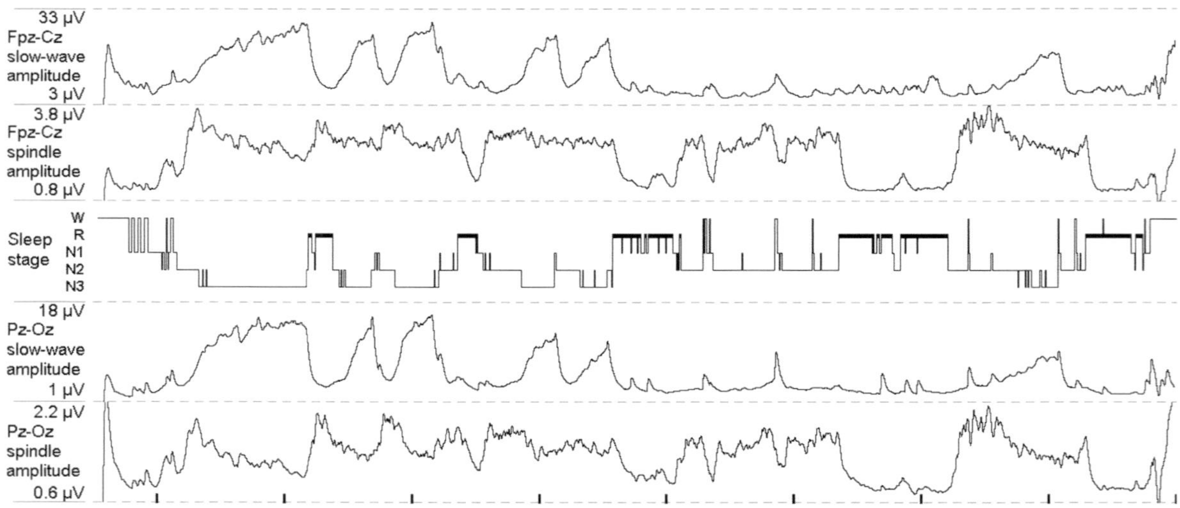

Fig. 5. Whole-night amplitude plots as in Fig. 1 but now after temazepam administration. Same subject, same computations. Traces 1 and 2 were obtained from Fpz-Cz EEG, as in Fig. 1. Extra traces 4 and 5 were obtained from the Pz-Oz derivation. Calibrations are on the left and differ between traces. Note the spindle activity in the first REM period. Note also the peaks in all plots during some wakefulness periods, due to several artefacts.

Therefore, the activity repeats itself: it is rhythmic and concentrates around a specific frequency. That frequency depends on the 'wiring' and is largely fixed. Sleep affects the gain of the loop, that is the fraction of the neuronal activity that is propagated. The larger the gain, the more of the rhythm propagates, which iteratively accumulates higher amplitudes in the loop. Deepening sleep corresponds to an increasing gain of the 1 Hz loop, which results in larger slow-wave amplitudes. The thalamic switch that blocks environmental input (sight, hearing etc.) increases the gain of the 14 Hz loop (Steriade et al., 1990), which results in larger spindle amplitudes. Therefore, measuring the rhythmic amplitude as in Figs. 1 and 5 is indeed useful for tracking these sleep processes. However, EEG amplitude is also affected by many non-sleep-related factors such as artefacts, anatomy, external neuronal drive and electrode distance. Neuro-loop analysis specifically measures only the sleep-related loop gain, independent of the amplitude of the rhythms.

Neuro-loop gain is computed as follows (Kemp et al., 2000). A resonance filter constantly tracks the rhythmic component of the recorded EEG. Between consecutive EEG samples (that is during a few milliseconds), the filter keeps swinging undamped and at the same frequency. In this way, the filter predicts the rhythm that is to be expected in the next EEG sample. However, this expected rhythm will only reach that next EEG sample if it is actually propagated by the neuro-loop. If the loop is inhibited, that is the loop gain is close to zero, the rhythm will not propagate and the next sample will not contain the expected rhythm. If the gain is close to one, the expected rhythm will indeed appear. Therefore, the actual loop gain can be obtained by comparing the predicted rhythm to the actual EEG at each sample. The computation is simple: the product of the EEG sample and the predicted rhythm is divided by the square of the predicted rhythm. The accuracy of the algorithm is improved by smoothing numerator and denominator over one or more seconds, before their division. The loop gain is commonly expressed as a percentage and equals the fraction (0–100%) of the rhythm that is propagated by the neuronal loop, that is the fraction that continues in the next EEG sample. Because of the latter, loop-gain analysis is also called microcontinuity analysis.

Figure 6 shows slow-wave and spindle loop gains at frontal and occipital scalp locations. Parameters are as in the original publication (Kemp et al., 2000), while the spindle resonance filter was set to 14 Hz with 3.5 Hz bandwidth. Compared with amplitude analysis (Fig. 5), loop-gain analysis is more sensitive to sleep and less sensitive to artefacts (see also Kemp et al., 1992). In fact, the slow-wave gain already increases during drowsiness. Also, although frontal amplitudes are much larger than occipital ones, both locations have the same loop gains. This has physiological implications and further supports analysing occipital rather than frontal EEG, thus reducing artefact sensitivity. One can reproduce these plots because the recording is in the Physionet database, the analysis software (micront.zip) can be downloaded from www.edfplus.info and the analysis results are saved in EDF files that can be displayed using any EDF(+) viewer.

Slow-wave loop analysis has demonstrated that the decrease in slow-wave power with increasing age is indeed partly due to a decrease of physiological sleep depth, that is a decrease of the slow-wave loop gain (Mourtazaev et al., 1995). In contrast, the same study showed that women have larger slow-wave power because of differences in anatomy, while their slow-wave loops have the same gain as in men. Thalamic input blocking (which activates the spindle-loop, i.e. sets its gain close to one) is a prerequisite to build up deep sleep. In fact, loop analysis has demonstrated that the temazepam-induced decrease in slow-wave sleep is partly compensated by temazepam-induced thalamic blocking (Kemp and Zwinderman, 2000). The analysis also showed that subjective sleep quality increases with both spindle time and slow-wave time. These results could not be reproduced using amplitude analysis.

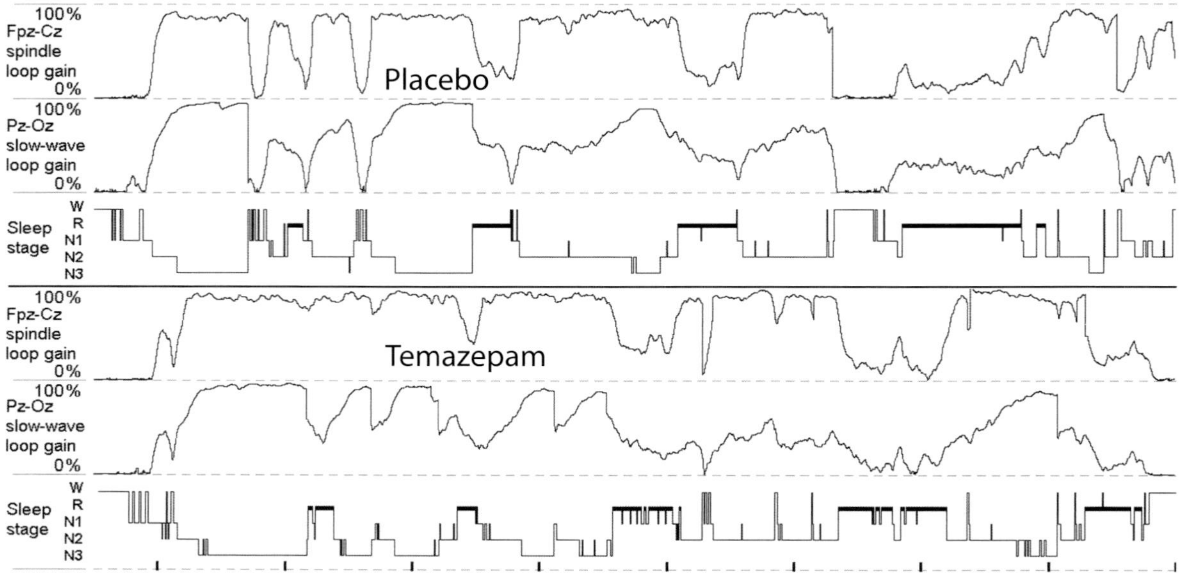

Fig. 6. Whole-night spindle and slow-wave loop gain computed from Fpz-Cz and Pz-Oz EEG, respectively, with corresponding hypnogram. Top and bottom halves of the figure are without and with temazepam administration, respectively. Resonance filters equal those in Figs. 1 and 5. Note that the traces have identical calibrations and are hardly affected by the artefacts during wakefulness.

Topographic analysis

Slow waves and sleep spindles reflect just two of the different sleep-related physiological processes. Those processes have different locations in the brain and can thus be characterized more completely by topographic analysis of the EEG. Such analyses have recently revealed local and functional sleep processes that respond to correspondingly local wake function evoked by sleep deprivation, learning and cognitive tasks.

Topographic studies typically record from 128 or 256 EEG electrodes, may include multi-channel magneto-encephalography and may be integrated with (functional) MRI. A complication is that an EEG signal is the voltage difference between two locations, while a topographic representation should indicate one local potential. This can be solved for each location by averaging all (typically 127 or 255) EEG signals that have that location in common. In this way, the local potential is retained while the other potentials (largely) cancel each other out. Finally, interpolation between the various locations results in a topographic map of scalp EEG potentials.

This map is a blurred projection of the underlying cortical EEG map. The blurring is caused by volume conduction of ionic currents through the skull to the highly conductive scalp, which makes cortical activity spread to neighbouring scalp electrodes and further. Similar to optical deblurring, the cortical EEG map can be reconstructed from the scalp EEG map by contrasting local potentials to neighbouring ones. The reconstruction is based on an electro-anatomical model of the skull and scalp. In this way, spatial resolution is much improved, which is a substantial advantage over single-channel EEG studies. Sampling by, for

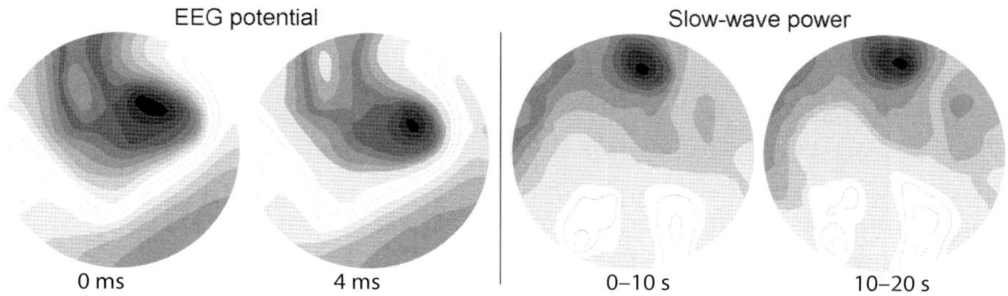

Fig. 7. Left: EEG potential distributions at 0 and at 4 ms. Right: slow-wave power distribution from two subsequent 10-s epochs. Darker colours indicate larger potential and power, respectively. Note the fronto-central EEG dipole and the relatively large frontal slow-wave power, respectively.

instance, 250 Hz thus results in a movie of 'cortical' potential maps every 4 ms (Fig. 7, left).

This movie offers the possibility to directly analyse various kinds of correlation or propagation of brain activity between locations. However, REM and non-REM dynamics are relatively slow and often correspond to certain frequency bands in the EEG. Therefore, many applications in sleep research apply Fourier analysis to fragments of, for example 10 s of the movie. During such a fragment, each local potential represents a 10-s 'cortical' signal and the Fourier analysis extracts the various frequency components in that signal. As described in the section on amplitude analysis, summation of slow-wave or spindle frequency components results in the average EEG amplitude of slow waves or spindles during that 10 s period and at that location. Repeating this for every location results in one topographic map every 10 s that shows the scalp distribution of that average amplitude (Fig. 7, right).

Discussion

Sleep is usually measured by either human scoring or computerized amplitude analysis. Human scoring adapts better to individual EXG characteristics and artefacts but it is less accurate because of the human interpretation of scoring rules, the small number (five or six) of detectable sleep states and the 30 s analysis interval. It is also laborious and does not allow separate analysis of sleep spindles, slow waves, submental EMG and so on. Amplitude analysis does not suffer from any of these limitations but is more sensitive to artefacts and not good at detecting sawtooth and vertex waves, K-complexes and eye movements.

New computer methods are being published or marketed every year and dozens are available now. Their value can be partly judged based on this contribution. Automatic methods that mimic human scoring may save labour but are a bad combination of limited accuracy and sensitivity to artefacts. They are reliable only if a human specialist rejects artefacts, sets analysis parameters such as detection thresholds or even corrects the analyses on an epoch-by-epoch basis (Anderer et al., 2005).

Some dispute still exists on the desirability of combining features such as alpha rhythm, sleep spindles, eye movements and slow waves as is done in human scoring or in artificial neural networks. Neurophysiologists recognize two separate processes during non-REM sleep: thalamic blocking of sensory input followed by deepening of sleep, the two processes being reflected by sleep spindles and slow waves, respectively. This is a strong argument for separate analysis of the two. In fact, we mentioned some new results that could only be obtained by separate slow-wave and spindle plots. Also the submental EMG should be analysed separately, since it can drop while large slow waves are still present, several minutes before REM sleep starts (Fig. 1). Apparently, different EXG features can reflect different sleep processes and should therefore be analysed separately (Kemp, 1993). In fact, REM and non-REM sleep may not be mutually exclusive states as was illustrated by the temazepam-induced spindles during traditional REM sleep (Fig. 5). A more realistic view is probably that thalamic blocking enables slow-wave sleep to build up, while the muscle drop should precede REM sleep.

New methods can be judged based on their results. However, many new methods are not fully specified, which means that they cannot be reproduced independently and therefore cannot be tested. The remaining ones were seldom compared to amplitude analysis. Education in, and availability of, amplitude analysis based on bandpass filtering or Fourier analysis is common. Therefore, investing in understanding and implementation of a new method only makes sense if it beats amplitude analysis in at least one good study. Also, investing in a new method is only attractive if it results in new knowledge. In reality, the results of most new methods are not new and/or could also have been obtained by amplitude analysis. There are a few exceptions, of which two were discussed here. Both are successful mainly because they exploit additional information. Topographic analysis measures at more locations, uses an electro-anatomical model of the scalp and can be integrated with MRI. Neuro-loop analysis uses a physiological model of slow-wave and spindle oscillation and thus quantifies a physiologically realistic parameter. It appears that integration of more measurements and physiological models can result in new knowledge.

Finally, computer analyses are objective and some have resulted in new knowledge. New results need interpretation by a human expert who knows the limitations and pitfalls of the method in relation to the EXG characteristics. Artefacts are a major obstacle, which means that constant attention to recording quality is very important.

References

AASM FAQs (2010). Items G1 and V5, on www.aasmnet.org. American Academy of Sleep Medicine.

Anderer, P., Gruber, G., Parapatics, S., Woertz, M., Miazhynskaia, T., & Klösch, G., et al. (2005). An E-health solution for automatic sleep classification according to Rechtschaffen and Kales: Validation study of the Somnolyzer 24 × 7 utilizing the Siesta database. *Neuropsychobiology*, *51*, 115–133.

Ferri, R., Manconi, M., Plazzi, G., Bruni, O., Vandi, S., & Montagna, P., et al. (2008). A quantitative statistical analysis of the submentalis muscle EMG amplitude during sleep in normal controls and patients with REM sleep behavior disorder. *Journal of Sleep Research*, *17*, 89–100.

Happe, S., Anderer, P., Gruber, G., Klösch, G., Saletu, B., & Zeitlhofer, J. (2002). Scalp topography of the spontaneous K-complex and of delta-waves in human sleep. *Brain Topography*, *15*, 43–49.

Huigen, E., Peper, A., & Grimbergen, C. A. (2002). Investigation into the origin of the noise of surface electrodes. *Medical and Biological Engineering and Computing*, *40*, 332–338.

Iber, C., Ancoli-Israel, S., Chesson, A. L., & Quan, S. F. for the American Academy of Sleep Medicine (2007). *The AASM manual for the scoring of sleep and associated events: Rules, terminology and technical specifications*. Westchester: American Academy of Sleep Medicine.

Jacobson, A., Kales, A., Lehmann, D., & Hoedemaker, F. S. (1964). Muscle tonus in human subjects during sleep and dreaming. *Experimental Neurology*, *10*, 418–424.

Jasper, H. H. (1958). Report of the committee on methods of clinical examination in electroencephalography. *Electroencephalography and Clinical Neurophysiology*, *10*, 370–371.

Kemp, B. (1993). A proposal for computer-based sleep/wake analysis. *Journal of Sleep Research*, *2*, 179–185.

Kemp, B., & Olivan, J. (2003). European data format 'plus' (EDF+), an EDF alike standard format for the exchange of physiological data. *Clinical Neurophysiology*, *114*, 1755–1761.

Kemp, B., & Zwinderman, K. (2000). The effects of temazepam on sleep quality, EEG slow waves and sleep spindles are correlated. *Clinical Neurophysiology*, *111*(Suppl. 1); S76.

Kemp, B., Värri, A., Rosa, A. C., Nielsen, K. D., & Gade, J. (1992). A simple format for exchange of digitized polygraphic recordings. *Electroencephalography and Clinical Neurophysiology*, *82*, 391–393.

Kemp, B., Zwinderman, A. H., Tuk, B., Kamphuisen, H. A. C., & Oberyé, J. J. L. (2000). Analysis of a sleep-dependent neuronal feedback loop: the slow-wave microcontinuity of the EEG. *IEEE Transactions on Biomedical Engineering*, *47*(9); 1185–1194.

Mourtazaev, M. S., Kemp, B., Zwinderman, A. H., & Kamphuisen, H. A. C. (1995). Age and gender affect different characteristics of slow-waves in the sleep EEG. *Sleep*, *18*, 557–564.

Rechtschaffen, A., & Kales, A. (1968). *A manual of standardized terminology, techniques and scoring system for sleep stages of human subjects*. Bethesda: U.S. National Institute of Neurological Diseases and Blindness, Neurological Information Network, Publication no. 204 of the National Institutes of Health (U.S.).

Steriade, M., Gloor, P., Llinás, R. R., Lopes da Silva, F. H., & Mesulam, M. M. (1990). Basic mechanisms of cerebral rhythmic activities. *Electroencephalography and Clinical Neurophysiology*, *76*, 481–508.

Tallgren, P., Vanhatalo, S., Kaila, K., & Voipio, J. (2005). Evaluation of commercially available electrodes and gels for recording of slow EEG potentials. *Clinical Neurophysiology*, *116*, 799–806.

G. A. Kerkhof and H. P. A. Van Dongen (Eds.)
Progress in Brain Research, Vol. 185
ISSN: 0079-6123

CHAPTER 3

Measurement of cognition in studies of sleep deprivation

Paul Whitney[†,*] and John M. Hinson[†,1]

[†]*Department of Psychology, Washington State University, Pullman, WA, USA*

Abstract: Controlled laboratory studies of the effects of sleep deprivation on cognition have the potential to further our understanding of why some complex tasks are more affected by lack of sleep than other tasks. However, apparently simple cognitive tasks reflect multiple cognitive processes at once. Some of the component processes involved in a task may be more affected by sleep deprivation than others. Thus, interpreting measures of overall performance without consideration of the specific task requirements can lead to misleading conclusions. Using examples from studies of attention, working memory and executive functioning, we demonstrate the importance of analysing how different task components contribute to performance and how the nature of the stimulus content can influence outcomes of sleep deprivation studies. Recent developments in cognitive neuropsychology may help sleep researchers conduct more precise tests of fatigue effects on cognition. In turn, studies of sleep and cognition hold promise as a strategy for the development of better general models of how the cognitive system adjusts dynamically to impairments in processing.

Keywords: Task impurity problem; task analysis; attention; working memory; executive function

Introduction

Given the well-documented role of sleep deprivation (SD) in catastrophic failures of human performance, it is not surprising that there is a long history of research devoted to revealing which mental abilities are most compromised under conditions of extended wakefulness (e.g. Harrison and Horne, 2000; Samkoff and Jacques, 1991). Because naturalistic operational environments typically involve a complex interplay of factors, a sensible strategy to try to understand the sources of performance errors caused by SD is to use measures of cognitive ability that isolate particular functions such as attention, memory or decision making. Basic research on cognitive effects of sleep loss has the potential to help us understand why some real-world tasks are affected more than

* Corresponding author.
Tel.: (+) 509-335-3854; Fax: (+) 509-335-8986.
E-mails: pwhitney@wsu.edu
hinson@wsu.edu

DOI:10.1016/B978-0-444-53702-7.00003-8

others, and apply the findings to designing conditions so that errors in performance are minimized and safety enhanced.

One challenge to this ambitious research agenda is the difficulty of scaling up from simple laboratory measures of cognitive ability to predict complex job performance (e.g. Hursh et al., 2004). Another challenge, and the focus of this chapter, is that even apparently simple measures of cognitive performance typically involve multiple processes that may be differentially affected by SD. Thus, researchers turn to more basic measures of cognitive function in order to disentangle the reasons for SD effects on complex task performance, but the basic laboratory measures of cognition are themselves not pure measures of a single cognitive ability. Our goal for this chapter is to demonstrate the importance of the *task impurity problem*, viz., that any cognitive task involves a number of interrelated processes that must be distinguished to understand the causal factors determining actual performance in any situation. Without careful attention to the task impurity problem researchers may come to misleading conclusions about what cognitive abilities are most affected by SD, which in turn will further complicate the challenge of using the data on basic cognitive effects of SD to reduce errors in complex natural environments.

A wide range of cognitive measures has been used with people performing under conditions of both acute, total SD and partial sleep restriction. From this research, it is not only clear that the effects of sleep loss on human cognition are substantial and widespread but also selective (e.g. Alhola and Polo-Kantola, 2007; Lim and Dinges, 2008, 2010). Two separate meta-analyses of SD effects on cognition have found a general trend that the greatest effects of SD are obtained on relatively simple attentional tasks that require vigilance, with substantial effects also found on more complex tests of attention and working memory (WM) that require the manipulation of information in the focus of attention (Lim and Dinges, 2010; Pilcher and Huffcutt, 1996). In general, lesser effects, and sometimes no effects, are obtained on complex measures of cognition such as reasoning or problem solving (e.g. Drummond et al., 2005). However, the effects are stronger and more general across cognitive domains when SD lasts longer than approximately 48 h.

It is clear that incidental reductions in speed of responding, interpreted as lapses of sustained attention typically measured using the psychomotor vigilance test (PVT), are a major contributor to performance decrements on tasks that require vigilance (e.g. driving). However, there are several reasons to believe that there is more to understanding SD effects on cognition than tracking the downstream effects of lapses of attention. Many operational environments that require sustained attention allow for more strategic intervention and shifts between task elements than is true of laboratory tests of vigilance (Matthews et al., 2010). Therefore, understanding how problems in vigilant attention scale up to performance problems in natural operational environments will require knowledge of SD effects on strategic and compensatory adaptations to challenges to attentional systems (cf. Boonstra et al., 2007). Many studies in the SD literature have investigated such attentional control processes, and as Lim and Dinges (2010) found in their meta-analysis, SD effects in this domain are substantial.

Most, although not all, studies of SD and attentional control have been based on the belief that the prefrontal cortex (PFC) is especially vulnerable to SD effects (e.g. Harrison and Horne, 2000). Much of this research has used batteries of well-established cognitive and neuropsychological measures to look for patterns in the types of tests that are most sensitive to the effects of SD (e.g. Harrison et al., 2000; Pace-Schott et al., 2009). A comprehensive task analysis of all the various measures of cognition used in studies of SD is beyond the scope of this chapter, but we can illustrate the importance of the task impurity problem, and offer some guidelines for task analysis, using examples from the interrelated domains of attention, WM and executive function. These abilities are often considered to be closely associated with the PFC, and measures of these abilities are widely employed in SD studies.

Attention and choice reaction time tasks

Tests of vigilance such as the PVT generally require only a simple stimulus detection response, and the challenge to performance is to maintain attention over time. As noted above, the ability to maintain vigilance is greatly reduced by SD, but substantial effects of SD are also obtained on choice reaction time (RT) tasks that lack the vigilance requirements of the PVT. The nature of the choice RT tasks varies across studies, but what they have in common is the requirement that the subject allocates attention to a stimulus and extracts information quickly in order to choose one response or another. One typical implementation is to present a stimulus and require the person to make one of two possible responses indicating what type of stimulus was presented, for example one response to indicate the number 1 was presented and a different response to indicate the number 2 was presented (e.g. Frey et al., 2004; Karakorpi et al., 2006).

Another common choice RT procedure is to present two stimuli and require the person to decide quickly whether the stimuli match on some dimension, for example whether two figures are visually identical (e.g. Alchanatis et al., 2005; Rocklage et al., 2009). In the literature on SD effects, these choice RT measures are often referred to as tests of *complex attention* or *decision making*. Because these speeded tasks are quite sensitive to SD the collective results are sometimes characterized as supporting the hypothesis that SD results in general cognitive slowing (cf. Alhola and Polo-Kantola, 2007; Lim and Dinges, 2010; Sagaspe et al., 2006). In turn, some investigators have suggested that problems in higher order cognition, including the WM and executive functions discussed below, could be a consequence of the general decline in speed of processing (e.g. Verstraeten, 2007). Note that in using the term speed of processing, we are referring here to slower RTs across a range of choice tasks rather than performance on a few standardized tests, such as digit symbol substitution, that have been labelled in the psychometric and neuropsychological literatures as 'speed of processing tests'. Lim and Dinges found in their meta-analysis that SD effects on the digit symbol substitution task tend to be small. We regard this as another example of the trend towards preservation of performance when complex tasks are performed under SD conditions. The digit symbol task is actually a very complex measure involving motor speed, response selection, WM and learning novel associations (Yoran-Hegesh et al., 2009).

There is no doubt that SD results in slower (and sometimes less accurate) performance on a wide range of choice RT tasks. However, that general finding should not be equated with the theoretical claim that choice RT tasks assess undifferentiated abilities of 'complex attention' or 'cognitive processing speed'. Performance on choice RT tasks is dependent on the efficient execution of several different cognitive processes that are dissociable both functionally and neuroanatomically (Posner, 1978; Posner and Rueda, 2002). At a minimum, typical choice RT paradigms require orienting and stimulus detection, accrual of stimulus information relevant to the decision, decision and response selection, and motor programming. Several different neural networks are invoked to provide attentional control to these processes. Not surprisingly then, cognitive slowing on choice RT tasks is observed in a wide range of neurological disorders, as well as in the aging brain and the fatigued brain. In commenting on the ubiquity of evidence for cognitive slowing, Posner and Rueda (2002) noted: 'There is probably no single reason why generalized slowing is found in so many disorders. Studies of neuroimaging have shown us that most chronometric tasks, even quite simple ones, involve activation of a number of separate neural generators' (p. 970).

Recent evidence on the sources of performance in choice RT tasks only serves to reinforce Posner and Rueda's conclusions. For example, whether or not one finds age-related slowing on choice RT tasks depends in part on whether the older adults can use attentional strategies that make use of context and background knowledge to assist their encoding of information from a stimulus (e.g. Gold et al., 2009). In addition, neuroimaging data suggest that slower speed of processing in older adults can be due to problems with stimulus feature analysis soon after stimulus presentation or to the later process of selecting relevant information for encoding into WM (Zanto et al., 2010). The implications of these findings for sleep researchers are that declines in performance on choice RT can sometimes be masked by effective use of attentional allocation strategies, and declines may be obtained with some stimuli and not others. Moreover, even apparently elementary cognitive tasks can have multiple potential sources of performance decrements.

There are multiple strategies for isolating specific components of choice RT tasks reported in the cognitive literature (e.g. Posner, 1978; Ratcliff, 1988; Whitney et al., 2001). In the context of SD research, a recent example of decomposing choice RT components was reported by Ratcliff and Van Dongen (2009). They used Ratcliff's (1988) diffusion model to characterize performance on a numerosity discrimination task in which subjects quickly judged displays of asterisks as containing a small (50 or less) or large (greater than 50) number of stimuli. The diffusion model decomposes accuracy and RT on two-choice paradigms into separate processes including the rate of accumulation of information needed for a decision, the decision criterion setting and non-decision task components such as response execution. Ratcliff and Van Dongen found that SD subjects showed substantial decreases in the ability to extract decision-related information from a stimulus, but no change in the duration of response execution processes. It is important to note, however, that their elegant task decomposition study leaves open an important question about whether the effect of SD on the rate of information accrual generalizes to other types of decisions besides the numerosity judgement task. There may be a general effect of SD on information accrual, but it is also possible that judgements that are less perceptually driven and based on more habitually used pathways (such as semantic encoding of words) would produce a different pattern of results than the numerosity task. Thus, it is important to consider not only how different task components may contribute to performance but also the nature of the stimulus content. The importance of task content as well as task processes is a theme that will be repeated as we turn to the topic of WM.

Working memory

The notion that human cognition is very dependent on a WM system for the maintenance and manipulation of information has a long history in general models of cognition (e.g. Anderson, 1983; Baddeley, 1986; Norman and Shallice, 1986). Although there is no single generally accepted model of WM, there is agreement that all models of WM must be able to address some key issues. Perhaps the most central is the general bottleneck in capacity for maintaining information in the focus of attention, while at the same time there are also modality specific (e.g. verbal and visual-spatial) processing limitations (Miyake and Shah, 1999). The concept of WM is also closely tied to the executive control functions of cognition because the information that is actively maintained in WM largely determines the next set of cognitive operations to be executed (e.g. the role of WM in the ACT-R model; Anderson, 2004).

Because the concept of WM plays a central role in explaining human performance, a number of studies have investigated SD effects on WM using a variety of tasks including memory-scanning tasks, short-term recall tasks and the N-back task (e.g. Mu et al., 2005; Smith et al., 2002). Global performance on all WM tasks can be influenced by the process of getting information into WM and decision and response processes in addition to maintenance and manipulation of information in WM. Interpreting performance decrements on these tasks as reflecting problems with WM requires careful consideration of the task components and the use of indices of performance that isolate the processes of interest.

The task impurity problem in WM tasks can easily be demonstrated with a memory-scanning task based on the classic studies by Sternberg (1966, 1969). Variants of this task have been used in several studies of SD effects on WM (e.g. Mu et al., 2005; Nilsson et al., 2005; Tucker et al., 2010). On each trial of the Sternberg task the subject is given a memory set with digits or letters as stimuli, with varying memory set sizes, typically from two to six items. The memory set is removed from view and a probe stimulus is presented. The task is to decide as quickly as possible whether the probe item came from the memory set. RTs on the task are a linear increasing function of the size of the memory set. The slope of the RT function over set size is a relatively pure measure of the efficiency of scanning WM. In contrast, overall mean RT on Sternberg trials also contain the time to encode the probe, make a decision and execute the response. Nevertheless, some studies cited as showing that SD impairs WM have either failed to manipulate set size or used a control condition in which both stimulus encoding and the memory load varied between conditions (e.g. Mu et al., 2005).

Recent data from Tucker et al. (2010) confirm the risk in using overall performance on the memory-scanning task as an index of WM functions. Mean RTs of SD subjects were much longer than baseline, and since the Sternberg task is considered a classic WM task, it would be tempting to conclude that WM is substantially impaired by SD. However, Tucker et al. decomposed the function relating RT to set size into memory scanning (slope) and non-WM (intercept) components. The results were striking. There was no effect of SD on the memory-scanning rate. The effect on mean RT in the Sternberg task was entirely in the non-WM aspects of the task (see Fig. 1).

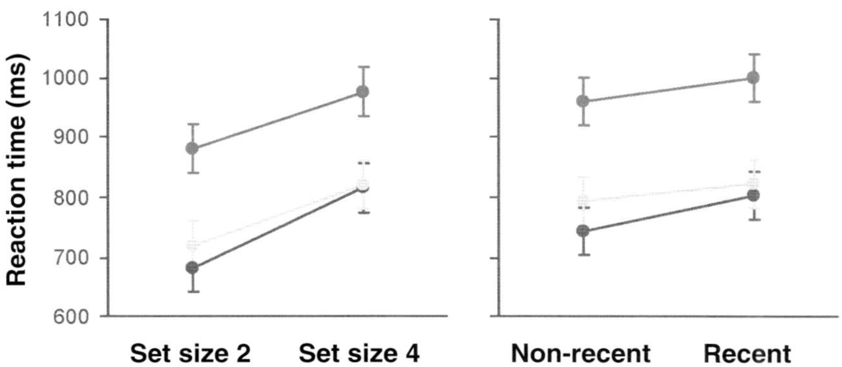

Fig. 1. Effects of SD on reaction times in a modified Sternberg task. $N = 11$ healthy young adults performed the task at baseline (black), after 51 h of total SD (dark grey), and following two nights of recovery sleep (light grey). See the main text for details on the task. The left panel shows reaction times (mean ± standard error) for memory sets containing two items versus four items; the slopes of the lines represent working memory scanning efficiency. The right panel shows reaction times (mean ± standard error) for negative probes not seen recently versus negative probes seen recently (i.e. in the previous trial); the differences in reaction times represent the ability to resist proactive interference. Sleep deprivation caused an overall increase in reaction times regardless of set size or probe recency. However, working memory scanning efficiency and resistance to proactive interference were not significantly affected by sleep deprivation. Data from Tucker et al. (2010).

Because WM tasks involve cognitive processes other than WM, SD effects on WM tasks can be due to non-WM sources. So, while a battery of WM tests may all show SD effects, which may produce an estimate of a substantial effect of SD on WM in a meta-analysis, the effect is not necessarily a WM effect. Only by using task analysis and extraction of the appropriate index to isolate WM processes can we draw conclusions about SD effects on WM.

It is also important to note that the Tucker et al. finding of preserved WM function under SD was obtained with verbal WM. There is evidence that somewhat different results are obtained when visual-spatial stimuli must be maintained. Chee and Chuah (2007) conducted a neuroimaging study in which the spatial positions of visual stimuli had to be maintained in WM. They systematically varied the WM load and found two types of SD-induced deficits. First, SD resulted in poorer performance even under low load conditions and this deficit was based on degraded perceptual processing. Second, there was an additional load-dependent process at work. The people least able to maintain performance after SD showed a reduced ability to inhibit irrelevant activation, which could make visual-spatial WM less effective.

The Chee and Chuah (2007) results provide a clear example that problems with early stimulus processing can have a downstream effect in WM tasks. However, unlike Tucker et al., they also found evidence for SD-induced processing deficits that could have a direct effect on WM. Their data are a useful reminder that WM is a complex system, and there are a number of examples in the literature of dissociations between verbal and visual-spatial WM (see Baddeley, 1986). In addition, when people are engaged in a complex cognitive task, WM must be updated regularly to maintain relevant information and purge irrelevant information. The updating processes of WM have seldom been specifically targeted for investigation by SD researchers. However, WM updating is closely tied to the related concept of executive function (cf. Killgore et al., 2009a, 2009b; Miyake et al., 2001), and executive function is the focus of a number of SD studies. Unfortunately, task impurity is even more problematic in the study of executive function than in the study of attention and WM.

Executive functioning

Executive functions are those higher cognitive processes that coordinate more basic aspects of cognition to allow for purposeful, goal-directed behaviour. Goal maintenance, set shifting, mental flexibility and inhibition are examples of cognitive abilities that are widely viewed as executive functions (see Chan et al., 2008; Jurado and Rosselli, 2007; Suchy, 2009, for excellent reviews of this literature). Executive functions are of particular interest to sleep researchers for two reasons. First, one of the prominent accounts of SD effects on cognition suggests that the PFC is particularly sensitive to SD (e.g. Harrison et al., 2000), and tests of executive function are strongly, although not exclusively, associated with frontal lobe functioning (Suchy, 2009). Second, if executive functioning is substantially affected by SD that may help relate the cognitive effects of SD to errors in complex operational environments.

In studies of SD effects on executive functioning, researchers have often administered tasks originally developed as tests of executive functioning in patients with damage to the PFC (e.g. Binks et al., 1999; Horne, 1988; Killgore et al., 2009a; Pace-Schott et al., 2009). Several neuropsychological tests of executive function used in SD research are shown in Table 1 with a description of the putative executive functions measured and examples of non-executive processes that also contribute to performance. Note that *all* of these executive tasks are necessarily dependent on attentional and stimulus encoding processes.

The neuropsychological battery approach has several notable strengths. The tests have known psychometric properties and they are normed so that absolute levels of performance are interpretable. Further, by using a battery of these tests

Table 1. Some common tests of executive functions

Test	Executive functions	Non-executive components
Wisconsin Card Sorting Test	Set shifting, inhibition	Encoding, attention, vigilance, visual-spatial processing
Verbal Fluency	Cognitive flexibility, inhibition	Encoding, attention, semantic memory
Stroop	Inhibition	Encoding, attention, word processing speed
Tower of London	Planning, inhibition	Encoding, attention, short-term memory; visual-spatial processing
Iowa Gambling Task	Emotional decision making	Encoding, attention, reversal learning, memory

researchers have the opportunity to detect problems across a wide range of executive functions. The downside of the breadth of measurement that these neuropsychological tests afford is that the task impurity problem affects their interpretation in two ways. It is difficult to determine which specific executive abilities are affected, and it is difficult to determine if an effect of SD on a test is due to executive or non-executive processes. In this context, it is interesting to note that results from SD studies of executive function are quite mixed, with reports of substantial effects of SD (e.g. Harrison and Horne, 1998; Nilsson et al., 2005) and reports of no effect of SD (e.g. Pace-Schott et al., 2009; Sagaspe et al., 2006). Differences in testing procedures and manipulation of sleep can account for some inconsistencies, but there are also reports of a mixed pattern of results within the same study depending on the executive test considered (e.g. Killgore et al., 2009b).

Neuropsychological tests of executive function are clinically meaningful and diagnostically useful. Yet, these tests are based on loosely defined constructs, involving an unspecified mixture of different cognitive processes. The result is that on a given neuropsychological test two people can show the same degree of deficit in performance, but for very different reasons (Jurado and Rosselli, 2007). The complications associated with assessing executive functioning make it difficult to untangle the mixed pattern of results in SD studies. However, progress is being made in defining and measuring executive functions that may make it possible to conduct more precise and interpretable tests of SD effects on executive functioning. One approach to better defining executive functions has used factor analysis to extract latent variables to represent core dimensions. For example, Miyake et al. (2000) used latent variable analysis to distill a wide range of executive tests into three executive factors: shifting, updating and inhibition. This three-factor model has proven useful in studies of the effects of changes in executive functioning across the lifespan (e.g. Marcovitch and Zelazo, 2009). While this general approach helps to better define domains of executive functioning, the latent dimensions of executive functioning obtained vary somewhat with the tasks chosen (e.g. de Frias et al., 2009). Also, the factor model may change after SD, as has been found with other task batteries (e.g. Frey et al., 2004). The ultimate value of the latent variable approach in separating executive from non-executive contributions to task performance is still uncertain.

Another approach to defining and measuring executive functioning is to use experimental tasks that are designed to isolate specific cognitive control functions. Two aspects of executive functioning that have received considerable attention are inhibition and goal maintenance. The concept of inhibition is invoked as a hypothetical control mechanism for a number of widely used cognitive tasks. Of particular interest are tasks that require withholding a prepotent response, such as go/no go and stop-signal tasks, and tasks that require overcoming interference from previous responses or mental representations of previously presented stimuli (Aron, 2007; Jonides et al., 2000; Tipper,

2001). In contrast to the generic view of inhibition that has emerged from clinical neuropsychology, the evidence suggests there may be multiple processes involved in overcoming response conflicts and interference. For inhibition of behaviour, as when subjects must interrupt the execution of a response in the go/no go or stop-signal tasks, neural networks that allow for inhibition of a prepotent response vary depending on the specific task requirements (e.g. Simmonds et al., 2008), but there is also some overlap of the brain pathways involved in tasks that require response inhibition (Zheng et al., 2008). The nature of inhibition of mental representations is less clear. MacLeod et al. (2003) argued that the effects of attentional interference in many tasks can be accounted for without using inhibition as an explanatory mechanism. However, there is some evidence from brain lesion studies that the brain regions associated with inhibition of prepotent responses may be involved in controlling interference among competing items in memory (Aron, 2007).

For sleep researchers, a lesson from the cognitive neuroscience of inhibition is that we should assume neither that all potential sources of interference in performance are resolved by a single executive inhibitory function nor that different implementations of the same general task have the same cognitive requirements. For example, Tucker et al. (2010) used several converging measures of susceptibility to interference from items recently processed in WM and found no evidence that interference effects increase with SD. This could mean that active inhibitory control mechanisms are relatively well maintained under SD, or this result could indicate simply that the passive decay of activation of concepts no longer in the focus of attention proceeds at a similar rate regardless of sleep state. Likewise, the results of studies of response inhibition must be interpreted in light of the specific requirements of the task employed. For example, some go/no go tasks have a WM component, and some do not (Simmonds et al., 2008). Despite the complexities, however, our increasing understanding of interference resolution and inhibitory control holds promise as a fruitful avenue for exploring SD effects on executive functioning.

An equally fruitful avenue of investigation may emerge from studies of goal maintenance and cognitive control. For example, Braver and colleagues (Braver and Barch, 2006; Braver et al., 2009) have proposed a fundamental distinction between proactive and reactive modes of cognitive control. In proactive control, contextual information related to current goals is actively maintained in the focus of attention and this information biases the processing of new information towards the most goal relevant stimuli. In reactive control, the processing of incoming information is not biased by the goal context, but goal-related information is retrieved and used as needed to resolve response conflicts.

The theory that there are dual mechanisms of control was developed using a very simple continuous performance task in which subjects are to respond if they see the letter X only when preceded by the letter A. With any other pairing of letters, the person is to withhold a response. In the typical design, the letter A is usually followed by an X. When a delay is introduced between the context letter and the test letter, older adults tend to make errors of commission by responding to trials in which X follows a letter other than A. Compared to younger adults, older adults show reduced prefrontal activation during the cue and delay period but increased activation when the probe is presented. Thus, younger adults appear to use a proactive strategy of maintaining the context letter over the delay and older adults react to the probe by trying to retrieve the most recent context information needed to control their task behaviour (Braver et al., 2009). Interestingly, if incentives are used that increase attentional focus on the probe letter at the expense of attention to the context letter, younger adults can be induced to shift to a reactive strategy.

Although laboratory tests such as the AX continuous performance test might help us isolate well-defined executive functions, a potential criticism of this approach is that there is little evidence for the ecological validity of these tasks for predicting complex task performance in natural situations. Of course, that problem is not unique to laboratory tests. Even though many standard neuropsychological instruments have been in use for decades, data supporting the ecological validity of neuropsychological tests is scant (Jurado and Rosselli, 2007). In fact, one of the ways that research on SD effects on executive functioning could have general implications for cognitive neuropsychology is that SD may be a tractable context for assessing whether laboratory task performance scales up to predict performance on more complex natural tasks. That is, in the laboratory SD can be used as an experimentally controlled method of inducing a neurological deficit. Unlike the progressive and irreversible changes in neurological functioning that are typically assessed or diagnosed by the clinical neuropsychologist using executive functioning tests, neurological functioning impaired by SD is reversible. Current executive function tests, developed over years of careful effort, still lack sufficient ecological validity to predict functional problems in everyday life for many neurological populations (e.g. Burgess et al., 1998; Hanna-Pladdy, 2007; Wood and Liossi, 2006). SD research may, indirectly, be a good way to improve the ecological validity of executive function tests.

Conclusions and recommendations

One of the more compelling controversies in the history of psychology and linguistics was generated by Benjamin Whorf's claim that human cognition is completely dependent on distinctions that are represented in a person's language, an idea known as linguistic determinism (Whorf, 1956). His strong account of linguistic determinism has been falsified. For example, if a language has only two colour names, the users of that language perceive differences in colour that are not distinguished by the two colour names (Heider, 1972). Nevertheless, there are many demonstrations of a weaker version of linguistic determinism: language affects and shapes thought (Hunt and Agnoli, 1991). Many of the problems with measurement of cognition that we have reviewed in this chapter resemble a form of linguistic determinism. Particular tasks become labelled in the professional literature as 'WM tasks' or 'executive tasks' and they become part of test batteries in which performance is interpreted as reflecting only the attribute captured by the verbal label. Those verbal labels can blind the user to the problem of task impurity, and to the fact that performance decrements may, in some cases, be due to processes other than those the investigator intends to assess.

The interpretive problems created by task impurity cannot be completely overcome by factor analysis or meta-analysis. Instead, task analysis is required. We recommend that investigators keep three points in mind in choosing and interpreting their tests of cognitive functioning. First, consider the *processing* components of the task. Are there means for extracting indices of performance that isolate the process of interest from other processes? Second, consider *content* as well as process. To what extent might variations in performance on a given task reflect the stimulus class (e.g. visual-spatial vs. verbal) used? Third, consider that performance changes with SD could reflect *qualitative differences* and not just quantitative differences. Could the subjects be changing task strategies or recruiting different neural networks to try and compensate for processing deficits? Our understanding of the dynamic adjustments people make to deal with cognitive challenges is rudimentary at both the functional and neurological levels of analysis. A fourth, and final consideration, is the distinct contribution of hot (i.e. affective) processing, and possible interaction of hot and cold (i.e. non-affective) cognitive processes in human performance. While this chapter has focused on cold cognition, there is no doubt that SD influences mood and affective reactions to stimuli. It is also clear than hot cognitive pathways can influence the function of cold cognition, particularly in the domains of memory and decision making (e.g. Seymour and

Dolan, 2008). The cognitive challenges presented by SD may be an excellent context in which to build better theories of such cognitive dynamics.

References

Alchanatis, M., Zias, N., Deligiorgis, N., Amfilochiou, A., Dionellis, G., & Orphanidou, D. (2005). Sleep apnea-related cognitive deficits and intelligence: An implication of cognitive reserve theory. *Journal of Sleep Research*, *14*(1); 69–75.

Alhola, P., & Polo-Kantola, P. (2007). Sleep deprivation: Impact on cognitive performance. *Neuropsychiatric Disease and Treatment*, *3*(5); 553–567.

Anderson, J. R. (1983). *The architecture of cognition.* Harvard University Press, Cambridge, MA.

Anderson, J. R. (2004). Human symbol manipulation within an integrated cognitive architecture. *Cognitive Science: A Multidisciplinary Journal. 2004 Rumelhart Prize Special Issue Honoring John R. Anderson: Theoretical Advances and Applications of Unified Computational Models*, *29*(3), 313–341.

Aron, A. R. (2007). The neural basis of inhibition in cognitive control. *Neuroscientist*, *13*(3); 214–228.

Baddeley, A. (1986). *Working memory.* Clarendon Press /Oxford University Press, Oxford.

Binks, P. G., Waters, W. F., & Hurry, M. (1999). Short-term total sleep deprivations does not selectively impair higher cortical functioning. *Sleep*, *22*(3); 328–334.

Boonstra, T. W., Stins, J. F., Daffertshofer, A., & Beek, P. J. (2007). Effects of sleep deprivation on neural functioning: An integrative review. *Cellular and Molecular Life Sciences*, *64* (7); 934–946.

Braver, T. S., & Barch, D. M. (2006). Extracting core components of cognitive control. *Trends in Cognitive Sciences*, *10* (12); 529–532 Epub 2006 Oct 30.

Braver, T. S., Paxton, J. L., Locke, H. S., & Barch, D. M. (2009). Flexible neural mechanisms of cognitive control within human prefrontal cortex. *Proceedings of the National Academy of Sciences of the United States of America*, *106* (18); 7351–7356 Epub 2009 Apr 20.

Burgess, P. W., Alderman, N., Evans, J., Emslie, H., & Wilson, B. A. (1998). The ecological validity of tests of executive function. *Journal of International Neuropsychological Society*, *4*(6); 547–558.

Chan, R. C., Shum, D., Toulopoulou, T., & Chen, E. Y. (2008). Assessment of executive functions: Review of instruments and identification of critical issues. *Archives of Clinical Neuropsychology*, *23*(2); 201–216 Epub 2007 Dec 21.

Chee, M. W., & Chuah, Y. M. (2007). Functional neuroimaging and behavioral correlates of capacity decline in visual short-term memory after sleep deprivation. *Proceedings of the National Academy of Sciences of the United States of America*, *104*(22); 9487–9492 Epub 2007 May 21.

de Frias, C. M., Dixon, R. A., & Strauss, E. (2009). Characterizing executive functioning in older special populations: From cognitively elite to cognitively impaired. *Neuropsychology*, *23*(6); 778–791.

Drummond, S. P., Brown, G. G., Salamat, J. S., & Gillin, J. C. (2005). Increasing task difficulty increases the cerebral compensatory response to total sleep deprivation. *Sleep*, *1*(27); 445–451.

Frey, D. J., Badia, P., & Wright Jr., K. P. (2004). Inter- and intra-individual variability in performance near the circadian nadir during sleep deprivation. *Journal of Sleep Research*, *13*(4); 305–315.

Gold, B. T., Andersen, A. H., Jicha, G. A., & Smith, C. D. (2009). Aging influences the neural correlates of lexical decision but not automatic semantic priming. *Cerebral Cortex*, *19* (11); 2671–2679 Epub 2009 Mar 8.

Hanna-Pladdy, B. (2007). Dysexecutive syndromes in neurologic disease. *Journal of Neurologic Physical Therapy*, *31* (3); 119–127.

Harrison, Y., & Horne, J. A. (1998). Sleep loss impairs short and novel language tasks having a prefrontal focus. *Journal of Sleep Research*, *7*(2); 95–100.

Harrison, Y., & Horne, J. A. (2000). The impact of sleep deprivation on decision making: A review. *Journal of Experimental Psychology Applied*, *6*(3); 236–249.

Harrison, Y., Horne, J. A., & Rothwell, A. (2000). Prefrontal neuropsychological effects of sleep deprivation in young adults – a model for healthy aging? *Sleep*, *23*(8); 1067–1073.

Heider, E. R. (1972). Universals in color naming and memory. *Journal of Experimental Psychology*, *93*(1); 10–20.

Horne, J. A. (1988). Sleep loss and "divergent" thinking ability. *Sleep*, *11*(6); 528–536.

Hunt, E., & Agnoli, F. (1991). The Whorfian hypothesis: A cognitive psychology perspective. *Psychological Review*, *98* (3); 377–389.

Hursh, S. R., Redmond, D. P., Johnson, M. L., Thorne, D. R., Belenky, G., & Balkin, T. J., et al. (2004). Fatigue models for applied research in warfighting. *Aviation Space and Environmental Medicine*, *75*(3); Suppl. A44–A53, discussion A54–A60.

Jonides, J., Marshuetz, C., Smith, E. E., Reuter-Lorenz, P. A., Koeppe, R. A., & Hartley, A. (2000). Age differences in behavior and PET activation reveal differences in interference resolution in verbal working memory. *Journal of Cognitive Neuroscience*, *12*(1); 188–196.

Jurado, M. B., & Rosselli, M. (2007). The elusive nature of executive functions: A review of our current understanding. *Neuropsychological Review*, *17*(3); 213–233 Epub 2007 Sep 5.

Karakorpi, M., Alhola, P., Urrila, A. S., Kylmata, M., Portin, R., & Kalleinen, N., et al. (2006). Hormone treatment gives no benefit against cognitive changes caused by acute sleep deprivation in postmenopausal women. *Neuropsychopharmacology*, *31*(9); 2079–2088 Epub 2006 Mar 15.

Killgore, W. D., Kahn-Greene, E. T., Grugle, N. L., Killgore, D. B., & Balkin, T. J. (2009a). Sustaining executive functions during sleep deprivation: A comparison of caffeine, dextroamphetamine, and modafinil. *Sleep*, *32*(2); 205–216.

Killgore, W. D., Grugle, N. L., Reichardt, R. M., Killgore, D. B., & Balkin, T. J. (2009b). Executive functions and the ability to sustain vigilance during sleep loss. *Aviation Space and Environmental Medicine*, *80*(2); 81–87.

Lim, J., & Dinges, D. F. (2008). Sleep deprivation and vigilant attention. *Annals of the New York Academy of Sciences*, *1129*, 305–322.

Lim, J., & Dinges, D. F. (2010). A meta-analysis of the impact of short-term sleep deprivation on cognitive variables. *Psychological Bulletin*, *136*(3); 375–389.

MacLeod, C. M., Dodd, M. D., Sheard, E. D., Wilson, D. E., & Bibi, U. (2003). Ross, B. H. (Ed.), *The psychology of learning and motivation: Advances in research and theory*. *Vol. 43*, Elsevier Science, New York, pp. 163–214.

Marcovitch, S., & Zelazo, P. D. (2009). A hierarchical competing systems model of the emergence and early development of executive function. *Developmental Science*, *12*(1); 1–18.

Matthews, G., Warm, J. S., Reinerman-Jones, L. E., Langheim, L. K., Washbun, D. A., & Tripp, L. (2010). Task engagement, cerebral blood flow velocity, and diagnostic monitoring for sustained attention. *Journal of Experimental Psychology Applied*, *16*(2); 187–203.

Miyake, A., & Shah, P. (1999). *Models of working memory*. Cambridge University Press, Cambridge, UK.

Miyake, A., Friedman, N. P., Emerson, M. J., Witzki, A. H., Howerter, A., & Wager, T. D. (2000). The unity and diversity of executive functions and their contributions to complex "Frontal Lobe" tasks: A latent variable analysis. *Cognitive Psychology*, *41*(1); 49–100.

Miyake, A., Friedman, N. P., Rettinger, D. A., Shah, P., & Hegarty, M. (2001). How are visuospatial working memory, executive functioning, and spatial abilities related? A latent-variable analysis. *Journal of Experimental Psychology: General*, *130*(4); 621–640.

Mu, Q., Mishory, A., Johnson, K. A., Nahas, Z., Kozel, F. A., & Yamanaka, K., et al. (2005). Decreased brain activation during a working memory task at rested baseline is associated with vulnerability to sleep deprivation. *Sleep*, *28*(4); 433–446.

Nilsson, J. P., Soderstrom, M., Karlsson, A. U., Lekander, M., Akerstedt, T., & Lindroth, N. E., et al. (2005). Less effective executive functioning after one night's sleep deprivation. *Journal of Sleep Research*, *14*(1); 1–6.

Norman, D. A., & Shallice, T. (1986). Attention to action: Willed and automatic control of behavior. In: Davidson, R., Schwartz, G., Shapiro, D. (Eds.), *Consciousness and self regulation*. Plenum, New York, pp. 1–18.

Pace-Schott, E. F., Hutcherson, C. A., Bemporad, B., Morgan, A., Kumar, A., & Hobson, J. A., et al. (2009). Failure to find executive function deficits following one night's total sleep deprivation in university students under naturalistic conditions. *Behavioral Sleep Medicine*, *7*(3); 136–163.

Pilcher, J. J., & Huffcutt, A. I. (1996). Effects of sleep deprivation on performance: A meta-analysis. *Sleep*, *19*(4); 318–326.

Posner, M. I. (1978). *Chronometric explorations of mind*. Lawrence Erlbaum, Oxford.

Posner, M. I., & Rueda, M. R. (2002). Mental chronometry in the study of individual and group differences. *Journal of Clinical and Experimental Neuropsychology*, *24*(7); 968–976.

Ratcliff, R. (1988). Continuous versus discrete information processing modeling accumulation of partial information. *Psychological Review*, *95*(2); 238–255.

Ratcliff, R., & Van Dongen, H. P. (2009). Sleep deprivation affects multiple distinct cognitive processes. *Psychonomic Bulletin Review*, *16*(4); 742–751.

Rocklage, M., Williams, V., Pacheco, J., & Schnyer, D. M. (2009). White matter differences predict cognitive vulnerability to sleep deprivation. *Sleep*, *32*(8); 1100–1103.

Sagaspe, P., Sanchez-Ortuno, M., Charles, A., Taillard, J., Valtat, C., & Bioulac, B., et al. (2006). Effects of sleep deprivation on Color-Word, Emotional, and Specific Stroop interference and on self-reported anxiety. *Brain and Cognition*, *60* (1); 76–87 Epub 2005 Nov 28.

Samkoff, J. S., & Jacques, C. H. (1991). A review of studies concerning effects of sleep deprivation and fatigue on residents' performance. *Academic Medicine*, *66*(11); 687–693.

Seymour, B., & Dolan, R. (2008). Emotion, decision making, and the amygdale. *Neuron*, *58*(5); 662–671.

Simmonds, D. J., Pekar, J. J., & Mostofsky, S. H. (2008). Meta-analysis of go/no-go tasks demonstrating that fMRI activation associated with response inhibition is task-dependent. *Neuropsychologia*, *46*(1); 224–232 Epub 2007 Jul 28.

Smith, M. E., McEvoy, L. K., & Gevins, A. (2002). The impact of moderate sleep loss on neurophysiologic signals during working-memory task performance. *Sleep*, *25*(7); 784–794.

Sternberg, S. (1966). High-speed scanning in human memory. *Science*, *153*(736); 652–654.

Sternberg, S. (1969). Memory-scanning: Mental processes revealed by reaction-time experiments. *American Scientist*, *57*(4); 421–457.

Suchy, Y. (2009). Executive functioning: Overview, assessment, and research issues for non-neuropsychologists. *Annals of Behavioral Medicine*, *37*(2); 106–116 Epub 2009 May 20.

Tipper, S. P. (2001). Does negative priming reflect inhibitory mechanisms? A review and integration of conflicting views. *Quarterly Journal of Experimental Psychology A*, *54*(2); 321–343.

Tucker, A. M., Whitney, P., Belenky, G., Hinson, J. M., & Van Dongen, H. P. (2010). Effects of sleep deprivation on dissociated components of executive functioning. *Sleep*, *33*(1); 47–57.

Verstraeten, E. (2007). Neurocognitive effects of obstructive sleep apnea syndrome. *Current Neurology and Neuroscience Reports*, *7*(2); 161–166.

Whitney, P., Arnett, P., Driver, A., & Budd, D. (2001). Measuring central executive function: What's in a reading span? *Brain and Cognition*, *45*(1); 1–14.

Whorf, B. L. (1956). *Language, thought, and reality.* MIT Press, Cambridge, MA.

Wood, R. L., & Liossi, C. (2006). The ecological validity of executive tests in a severely brain injured sample. *Archives of Clinical Neuropsychology*, *21*(5); 429–437.

Yoran-Hegesh, R., Kertzman, S., Vishne, T., Weizman, A., & Kolter, M. (2009). Neuropsychological mechanisms of Digit Symbol Substitution Test impairment in Asperger Disorder. *Psychiatry Research*, *166*(1); 35–45 Epub 2009 Feb 11.

Zanto, T. P., Toy, B., & Gazzaley, A. (2010). Delays in neural processing during working memory encoding in normal aging. *Neuropsychologia*, *48*(1); 13–25.

Zheng, D., Oka, T., Bokura, H., & Yamaguchi, S. (2008). The key locus of common response inhibition network for no-go and stop signals. *Journal of Cognitive Neuroscience*, *20*(8); 1434–1442.

G. A. Kerkhof and H. P. A. Van Dongen (Eds.)
Progress in Brain Research, Vol. 185
ISSN: 0079-6123

CHAPTER 4

Sleep, memory and emotion

Matthew P. Walker*

Sleep and Neuroimaging Laboratory, Department of Psychology, Helen Wills Neuroscience Institute, University of California, Berkeley, CA, USA

Abstract: As critical as waking brain function is to cognition, an extensive literature now indicates that sleep supports equally important, different, yet complementary operations. This review will consider recent and emerging findings implicating sleep, and specific sleep-stage physiologies, in the modulation, regulation and even preparation of cognitive and emotional brain processes. First, evidence for the role of sleep in memory processing will be discussed, principally focusing on declarative memory. Second, at a neural level, several mechanistic models of sleep-dependent plasticity underlying these effects will be reviewed, with a synthesis of these features offered that may explain the ordered structure of sleep, and the orderly evolution of memory stages. Third, accumulating evidence for the role of sleep in associative memory processing will be discussed, suggesting that the long-term goal of sleep may not be the strengthening of individually memory items, but, instead, their abstracted assimilation into a schema of generalized knowledge. Forth, the newly emerging benefit of sleep in regulating emotional brain reactivity will be considered. Finally, and building on this latter topic, a novel hypothesis and framework of sleep-dependent affective brain processing will be proposed, culminating in testable predictions and translational implications for mood disorders.

Keywords: Sleep; emotion; affect; memory; encoding; consolidation; integration; SWS; REM; reactivation

Introduction

Despite the vast amount of time this state takes from our lives, we still lack any consensus function for sleep. In part, this is perhaps because sleep, like its counterpart wakefulness, may serve not one but many functions, for brain and body alike. Centrally, sleep is a brain phenomenon, and over the past 20 years, an exciting revival has taken place within the neurosciences, focusing on the question of why we sleep, and specifically targeting the role of sleep in a number of cognitive and emotional processes. This chapter aims to provide a synthesis of these recent findings in humans, with the goal of extracting

* Corresponding author.
Tel.: (+) 510 642 5292; Fax: (+) 510 642 5293.
E-mail: mpwalker@berkeley.edu

DOI:10.1016/B978-0-444-53702-7.00004-X

consistent themes across domains of brain function that appear to be regulated by sleep. 'Memory processing and brain plasticity' section will explore the role of sleep in memory and brain plasticity, and also examine competing models of sleep-dependent learning. 'Association, integration and creativity' section will address the role of sleep beyond memory consolidation, in processes of association, integration and creativity. Finally, 'Emotional regulation' section will discuss the more recent and emerging role for sleep in emotional and affective brain regulation.

Memory processing and brain plasticity

When considering the role of sleep in memory processing, it is pertinent to appreciate that memories *evolve* (Walker and Stickgold, 2006). Specifically, memories pass through discrete stages in their 'lifespan'. The conception of a memory begins with the process of encoding, resulting in an initial stored representation of an experience within the brain. However, it is now understood that a vast number of post-encoding memory processes can take place. For memories to persist over the longer time course of minutes to years, an offline, non-conscious operation of consolidation appears to be necessary, affording memories greater resistance to decay (a process of stabilization), or even improved recollection (a process of enhancement). Sleep has been implicated in both the encoding and consolidation of memory.

Sleep and memory encoding

In contrast to the role of sleep after learning promoting offline consolidation (discussed below), emerging evidence indicates an important need for sleep before learning in preparing specific brain networks for initial encoding of information. One of the earliest human studies to report the effects of sleep and sleep deprivation on declarative memory encoding was by Morris et al. (1960), indicating that 'temporal memory' (memory for when events occur) was significantly disrupted by a night of pre-training sleep loss. These findings have been revisited in a more rigorous study by Harrison and Horne (2000), again using the temporal memory paradigm. Significant impairments in retention were evident in a group of subjects deprived of sleep for 36 h, scoring significantly lower than controls, even in a subgroup that received caffeine to overcome non-specific effects of lower alertness. Furthermore, the sleep-deprived subjects displayed significantly worse insight into their memory encoding performance, resulting in lower predictive ability of performance.

Pioneering work by Drummond and colleagues has examined the neural basis of similar memory impairments using fMRI, investigating the effects of 35 h of total sleep deprivation on verbal learning (Drummond et al., 2000). In those who were sleep deprived, regions of the medial temporal lobe (MTL) were significantly less active during learning, relative to a control group that had slept, while the prefrontal cortex actually expressed greater activation. Most interesting, the parietal lobes, which were not activated in the control group during learning, were significantly active in the deprivation group. Such findings suggest that inadequate sleep (at least following one night) prior to learning produces bi-directional changes in episodic encoding activity, involving the inability of the MTL to engage normally during learning, combined with potential compensation attempts by prefrontal regions, which in turn may facilitate recruitment of parietal lobe function (Drummond and Brown, 2001).

The impact of sleep deprivation on memory formation may be especially pronounced for emotional material. We have investigated the impact of sleep deprivation on the encoding of emotionally negative, positive and neutral words (Walker and Stickgold, 2006). When combined across all stimulus types, subjects in the sleep-deprived condition exhibited a striking 40% reduction in the ability to form new human memories under conditions of sleep deprivation. When these data were separated into the three affective categories (negative, positive or neutral), the magnitude of encoding impairment differed. In those that had slept, both positive and negative stimuli were associated with superior retention levels relative to the neutral condition, consonant with the notion that emotion facilitates memory encoding. However, there was severe disruption of encoding and hence later retention for neutral and especially positive emotional memory in the sleep-deprived group. In contrast, a relative resistance of negative emotional memory was observed in the deprivation group. These data suggest that, while the effects of sleep deprivation are directionally consistent across memory sub-categories, the most profound impact is on the encoding of positive emotional stimuli, and to a lesser degree, emotionally neutral stimuli. In contrast, the encoding of negative memory appears to be more resistant to the effects of prior sleep loss, at least following one night.

The impact of sleep deprivation on the neural dynamics associated with declarative memory encoding has recently been examined using event-related fMRI (Yoo et al., 2007a). In addition to performance impairments under condition of sleep deprivation, and relative to a control group that slept, a highly significant and selective deficit was identified in bilateral regions of the hippocampus – a structure known to be critical for learning new episodic information. When taken together, this collection of findings indicate the critical need for sleep before learning in preparing key neural structures for efficient next-day learning. Without adequate sleep, hippocampal function becomes markedly disrupted, resulting in the decreased ability for recording new experiences, the extent of which appears to be further governed by alterations in prefrontal encoding dynamics.

Sleep and memory consolidation

Using a variety of behavioural paradigms, evidence for the role of sleep in memory consolidation has now been reported across a diverse range of phylogeny. Perhaps the earliest reference to the beneficial impact of sleep on memory is by the Roman rhetoritician, Quintilian, stating that

> ...[it] is a curious fact, of which the reason is not obvious, that the interval of a single night will greatly increase the strength of the memory... Whatever the cause, things which could not be recalled on the spot are easily coordinated the next day, and time itself, which is generally accounted one of the causes of forgetfulness, actually serves to strengthen the memory.

A robust and consistent literature has demonstrated the need for sleep after learning in the subsequent consolidation and enhancement of procedural memories; the evidence for which has recently been reviewed elsewhere (Walker and Stickgold, 2006). Early work focusing on the role for sleep in declarative memory processing was somewhat less consistent, but more recent findings have now begun to reveal a robust beneficial effect of sleep on the consolidation of declarative memory – our focus here.

Several reports by Born and his colleagues have shown offline improvement on a word-pair associates task following sleep, attributed to early night sleep, rich in SWS (Diekelmann and Born, 2010). More recently, the same group has demonstrated that, in addition to classically defined slow delta waves (0.5–4 Hz), the very slow cortical oscillation (<1 Hz) appears to be important for the consolidation of declarative memories. Following learning of a word-pair list, a technique called ‘direct current stimulation’ was used to induce slow oscillation-like field potentials in the prefrontal cortex (in this case, at 0.75 Hz) during early night SWS (Diekelmann and Born, 2010). Direct current stimulation not only increased the amount of slow oscillations during the simulation period (and for some time after) but also enhanced next-day word-pair retention, suggesting a critical role for SWS neurophysiology in the offline consolidation of episodic facts.

Rather than simply testing memory recall, Ellenbogen et al. (2006) have since revealed the extent of sleep's ability to protect declarative memories using experimentally induced learning disruption. Taking advantage of a classic interference technique called the A-B–A-C paradigm, subjects first learned unrelated word-paired associates, designated as list A-B (e.g. leaf-wheel etc.). After sleep at night, or wakefulness during the day, half of the subjects in each group learned a new, interfering list containing a new associate paired with the first word, designated as list A-C (e.g. leaf-nail etc.), before being tested on the original A-B list (e.g. leaf-wheel etc.). In the groups that did not experience the interfering challenge – simply being trained and then tested on list A-B – sleep provided a modest benefit to memory recollection (Fig. 1A). However, when testing the groups that were exposed to interfering list learning (list A-C) prior to recalling the original list (list A-B), a large and significant protective benefit was seen in those that slept (Fig. 1B). Thus, memories tested after a night of sleep were significantly more resistant to interference, whereas across a waking day, memories were far more susceptible to this antagonistic learning challenge. Yet, it was only by using an interfering challenge, the A-C list, that the true benefit of sleep's protection of memory was revealed, a benefit that would not necessarily have been evident in a standard study-test memory paradigm.

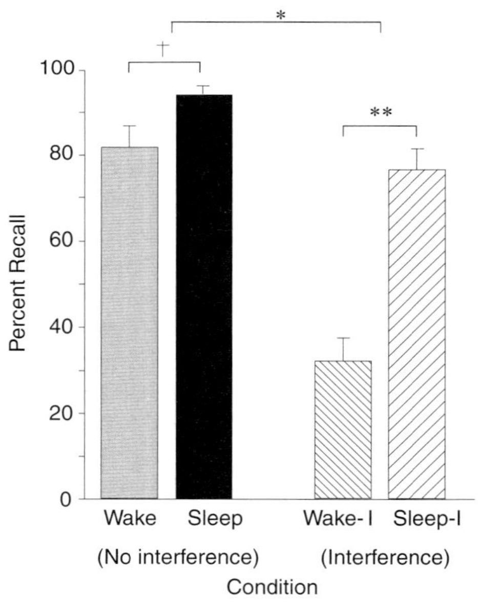

Fig. 1. Impact of sleep on the consolidation and stabilization of declarative memory. Percent correct recall for B words from the original A-B pair after a 12 h retention interval of either wake or sleep following no interference or interference learning (list A-C). $^{\dagger}p < 0.10$, $^{*}p < 0.05$, $^{**}p < 0.001$; error bars indicate s.e.m. Modified from Ellenbogen et al. (2007).

One mechanism proposed to underlie these effects on hippocampal-dependent learning tasks (and see next section) is the reactivation of memory representations at night. A considerable number of reports have investigated the firing patterns of large networks of individual neurons across the wake-sleep cycle in animals. The signature firing patterns of these hippocampal and cortical networks, expressed during waking performance of spatial tasks and novel experiences, appear to be 'replayed' during subsequent SWS (and in some studies, also REM) (Dave and Margoliash, 2000; Dave et al., 1998; Ji and Wilson, 2007; Jones and Wilson, 2005; Louie and Wilson, 2001; Poe et al., 2000; Ribeiro et al., 2004; Skaggs and McNaughton, 1996; Wilson and McNaughton, 1994). Homologous evidence has been reported in the human brain using a virtual maze task in combination with positron emission tomography (PET) scanning (Peigneux et al., 2004). Daytime learning was initially associated with hippocampal activity. Then, during post-training sleep, there was a re-emergence of hippocampal activation, specifically during SWS. Most compelling, however, the amount of SWS reactivation in the hippocampus was proportional to the amount of next-day task improvement, suggesting that this reactivation is associated with offline memory improvement.

Building on the framework that memories, particularly those involving the hippocampus, are reactivated at night during sleep, Rasch et al. (2007) have taken advantage of the classical psychology effect of cue-dependent recall and translated it into a sleep-dependent consolidation paradigm. It is well known that memory can be strongly modulated by smell; most of us have associated the smell of a certain perfume or cologne with a particular person, and when we encounter that same perfume again, it often results in the powerful cued recall of memories of that particular person. In this study, however, following learning of a spatial memory task that was paired with the smell of rose, the odour was not re-presented again at retrieval, but instead, during subsequent SWS that night – a time when consolidation was presumed to be occurring. Relative to a control condition where the odour was not presented again during SWS, the re-perfusion of the rose scent at night resulted in significantly improved recall the following day. Moreover, the re-presentation of the odour resulted in greater (re)activation of the hippocampus during SWS. These findings support the role of SWS in the consolidation of individual declarative memories, and may indicate an active reprocessing of hippocampal-bound information during SWS.

Models of sleep-dependent memory processing

Elucidating the neural mechanisms that control and promote sleep-dependent human memory consolidation remains an active topic of research, and debate. It is perhaps unlikely that multiple different memory systems, involving diverse cortical and/or subcortical networks, require the same underlying neural mechanisms for their modulation. Even if they do, it is not clear that this process would rely on just one type of sleep-stage physiology. At present, two intriguing models of sleep-dependent plasticity, relevant to declarative memory, have been offered to account for the overnight facilitation of recall, which build on different aspects of neural activity during sleep: (1) hippocampal-neocortical dialogue and (2) synaptic homeostasis hypothesis.

Hippocampal-neocortical dialogue

There is considerable agreement that structures within the MLT, most notably the hippocampal complex, are crucial for the formation and retrieval of new declarative memories. These structures are believed to guide the reinstatement of recently formed memories by binding together patterns of cortical activation that were present at the time of initial learning. A classical model of declarative memory consolidation suggests that information initially requires MTL binding, but over time, and by way of slow offline processes, is eventually integrated into neocortical circuits (Fig. 2).

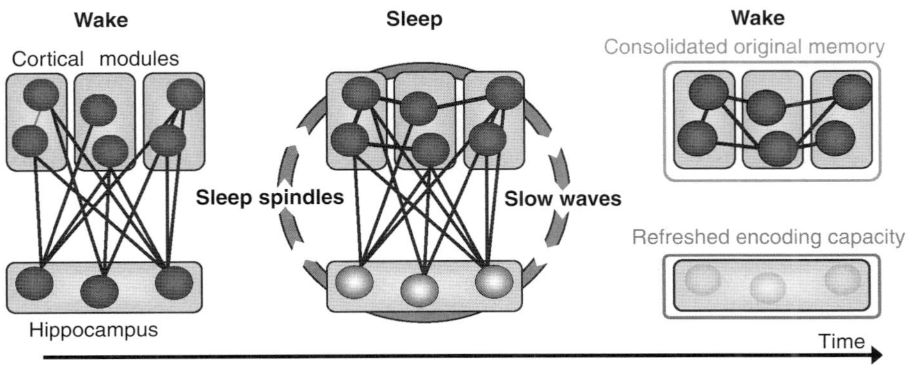

Fig. 2. Model of sleep-dependent hippocampal-neocortical memory consolidation. At encoding the hippocampus rapidly integrates information within distributed cortical modules. Successive sleep-dependent reactivation of this hippocampal-cortical network leads to progressive strengthening of cortico-cortical connections, which, over time, allow these memories to become independent of the hippocampus and gradually integrated with pre-existing cortical memories. (For interpretation of the references to colour in this figure legend, the reader is referred to the web version of this book.)

Neocortical structures thus become the eventual storage site for consolidated episodic memories through cross-cortical connections, and as a consequence, the MTL is not necessary for their retrieval. Therefore, the classical model of memory consolidation holds that neocortical structures become increasing important for the retention and retrieval of successfully consolidated episodic memories, while the corresponding contribution of the hippocampus progressively decreases. In addition to its role in binding distributed cortical memory components, the hippocampus plays a critical role in reactivating these networks, specifically during sleep. This process of reactivation would, over multiple sleep cycles across a night, and/or multiple occurrences of sleep over many nights, gradually strengthen the initially weak connections between neocortical sites, thereby reinforcing them (Fig. 2). Eventually, this strengthening would allow the original information to be activated in the cortex, independent of the hippocampus.

Interestingly, these models make two predictions about the impact of sleep on declarative memory. The first is that declarative memories from the day prior should be more resistant to interference the next day, due to the increased cortico-cortical connections formed during overnight consolidation (Fig. 1). It is precisely this behavioural effect that was reported in the study by Ellenbogen et al. (2006), showing greater post-sleep resistance to interference, using the A-B–A-C paradigm. A second and far less considered benefit of this sleep-dependent dialogue is the encoding capacity of the hippocampus (Fig. 2). If the strengthening of cortico-cortical connections takes place during sleep, albeit iteratively, then blocking sleep after hippocampal learning should negate this offline transfer, preventing the development of independence from (or 'refreshing' of) the hippocampus, and, by doing so, decrease the capacity for new hippocampal learning the next day. This second premise appears to accurately explain the findings discussed in the 'Sleep and memory encoding' section above (Yoo et al., 2007b), which describe a significant impairment of hippocampal encoding activity when sleep has not taken place (through deprivation), being associated with a decreased ability to form new episodic memories.

Two recent reports have provided further evidence in support of this sleep-dependent dialogue and neural transformation of declarative memory. In the first such report, Takashima et al. (2006) examined the benefit of daytime naps on episodic declarative memory consolidation. In addition to a long-term evaluation of memory over 3 months, there was also a short-term evaluation of memory across the first day, which included an intervening nap period (90 min) between training and testing of the original studied (remote) stimuli. Interestingly, the duration of NREM SWS during the intervening nap correlated positively with later recognition memory performance, yet negatively with retrieval-related activity in the hippocampus. Advancing on these findings, Maquet and colleagues have since demonstrated that one night of post-training sleep deprivation, even following recovery sleep, significantly impairs the normal modulation of hippocampal activity associated with episodic memory recollection (Gais et al., 2007). Furthermore, first-night sleep deprivation also prevented an increase in hippocampal connectivity with the medial prefrontal cortex (mPFC), a development that was only observed in those who sleep after learning.

No study has yet demonstrated that the neural signature of learning during the day is subsequently reactivated and driven by characteristics of SWS at night, and that the extent of these properties is consequently proportional to the degree of next-day recall and memory reorganization. Nevertheless, collectively, they offer an empirical foundation on which to entertain this possibility.

Synaptic homeostasis hypothesis

In recent years, an orthogonal theory of SWS and learning has emerged, which postulates a role for sleep in regulating the synaptic connectivity of the brain – principally the neocortex (Tononi and Cirelli, 2003, 2006). The model by Tononi and Cirelli considers NREM SWS, and specifically the magnitude of slow-wave activity (SWA) of SWS, as a brain state that promotes the *decrease* of synaptic connections, not their increase. Accordingly, plastic processes, such as learning and memory occurring during wakefulness, result in a net increase in synaptic strength in diffuse brain circuits. The role of subsequent SWS, therefore, and the slow oscillation in particular, is to selectively downscale or 'depotentiate' synaptic strength back to baseline levels, preventing synaptic over-potentiation, which would result in saturated brain plasticity. In doing so, this re-scaling would leave behind more efficient and refined memory representations the next day, affording improved recall. A number of human studies by Huber, Tononi and colleagues have provided evidence supporting their model. For example, it has been shown that learning of a motor-skill adaptation task during the day subsequently triggers locally specific increases in cortical SWA at night, the extent of which is proportional to both the amount of initial daytime learning and the degree of next-day improvement (Fig. 3) (Huber et al., 2004). Taken together with complementary cellular evidence demonstrating sleep-dependent reductions in synaptic strength (Liu et al., 2010), such findings are considered supportive of a homeostatic function of NREM slow waves in promoting synaptic downscaling.

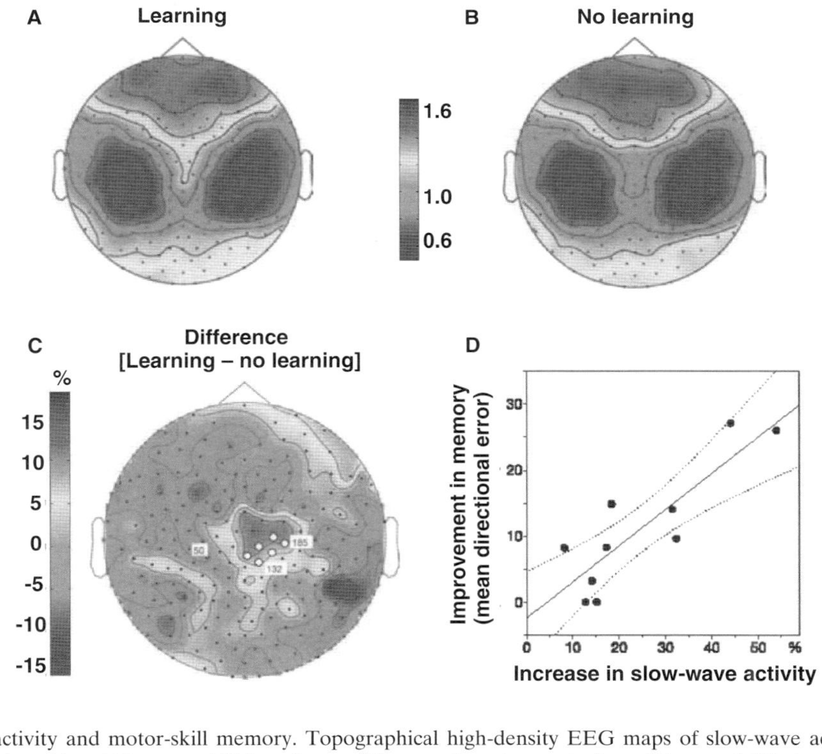

Fig. 3. Slow-wave activity and motor-skill memory. Topographical high-density EEG maps of slow-wave activity (SWA) during NREM sleep following either (A) motor-skill learning or (B) a non-learning control condition, and (C) the subtracted difference between SWA in the learning versus non-learning condition, demonstrating a local homeostatic increase above the learning-related central-parietal brain region. (D) The correlation between the amount of overnight improvement on the task (measured the next day) and the extent of increase in SWA across subjects. Modified from Huber et al., 2004. (For interpretation of the references to colour in this figure legend, the reader is referred to the web version of this book.)

How can the two concepts of neural reactivation (such as increased fMRI activity during SWS) and neural homeostasis (such as increased slow-wave EEG activity) be interpreted at a neural synaptic level? It could be argued that both these reported changes reflect *either* an increased neural reactivation or an increase in SWA associated with homeostasis and synaptic downscaling. Furthermore, both hypotheses, while distinctly different, mechanistically, could offer complementary benefits at the network level in terms of signal-to-noise ratio (SNR), and may account for overnight memory improvements. Specifically, homeostatic synaptic downscaling could result in the removal of superfluous neural connections, resulting in improved SNR. However, neural reactivation and strengthening of experience-dependent circuits, without removing redundant synaptic connects, may equally improve SNR. Therefore, both mechanisms, while different, could produce a similar outcome-enhanced fidelity of the memory representation. Presumably the combination of both would produce perhaps the most optimal and efficient memory trace, yet a careful delineation of these possibilities remains an important goal for future studies.

Interestingly, the homeostasis model would also predict that sleep deprivation, specifically the prevention of SWS, would also negate effective new learning the next day, due to over-potentiation of synaptic connections. Thus, any region that exhibits SWA, and is involved in representing memory (e.g. hippocampus), would display a corresponding inability to code further information beyond a normal waking duration (~16 h in humans). Such a premise may offer an alternative explanation to the marked hippocampal encoding deficits reported under conditions of sleep loss (Yoo et al., 2007b).

A role for sleep spindles?

Independent of both these models, which consider the role of SWS in memory processing, a number of reports have also described an association between learning and the hallmark feature of stage-2 NREM – sleep spindles; short (~1 s) synchronous bursts of activity expressed in the EEG in the 10–16 Hz frequency range. For example, following learning of a motor-skill memory task, Nishida and Walker (2007) have examined post-training sleep spindles over the motor cortex, evaluating the difference in spindle activity in the right, learning hemisphere (since subjects performance the task with their left non-dominant hand), relative to the left, non-learning hemisphere. Remarkably, when sleep-spindle power at electrode sites above the primary motor cortex of the non-learning hemisphere (left) were subtracted from those in the learning hemisphere (right), representing the within-subject, between-hemisphere difference in spindle activity following learning, a strong predictive relationship with the amount of memory improvement emerged.

Such findings indicate that the enhancement of specific memory representations is associated with electrophysiological events expressed at local, anatomically discrete locations of the brain. Contrasting with the proposed impact of SWS, the mechanistic benefit of sleep spindles may be related to their faster stimulating frequency; a range suggested to facilitate long-term potentiation (LTP; a foundational principle of synaptic strengthening in the brain), and not synaptic depression. This increase in spindle activity may represent a local, endogenous trigger of intrinsic synaptic plasticity, again corresponding topographically to the underlying memory representation (Nishida and Walker, 2007).

Increases in post-training spindle activity are not limited to procedural memory tasks. For example, Gais et al. have shown that there is significantly higher sleep-spindle density in subjects that underwent a daytime episodic learning session (encoding of word-pair associates) compared to a control group that did not perform the learning session. Moreover, the spindle density was associated with the proficiency of memory recalled the next day in the learning group (Gais et al., 2002).

Reconciling models

None of these models needs necessarily to be wrong. Instead, aspects of each may afford complementary and synergistically beneficial outcomes for memory. Clues to this possibility lie within the ordered structure of human sleep, with NREM SWS dominating early in the night, and stage-2 NREM and REM prevailing later in the night. When placed in this temporal framework, a progression of events emerges that may be optimal for the neuroplastic modulation of memory representations. From a reactivation perspective, the predominance of hippocampal-neocortical interaction would take place in the early SWS-rich phase of the night, leaving cortico-cortical connections on offer for later processing during stage-2 NREM and REM. Similarly, and even in coincidence, SWS may downscale cortical (and possibly subcortical) plasticity, and do so in a learning-dependent manner, again leaving only those representations (or aspects of these representations) which are strongest – including those strengthened by hippocampal-neocortical interplay – for processing during these latter periods of sleep, dominated by faster frequency oscillations.

This concept is analogous to the art of sculpture. During the day, through experience, substantial informational 'clay' is acquired on the cortical pedestal; some relevant, some not. Once accumulated, the next step is to carve out and select the strongest and most salient memory representations (statues) for the organisms – a mechanism that SWS, occurring first and predominately early in the night, may be ideally suited for. Following such downscaling and/or dynamic selection of memory through translocation, the remaining cortical representations – the rough outline of the sculpted form – may finally be strengthened by faster frequency oscillations, including those of sleep spindles (and potentially PGO-wave burst during REM), more associated with the potentiation of synaptic connections, not their depotentiation. This final step is akin to polishing and improving the detailed features of the memory statue, which, in terms of computational modelling, would offer improved signal-to-noise quality within the system. Such a cooperative mechanism, which appreciates the temporal order of the wake-sleep cycle (acquisition, followed by post-processing), and, within sleep, the ultradian pattern of sleep-stage progression across a night (selection and removal, followed by strengthening) would produce a network of stored information that is not only more efficient, but, for those representations remaining, more enhanced. Both these processes would predict improved recall of remodelled individual memories from the prior day and further afford the synaptic capacity for efficient acquisition of new 'information clay' the next day.

Association, integration and creativity

As critical as consolidation may be – an operation classically concerned with individual memory items – the association and integration of new experience into pre-existing networks of knowledge is equally, if not more, important. The resulting creation of associative webs of information offers numerous and powerful advantages. Indeed, the end goal of sleep-dependent memory processing may not be to enhance individual memories in isolation, but, instead, to integrate them into a common schema, and by doing so, facilitate the development of universal concepts; a process which forms the basis of generalized knowledge, and even creativity.

Association and integration

Perhaps the earliest demonstration that sleep may be involved in a form of memory generalization was by Fenn et al. (2003). Utilizing an artificial grammar task, subjects were trained and later tested on their ability to transfer phonological categories across different acoustic patterns. The task required forming new mappings from complex acoustical sounds to pre-existing linguistic categories, which then generalized to new stimuli. As such, it involved both a declarative process of forming specific memories associated with the learned stimuli, together with a procedural component involving mapping across the set of learned sounds that supports generalization to novel stimuli. During the initial training session there was a significant improvement in recognition performance on the task. However, when retested after a 12 h waking interval, performance had decayed. Yet, if subjects were retested following a night of sleep, this ability for memory generalization was restored. Supporting this concept, Dumay and Gaskell (2007) have also demonstrated that sleep, and not equivalent time awake, can integrate related but novel phonemes into pre-existing long-term lexical memory stores overnight.

In a related study by Gomez et al. (2006), infants were exposed to 'phrases' from an artificial language during a learning session – for example phrases like 'pel-wadim-jic' – until the infants became familiar (as indexed by look responses). However, these three syllable units had an embedded rule, which was that the first and last unit formed a relationship of non-adjacency; in this case, pel predicts jic. The infants were then retested several hours later, yet some infants took normally scheduled naps, while others were scheduled at a time when they would not sleep after learning. At later testing, infants again heard the recordings, along with novel phrases in which the predictive relationship between the first and last word was new. Infants who did not sleep recognized the phrases they had learned earlier, yet those who had slept demonstrated a generalization of the predictive relationship to new phrases, suggesting that the intervening process of sleep allowed the *re*interpretation of prior experience, and supported the abstraction of commonalities – that is the ability to detect a general pattern in new information.

Ellenbogen et al. have since tested this sleep-dependent hypothesis of integration by examining human relational memory – the ability to generalize previously acquired associations to novel situations. Participants initially learned five 'premise pairs' ($A > B$, $B > C$, $C > D$, $D > E$, $E > F$). Unknown to subjects, the pairs contained an embedded hierarchy ($A > B > C > D > E > F$). Following an offline delay of 20 min, 12 h across the day or 12 h containing a night of sleep, knowledge of this hierarchy was tested by examining relational judgements for novel 'inference' pairs, separated either by 1° of associative distance ($B > D$, $C > E$ pairs) or by 2° of associative distance ($B > E$ pair). Despite all groups achieving near identical premise-pair retention after the offline delay (i.e. the building blocks of the hierarchy), a striking dissociation was evident in the ability to make relational inference judgements. Subjects that were tested soon after learning in the 20 min group showed no evidence of inferential ability, performing at chance levels (Fig. 4A). In contrast, the 12 h groups displayed highly significant relational memory development. Most remarkable, however, if the 12 h period contained a night of sleep, a near 25% advantage in relational memory was seen for the most distantly connected inferential judgement (the $B > E$ pair; Fig. 4A). Together, these findings demonstrate that human memory integration takes time to develop, requiring slow, offline associative processes. Furthermore, sleep appears to preferentially facilitate this integration by enhancing hierarchical memory binding, biasing the development of the most distant/weak associative links amongst related yet separate memory items (Fig. 4B). It is also interesting to note a further advantage of this sleep-dependent assimilation process. When stored as individual premise pairs (top row, Fig. 4B), the size/number of items (bits) of information to code is 10 (A-B, B-C, C-D, D-E, E-F). However, when formed into a hierarchy, the informational load is compressed, reduced by nearly 50% to just six bits (A-B-C-D-E-F). Therefore, a supplementary benefit of sleep-dependent memory association may be the improved efficiency of memory storage, in addition to a more generalized representation.

Thus, the overnight strengthening and consolidation of individual item memories (reviewed above) may not be the ultimate objective of sleep-dependent memory processing, especially when considering that declarative (non-emotional) memories decay over the long term. It is then interesting to speculate whether sleep serves to facilitate two complementary objectives for declarative

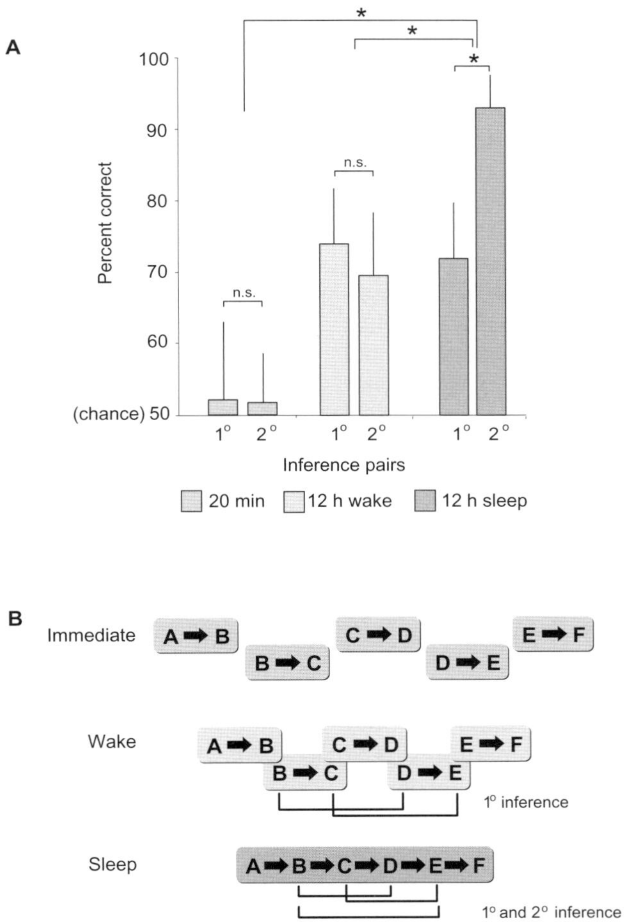

Fig. 4. Sleep-dependent integration of human relational memory. (A) Delayed inference (associative) memory performance (% correct) in a relational memory task following different offline delays. Immediate testing after just a 20 min offline delay demonstrated a lack of any inferential ability resulting in chance performance on both 1° (first order) and 2° and 2° (second order) associative judgements. Following a more extended 12 h delay, across the day (wake group), performance was significantly above chance across both the 1° and 2° inference judgements. However, following an equivalent 12 h offline delay, but containing a night of sleep (sleep group), significantly better performance was expressed on the more distant 2° inference judgement compared with the 1° judgement. (B) A conceptual model of the effects of sleep on memory integration. Immediately after learning, the representation of each premise is constituted as the choice of one item over another (A > B etc.), and these premises are isolated from one another despite having overlapping elements. After a 12 h period with no sleep, the premise representations are partially integrated by their overlapping elements, sufficient to support first-order transitive inferences. However, following a 12 h offline period with sleep, the premise representations are fully interleaved, supporting both first- and second-order transitive inferences. $^{*}p < 0.05$; error bars indicate s.e.m. (For interpretation of the references to colour in this figure legend, the reader is referred to the web version of this book.)

memory, which span different time courses. The first may be an initial process of consolidating individual item (episodic) memories that are novel, which may occur in the relative short term. Over a longer time course, however, and utilizing these recently consolidated item memories prior to their fading, sleep may begin the process of extraction (of meaning) and abstraction (building associational links with existing information), thereby creating more adaptive semantic networks (Walker and Stickgold, 2010). Ultimately, individual item memories would no longer be necessary for the goal that sleep is trying to achieve, and only the conceptual meaning of such experiences would remain. Whether the subsequent loss of item memories is passive, or whether sleep plays an active role in this process remains to be examined, but this is a testable hypothesis, that is *forgetting (individual items) is the price we pay for remembering (general rules)*.

Creativity

One potential advantage of testing associative connections and building cross-linked systems of knowledge is creativity – the ability to take existing pieces of information and combine them in novel ways that lead to greater understanding and offer new advantageous behavioural repertoires. The link between creativity and sleep, especially dreaming, has long been a topic of intense speculation. From the dreams of both August Kekulé, which led to the conception of a simple structure for benzene, and Dmitry Mendeleyev, which initiated the creation of the periodic table of elements, to the late-night dreaming of Otto Loewi, which inspired the experimental demonstration of neurochemical transmission, even scientific examples of creativity occurring during sleep are not uncommon.

Quantitative data have further demonstrated that solution performance on tests of cognitive flexibility using anagram word puzzles is more than 30% better following awakenings from REM sleep compared with NREM awakenings (Walker et al., 2002). Similarly, a study of semantic priming has demonstrated that, in contrast to the situation in waking, performance following REM sleep awakenings shows a greater priming effect by weakly related words than by strong primes, while strong priming exceeds weak priming in NREM sleep (Stickgold et al., 1999), again indicating the highly associative properties of the REM sleep brain. Even the study of mental activity (dreams) from REM sleep indicates that there is not a concrete episodic replay of daytime experiences, but instead, a much more associative process of semantic integration during sleep (Fosse et al., 2003).

Yet, the most striking experimental evidence of sleep-inspired insight is arguably that reported by Wagner et al. (2004). Using a mathematical 'Number Reduction Task', a process of sleep-dependent creative insight was elegantly demonstrated. Subjects analysed and worked through a series of 8-digit string problems, using specific addition rules. Following initial training, after various periods of wake or sleep, subjects returned for an additional series of trials. When retested after a night of sleep, subjects solved the task, using this 'standard' procedure, 16.5% faster. In contrast, subjects who did not sleep prior to retesting averaged less than a 6% improvement. However, hidden in the construction of the task was a much simpler way to solve the problem. On every trial, the last three response digits were the mirror image of the preceding three. As a result, the second response digit always provided the answer to the problem, and using such 'insight', subjects could stop after producing the second response digit. Most dramatically, nearly 60% of the subjects who slept for a night between training and retesting discovered this short cut the following morning. In contrast, no more than 25% of subjects in any of four different control groups who did not sleep had this insight. Sleeping after exposure to the problem therefore more than doubled the likelihood of solving it (although it is interesting to note that this insight was not present immediately following sleep, but took over 100 trials on average to emerge the next day).

In summary, substantial evidence now suggests that sleep serves a meta-level role in memory processing that moves far beyond the consolidation and strengthening of individual memories, and, instead, aims to intelligently assimilate and generalize these details offline. In doing so, sleep may offer the ability to test and build common informational schemas of knowledge, providing increasingly accurate statistic predictions about the world, and allowing for the discovery of novel, even creative next-day solution insights.

Emotional regulation

Despite substantial research focusing on the interaction between sleep and cognition, especially memory, the impact of sleep and sleep loss on affective and emotional regulation has received more limited research attention. This absence of investigation is perhaps surprising considering that nearly all psychiatric and neurological mood disorders express co-occurring abnormalities of sleep, suggesting an intimate relationship between sleep and emotion. Nevertheless, a number of recent studies evaluating subjective as well as objective measures of mood and affect, combined with insights from clinical domains, offer an emerging understanding for the critical role of sleep in regulating emotional brain function.

Affective reactivity

Together with impairments of attention and alertness, sleep deprivation is commonly associated with increased subjective reports of irritability and affective volatility (Horne, 1985). Using a sleep restriction paradigm (5 h/night), Dinges et al. (1997) have reported a progressive increase in emotional disturbance across a 1-week period on the basis of questionnaire mood scales. In addition, subjective descriptions in participants' daily journals also indicated increasing complaints of emotional difficulties. Zohar et al. (2005) have investigated the effects of sleep disruption on emotional reactivity to daytime work events in medical residents. Sleep loss was shown to amplify negative emotional consequences of disruptive daytime events while blunting the positive benefit associated with rewarding or goal-enhancing activities.

Although these findings help to characterize the behavioural irregularities imposed by sleep loss, evidence for the role of sleep in regulating our emotional brain is surprisingly scarce. To date, only one such study has investigated whether a lack of sleep inappropriately modulates human emotional brain reactivity (Yoo et al., 2007a). Healthy young participants were allowed to sleep normally prior to a functional MRI (fMRI) scanning session, or were sleep deprived for one night (accumulating approximately 35 h of wakefulness). During scanning, subjects performed an affective stimulus-viewing task involving the presentation of picture slides ranging in a gradient from emotionally neutral to increasingly negative and aversive.

While both groups expressed significant amygdala activation in response to increasingly negative picture stimuli, those in the sleep-deprived condition exhibited a remarkable +60% greater magnitude of amygdala reactivity, relative to the control group. In addition to this increased intensity of activation, there was also a threefold increase in the extent of amygdala volume recruited in response to the aversive stimuli in the sleep-deprived group. Perhaps most interestingly, relative to the sleep-control group, there was a significant loss of functional connectivity identified between the amygdala and the mPFC in those who were sleep deprived – a region known to have strong inhibitory projections and hence modulatory impact on the amygdala. In contrast, significantly greater connectivity in the deprivation group was observed between the amygdala and the autonomic-activating centres of the locus coeruleus.

Thus, without sleep, an amplified hyper-limbic reaction by the human amygdala was observed in response to negative emotional stimuli. Furthermore, this altered magnitude of limbic activity is associated with a loss of functional connectivity with the mPFC in the sleep-deprived condition; implying a failure of top-down inhibition by the prefrontal lobe. It would therefore appear that a night of sleep may 'reset' the correct affective brain reactivity to next-day emotional challenges by maintaining functional integrity of this mPFC-amygdala circuit and thus govern appropriate behavioural repertoires (e.g. optimal social judgements and rational decisions). Intriguingly, a similar pattern of anatomical dysfunction has been implicated in a number of psychiatric mood disorders which express co-occurring sleep abnormalities, directly raising the issues of whether such factors (sleep loss and clinical mood disorders) are causally related.

Emotional information processing

Sleep's role in declarative memory consolidation, rather than being absolute, may depend on more intricate aspects of the information being learned, such as novelty, meaning to extract, and also the affective salience of the material. Independent of the field of sleep and memory, there is a wealth of evidence demonstrating that memory processing is modulated by emotion. Experiences which evocate emotions not only encode more strongly but appear to persist and even improve over time as the delay between learning and testing increases (hours/days).

Although these findings indicate a strong influence of emotion on slow, time-dependent consolidation processes, based on the coincident neurophysiology that REM sleep provides and the neurobiological requirements of emotional memory processing, work has now begun to test a selective REM-dependent hypothesis of affective human memory consolidation. For example, Hu et al. (2006) have compared the consolidation of emotionally arousing and non-arousing picture stimuli following a 12 h period across a day or following a night of sleep. A specific emotional memory benefit was observed only following sleep and not across an equivalent time awake. Wagner et al. (2001) have also shown that sleep selectively favours the retention of previously learned emotional texts relative to neutral texts, and that this affective memory benefit is only present following late-night sleep (a time period rich in stage-2 NREM and REM sleep).

Using a nap paradigm, it has most recently been demonstrated that sleep, and specifically REM neurophysiology, may underlie this consolidation benefit (Nishida and Walker, 2007). Subjects performed two study sessions in which they learned emotionally negative and neutral picture stimuli: one 4 h prior, and one 15 min prior to a recognition memory test. In one group, participants slept (90 min nap) after the first study session, while in the other group, participants remained awake. Thus, items from the first (4 h) study sessions transitioned through different brain states in each group prior to testing, containing sleep in the nap group and no sleep in the no-nap group, yet experienced identical brain-state conditions following the second (15 min) study session prior to testing. No change in memory for emotional (or neutral) stimuli occurred across the offline delay in the no-nap group. However, a significant and selective offline enhancement of emotional memory was observed in the nap group, the extent of which was correlated with the amount of REM sleep and the speed of entry into REM (latency). Furthermore, spectral analysis of the EEG demonstrated that the magnitude of right-dominant prefrontal theta power during REM (activity in the frequency range of 4.0–7.0 Hz) exhibited a significant and positive relationship with the amount of emotional memory improvement.

These findings go beyond demonstrating that affective memories are preferentially enhanced across periods of sleep, and indicate that the extent of emotional memory improvement is associated with specific REM sleep characteristics – both quantity and quality. Corroborating these correlations, it has previously been hypothesized that REM sleep represents a brain state particularly amenable to emotional memory consolidation, based on its unique biology. Neurochemically, levels of limbic and forebrain acetylcholine (ACh) are markedly elevated during REM, reportedly quadruple those seen during NREM and double those measured in quite waking. Considering the known importance of ACh in the long-term consolidation of emotional learning, this pro-cholinergic REM state may result in a selective facilitation of affective memories, similar to that reported using experimental manipulations of ACh. Neurophysiologically, theta oscillations have been proposed as a carrier frequency allowing disparate brain regions that initially encode information to selectively interact offline, in a coupled relationship. By doing so, REM theta may afford the ability to promote the strengthening of specific memory representations across distributed networks.

A hypothesis of emotional memory: sleep to forget and sleep to remember, respectively

Beyond the strengthening of emotional memories, there may be an additional consequence of sleep-dependent affective modulation, and one that has significant implications for mood disorders – that is sleeping to forget. Based on the emerging interaction between sleep and emotion, below I outline a model of affective information processing that may offer brain-based explanatory insights regarding the impact of sleep abnormalities, particularly REM, for the initiation and/or maintenance of mood disturbance.

While there is abundant evidence to suggest that emotional experiences persist in our autobiographies over time, an equally remarkable but far less noted change is a reduction in the affective tone associated with their recall. The reason that affective experiences appear to be encoded and consolidated more preferentially than neutral memories is due to autonomic neurochemical reactions elicited at the time of the experience, creating what we commonly term an 'emotional memory'. However, the later recall of these experiences tends not to be associated with anywhere near the same magnitude of autonomic (re)activation as that elicited at the moment of learning/experience – suggesting that, over time, the affective 'blanket' previously enveloped around the memory during encoding has been removed, while the information contained within that experience (the memory) remains.

For example, neuroimaging studies have shown that initial exposure and learning of emotional stimuli is associated with substantially greater activation in the amygdala and hippocampus, relative to neutral stimuli (Dolcos et al., 2004, 2005; Kilpatrick and Cahill, 2003). In one of these studies (Dolcos et al., 2004), however, when participants were re-exposed to these same stimuli during recognition testing many months later, a change in the profile of activation occurred (Dolcos et al., 2005). Although the same magnitude of differential activity between emotional and neutral items was observed in the hippocampus, this was not true in the amygdala. Instead, the difference in amygdala (re)activity compared with neutral items had dissipated over time. This would support the idea that the strength of the memory (hippocampal-associated activity) remains at later recollection, yet the associated emotional reactivity to these items (amygdala activity) is reduced over time.

The hypothesis predicts that this decoupling preferentially takes place overnight, such that we sleep to forget the emotional tone, yet sleep to remember the tagged memory of that episode (Fig. 5). The model further argues that if this process is not achieved, the magnitude of visceral autonomic 'charge' remaining within autobiographical memory networks will persist, resulting in the potential condition of chronic anxiety. Based on the consistent relationship identified between REM and emotional processing, combined with its unique neurobiology, the hypothesis proposes that REM sleep provides an optimal biological state for achieving such affective 'therapy'. Specifically, increased activity within limbic and paralimbic structures (including the hippocampus and amygdala) during REM may first offer the ability for

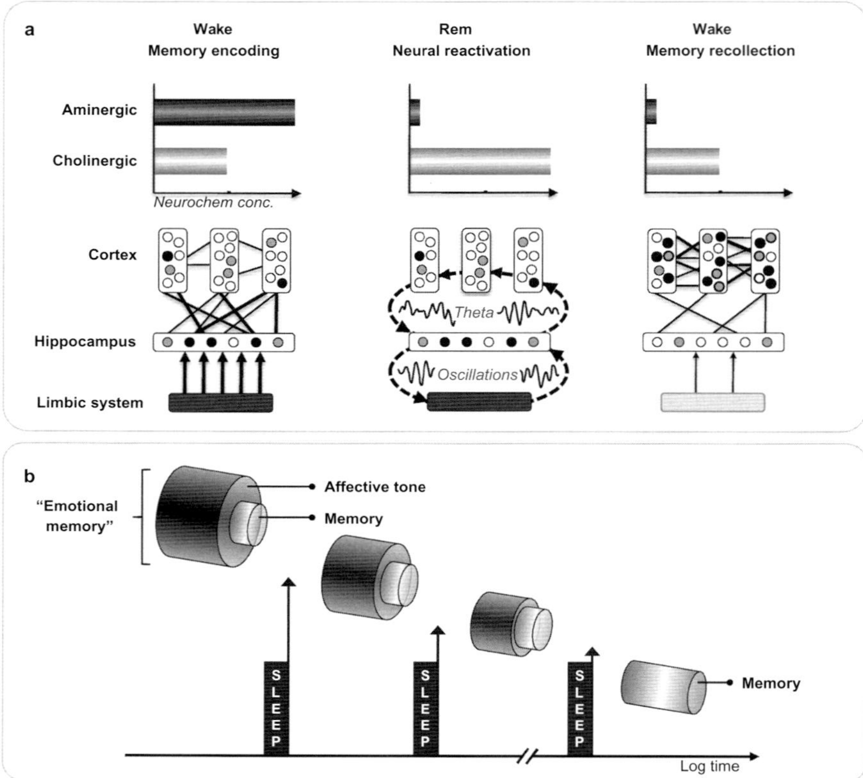

Fig. 5. The sleep to *forget* and sleep to *remember* (SFSR) model of emotional memory processing. (a) Neural dynamics. Waking formation of an episodic emotional memory involves the coordinated encoding of hippocampal-bound information within cortical modules, facilitated by the extended limbic system, including the amygdala, and modulated by high concentrations of aminergic neurochemistry. During subsequent REM sleep, these same neural structures are reactivated, the coordination of which is made possible by synchronous theta oscillations throughout these networks, supporting the ability to reprocess previously learned emotional experiences. However, this reactivation occurs in a neurochemical milieu devoid of aminergic modulation, and dominated by cholinergic neurochemistry. As a consequence, emotional memory reprocessing can achieve, on the one hand, a depotentiation of the affective tone initially associated with the event(s) at encoding, while on the other hand, a simultaneous and progressive neocortical consolidation of the information. The latter process of reactivation, resulting in next-day stronger cortico-cortical connections, additionally supports integration into previous acquired autobiographical experiences, further aiding the assimilation of the affective event(s) in the context of past knowledge, the conscious expression of which may contribute to the experience of dreaming. Cross-connectivity between structures before and after sleep is represented by number and thickness of lines. Circles within cortical and hippocampal structures represent information nodes; shade reflects extent of connectivity: strong (filled), moderate (grey) and weak (clear). Fill of limbic system and arrow thickness represents magnitude of co-activation with and influence on the hippocampus. (b) Conceptual outcome. Through multiple iterations of this REM mechanism across the night, and/or across multiple nights, the long-term consequence of such sleep-dependent reprocessing would allow for the strengthening and retention of salient information previously tagged as emotional at the time of learning. However, recall no longer maintains an affective, aminergic charge, allowing for post-sleep recollection with minimal autonomic reactivity (unlike encoding), thereby preventing a state of chronic anxiety.

reactivation of previously acquired affective experiences. Second, the neurophysiological signature of REM involving dominant theta oscillations within subcortical as well as cortical nodes may offer large-scale network cooperation at night, allowing the integration and, as a consequence, greater understanding of recently experienced emotional events in the context of pre-existing neocortically stored semantic memory. Third, these interactions during REM critically, and perhaps most importantly, take place within a brain that is devoid of aminergic neurochemical concentration, particularly noradrenergic input from the locus coeruleus; the influence of which has been linked to states of high stress and anxiety disorders.

In summary, the described neuroanatomical, neurophysiological and neurochemical conditions of REM sleep offer a unique biological theatre in which to achieve, on the one hand, a balanced neural potentiation of the informational core of emotional experiences (the memory), yet may also depotentiate and ultimately ameliorate the autonomic arousing charge originally acquired at the time of learning (the emotion), negating a long-term state of anxiety (Fig. 5).

The model also asserts that if the process of divorcing emotion from memory is not achieved across the first night following an emotional event, a repeat attempt would occur on the second night, since the strength of emotional 'tag' associated with the memory would remain high. Should this process fail a second time, the same events would continue to repeat across ensuing nights, potentially with an increasing progressive amount of REM in response. It is just such a cycle of REM-sleep dreaming (nightmares) that represents a diagnostic key feature of post-traumatic stress disorder (PTSD) (Lavie, 2001). It may not be coincidental, therefore, that these patients continue to display hyperarousal reactions to associated trauma cues, indicating that the process of separating the affective tone from the emotional experience has not been accomplished. The reason why such a REM mechanism may fail in PTSD remains unknown, although the exceptional magnitude of trauma-induced emotion at the time of learning may be so great that the system is incapable of initiating/completing one or both these processes, leaving some patients unable to depotentiate, integrate and hence 'overcome' the experience. Alternatively, it may be the hyperarousal status of the brain during REM sleep in these patients (Harvey et al., 2003; Pole, 2007; Strawn and Geracioti, 2008), potentially lacking sufficient aminergic demodulation, that prevents the processing and separation of emotion from memory. Indeed, this hypothesis has gained support from recent pharmacological studies in PTSD patients, demonstrating that nocturnal alpha-adrenergic blockade using prazosin (i.e. reducing adrenergic activity during sleep) both decreases trauma-dream symptomatology and restores characteristics of REM sleep (Raskind et al., 2007; Taylor et al., 2008).

This model also makes specific experimental predictions as to the fate of these two components – the memory and the emotion. As partially demonstrated, the first prediction would be that, over time, the veracity of the memory itself would improve, and the extent to which these [negative] emotional experiences are strengthened would be proportional to the amount of post-experience REM sleep obtained, as well as how quickly it is achieved (REM latency).

Secondly, using autonomic physiology measures, these same predictions would hold in the inverse direction for the magnitude of emotional reactivity induced at the time of recall. Together with the neuroimaging studies of emotional memory recall over time, and the psychological studies investigating the role of REM sleep dreaming in mood regulation, a recent fMRI study offers perhaps the strongest preliminary support of this sleep-dependent model of emotional memory processing (Sterpenich et al., 2007). The investigation demonstrated that subjects who were deprived of sleep the first night after learning arousing emotion picture slides showed not only reduced recall of the information (the sleep to remember component of the hypothesis) but also a lack of reduction in amygdala reactivity when re-exposed to these same emotional picture slide at recognition testing – as compared to a control group that did sleep (the sleep to forget component of the hypothesis).

Thirdly, the model predicts that a pathological increase in REM (as commonly occurs in depression) may disproportionately amplify the strength of negative memories so much that, despite concomitant attempts at ameliorating the associated affective tone, it would still create a perceived autobiographical history dominated by negative memory excess (which may also facilitate disadvantageous waking rumination). In contrast, the selective decrease of REM, as occurs with many anti-depressants, would predict a reduction of such negative memory consolidation and bias, although it may curtail the degree of affect decoupling that can occur. Long term, the balanced extent of accumulated REM should, therefore, not only correlate with the persistence, in memory, of the emotional experience, but also be associated with a decreased magnitude of autonomic response associated with recall – all of which are testable objectives for future research.

If such a hypothesis is correct, there would be translation implications for psychiatric and mood disorders. This would require a new appreciation for the palliative role of sleep in treatment regimes, and a consideration of whether altering sleep architecture to regulate the balance of emotion and memory of past experience is a useful and viable possibility.

Conclusions

While not fully complete, we will soon have a new taxonomy of sleep-dependent memory processing, and one that will supersede the polarized all-or-none views of the past. With such findings, we can come to a revised appreciation of how *both* wake and sleep unite in a symbiotic alliance to coordinate the encoding, consolidation and integration of our memories, the ultimate aim of which may be to create a generalized catalogue of stored knowledge that does not rely on the verbose retention of all previously learned facts.

Beyond memory and plasticity, a growing number of human neuroscience studies, set on a foundation of clinical insights, point to an exciting role for sleep in regulating affective brain function and emotional experience. Based on the remarkable neurobiology of sleep, and REM in particular, a unique capability for the overnight modulation of affective networks and previously encountered emotional experiences may be possible, redressing and maintaining the appropriate connectivity and hence next-day reactivity throughout limbic and associated autonomic systems.

Ultimately, the timeless maternal wisdom of mothers alike may have long held the answers to Allan Rechtschaffen's original question; that is '*you should sleep on a problem*', and when troubled '*get to bed, you'll feel better in the morning*'.

Acknowledgements

The author wishes to thank Edwin Robertson, Robert Stickgold, Allison Harvey, Ninad Gujar and Els van der Helm for thoughtful insights. This work was supported in part by grants from the National Institutes of Health (NIA AG31164); and the University of California, Berkeley.

References

Dave, A. S., & Margoliash, D. (2000). Song replay during sleep and computational rules for sensorimotor vocal learning. *Science*, *290*, 812–816.

Dave, A. S., Yu, A. C., & Margoliash, D. (1998). Behavioral state modulation of auditory activity in a vocal motor system. *Science*, *282*, 2250–2254.

Diekelmann, S., & Born, J. (2010). The memory function of sleep. *Nature Reviews Neuroscience*, *11*, 114–126.

Dinges, D. F., Pack, F., Williams, K., Gillen, K. A., Powell, J. W., & Ott, G. E., et al., (1997). Cumulative sleepiness, mood disturbance, and psychomotor vigilance performance decrements during a week of sleep restricted to 4–5 h per night. *Sleep*, *20*, 267–277.

Dolcos, F., LaBar, K. S., & Cabeza, R. (2004). Interaction between the amygdala and the medial temporal lobe memory system predicts better memory for emotional events. *Neuron*, *42*, 855–863.

Dolcos, F., LaBar, K. S., & Cabeza, R. (2005). Remembering one year later: Role of the amygdala and the medial temporal lobe memory system in retrieving emotional memories. *Proceedings of the National Academy of Sciences USA*, *102*, 2626–2631.

Drummond, S. P., & Brown, G. G. (2001). The effects of total sleep deprivation on cerebral responses to cognitive performance. *Neuropsychopharmacology*, *25*, S68–S73.

Drummond, S. P., Brown, G. G., Gillin, J. C., Stricker, J. L., Wong, E. C., & Buxton, R. B. (2000). Altered brain response to verbal learning following sleep deprivation. *Nature*, *403*, 655–657.

Dumay, N., & Gaskell, M. G. (2007). Sleep-associated changes in the mental representation of spoken words. *Psychological Science*, *18*, 35–39.

Ellenbogen, J. M., Hulbert, J. C., Stickgold, R., Dinges, D. F., & Thompson-Schill, S. L. (2006). Interfering with theories of sleep and memory: Sleep, declarative memory, and associative interference. *Current Biology*, *16*, 1290–1294.

Ellenbogen, J., Hu, P., Payne, J. D., Titone, D., & Walker, M. P. (2007). Human relational memory requires time and sleep. *The Proceedings of the National Academy of Sciences of the United States of America*, *104*, 7723–7728.

Fenn, K. M., Nusbaum, H. C., & Margoliash, D. (2003). Consolidation during sleep of perceptual learning of spoken language. *Nature*, *425*, 614–616.

Fosse, M. J., Fosse, R., Hobson, J. A., & Stickgold, R. J. (2003). Dreaming and episodic memory: A functional dissociation? *Journal of Cognitive Neuroscience*, *15*, 1–9.

Gais, S., Albouy, G., Boly, M., Dang-Vu, T. T., Darsaud, A., & Desseilles, M., et al., (2007). Sleep transforms the cerebral trace of declarative memories. *Proceedings of the National Academy of Sciences USA*, *104*, 18778–18783.

Gais, S., Molle, M., Helms, K., & Born, J. (2002). Learning-dependent increases in sleep spindle density. *Journal of Neuroscience*, *22*, 6830–6834.

Gomez, R. L., Bootzin, R. R., & Nadel, L. (2006). Naps promote abstraction in language-learning infants. *Psychological Science*, *17*, 670–674.

Harrison, Y., & Horne, J. A. (2000). Sleep loss and temporal memory. *Quarterly Journal of Experimental Psychology*, *53*, 271–279.

Harvey, A. G., Jones, C., & Schmidt, D. A. (2003). Sleep and posttraumatic stress disorder: A review. *Clinical Psychology Review*, *23*, 377–407.

Horne, J. A. (1985). Sleep function, with particular reference to sleep deprivation. *Annals of Clinical Research*, *17*, 199–208.

Hu, P., Stylos-Allen, M., & Walker, M. P. (2006). Sleep facilitates consolidation of emotionally arousing declarative memory. *Psychological Science*, *17*, 891–898.

Huber, R., Ghilardi, M. F., Massimini, M., & Tononi, G. (2004). Local sleep and learning. *Nature*, *430*, 78–81.

Ji, D., & Wilson, M. A. (2007). Coordinated memory replay in the visual cortex and hippocampus during sleep. *Nature Neuroscience*, *10*, 100–107.

Jones, M. W., & Wilson, M. A. (2005). Theta rhythms coordinate hippocampal-prefrontal interactions in a spatial memory task. *PLoS Biology*, *3*, e402.

Kilpatrick, L., & Cahill, L. (2003). Amygdala modulation of parahippocampal and frontal regions during emotionally influenced memory storage. *Neuroimage*, *20*, 2091–2099.

Lavie, P. (2001). Sleep disturbances in the wake of traumatic events. *New England Journal of Medicine*, *345*, 1825–1832.

Liu, Z. W., Faraguna, U., Cirelli, C., Tononi, G., & Gao, X. B. (2010). Direct evidence for wake-related increases and sleep-related decreases in synaptic strength in rodent cortex. *Journal of Neuroscience*, *30*, 8671–8675.

Louie, K., & Wilson, M. A. (2001). Temporally structured replay of awake hippocampal ensemble activity during rapid eye movement sleep. *Neuron*, *29*, 145–156.

Morris, G. O., Williams, H. L., & Lubin, A. (1960). Misperception and disorientation during sleep. *Archives of General Psychiatry*, *2*, 247–254.

Nishida, M., & Walker, M. P. (2007). Daytime naps, motor memory consolidation and regionally specific sleep spindles. *PLoS ONE*, *2*, e341.

Peigneux, P., Laureys, S., Fuchs, S., Collette, F., Perrin, F., & Reggers, J., et al., (2004). Are spatial memories strengthened in the human hippocampus during slow wave sleep? *Neuron*, *44*, 535–545.

Poe, G. R., Nitz, D. A., McNaughton, B. L., & Barnes, C. A. (2000). Experience-dependent phase-reversal of hippocampal neuron firing during REM sleep. *Brain Research*, *855*, 176–180.

Pole, N. (2007). The psychophysiology of posttraumatic stress disorder: A meta-analysis. *Psychological Bulletin*, *133*, 725–746.

Rasch, B., Buchel, C., Gais, S., & Born, J. (2007). Odor cues during slow-wave sleep prompt declarative memory consolidation. *Science*, *315*, 1426–1429.

Raskind, M. A., Peskind, E. R., Hoff, D. J., Hart, K. L., Holmes, H. A., & Warren, D., et al., (2007). A parallel group placebo controlled study of prazosin for trauma nightmares and sleep disturbance in combat veterans with post-traumatic stress disorder. *Biological Psychiatry*, *61*, 928–934.

Ribeiro, S., Gervasoni, D., Soares, E. S., Zhou, Y., Lin, S. C., & Pantoja, J., et al., (2004). Long-lasting novelty-induced neuronal reverberation during slow-wave sleep in multiple forebrain areas induction of hippocampal long-term potentiation during waking leads to increased extrahippocampal zif-268 expression during ensuing rapid-eye-movement sleep. *PLoS Biology*, *2*, E24.

Skaggs, W. E., & McNaughton, B. L. (1996). Replay of neuronal firing sequences in rat hippocampus during sleep following spatial experience. *Science*, *271*, 1870–1873.

Sterpenich, V., Albouy, G., Boly, M., Vandewalle, G., Darsaud, A., & Balteau, E., et al., (2007). Sleep-related hippocampo-cortical interplay during emotional memory recollection. *PLoS Biology*, *5*, e282.

Stickgold, R., Scott, L., Rittenhouse, C., & Hobson, J. A. (1999). Sleep-induced changes in associative memory. *Journal of Cognitive Neuroscience*, *11*, 182–193.

Strawn, J. R., & Geracioti Jr., T. D. (2008). Noradrenergic dysfunction and the psychopharmacology of posttraumatic stress disorder. *Depression and Anxiety*, *25*, 260–271.

Takashima, A., Petersson, K. M., Rutters, F., Tendolkar, I., Jensen, O., & Zwarts, M. J., et al., (2006). Declarative memory consolidation in humans: A prospective functional magnetic resonance imaging study. *Proceedings of the National Academy of Sciences USA*, *103*, 756–761.

Taylor, F. B., Martin, P., Thompson, C., Williams, J., Mellman, T. A., & Gross, C., et al., (2008). Prazosin effects on objective sleep measures and clinical symptoms in civilian trauma posttraumatic stress disorder: A placebo-controlled study. *Biological Psychiatry*, *63*, 629–632.

Tononi, G., & Cirelli, C. (2003). Sleep and synaptic homeostasis: A hypothesis. *Brain Research Bulletin*, *62*, 143–150.

Tononi, G., & Cirelli, C. (2006). Sleep function and synaptic homeostasis. *Sleep Medicine Reviews*, *10*, 49–62.

Wagner, U., Gais, S., & Born, J. (2001). Emotional memory formation is enhanced across sleep intervals with high amounts of rapid eye movement sleep. *Learning & Memory*, *8*, 112–119.

Wagner, U., Gais, S., Haider, H., Verleger, R., & Born, J. (2004). Sleep inspires insight. *Nature*, *427*, 352–355.

Walker, M. P., & Stickgold, R. (2006). Sleep, memory and plasticity. *Annual Review of Psychology*, *10*, 139–166.

Walker, M. P., & Stickgold, R. (2010). Overnight alchemy: Sleep-dependent memory evolution. *Nature Reviews Neuroscience*, *11*, 218.

Walker, M. P., Liston, C., Hobson, J. A., & Stickgold, R. (2002). Cognitive flexibility across the sleep-wake cycle: REM-sleep enhancement of anagram problem solving. *Brain Research. Cognitive Brain Research*, *14*, 317–324.

Wilson, M. A., & McNaughton, B. L. (1994). Reactivation of hippocampal ensemble memories during sleep. *Science*, *265*, 676–679.

Yoo, S. S., Gujar, N., Hu, P., Jolesz, F. A., & Walker, M. P. (2007a). The human emotional brain without sleep – A prefrontal amygdala disconnect. *Current Biology*, *17*, R877–878.

Yoo, S. S., Hu, P. T., Gujar, N., Jolesz, F. A., & Walker, M. P. (2007b). A deficit in the ability to form new human memories without sleep. *Nature Neuroscience*, *10*, 385–392.

Zohar, D., Tzischinsky, O., Epstein, R., & Lavie, P. (2005). The effects of sleep loss on medical residents' emotional reactions to work events: A cognitive-energy model. *Sleep*, *28*, 47–54.

G. A. Kerkhof and H. P. A. Van Dongen (Eds.)
Progress in Brain Research, Vol. 185
ISSN: 0079-6123

CHAPTER 5

How treatment affects cognitive deficits in patients with sleep disorders: methodological issues and results

Stephany Fulda[†,*] and Hartmut Schulz[‡]

[†]*Max Planck Institute for Psychiatry, Munich, Germany*
[‡]*Department of Educational Science and Psychology, Free University Berlin, Berlin, Germany*

Abstract: Sleep disorders are frequently associated with impaired performance although the type and extent of cognitive deficits varies widely between different types of sleep disorders. Treatment is expected to ameliorate these deficits. However, cognitive functioning and its change with treatment depend on numerous factors. In this chapter we discuss methodological issues, including test selection, and person-specific, task-specific and environmental factors that influence cognitive functioning. In addition, features of study design and sampling strategies are discussed. The chapter ends with a short overview of routes by which treatment may affect cognition in sleep-disordered patients.

Keywords: Cognitive functioning; attention; sleepiness; insomnia; sleep-related breathing disorders; CPAP; children; treatment

Introduction

Sleep disorders are frequently associated with impaired performance. The type and extent of impairment seems to vary widely between sleep disorders. It is most pronounced in disorders that are associated with daytime sleepiness such as narcolepsy and sleep-related breathing disorders (SRBD). Patients from these diagnostic categories not only complain of cognitive difficulties but also have a higher risk for accidents as an objective indicator of dysfunctioning (Philip, 2005). While insomniac patients may also complain about cognitive difficulties such as difficulty to concentrate or reduced attention, implications for cognitive functioning in daily life are less well studied

* Corresponding author.
Tel.: (+) 49 89 30622 226; Fax: (+) 49 89 30622 605.
E-mail: fulda@mpipsykl.mpg.de

DOI:10.1016/B978-0-444-53702-7.00005-1

(Szentkirályi et al., 2009), although some studies indicate higher accident rates in insomniacs (Léger and Bayon, 2010). Finally, there are sleep disorders where cognitive consequences are either largely unexplored, as in restless legs syndrome (RLS; Szentkirályi et al., 2009) or periodic leg movement disorders (PLMD), or presumably absent, as in different parasomnias. Circadian rhythm sleep disorders play a special role in the present context, since the majority of them (jet lag disorder, shift work disorder) are induced by planned or accidental disturbances of the usual sleep-wake schedule. In these cases, it is impossible to separate the effects of disturbed or curtailed sleep from those of the shifted sleep-wake schedule itself.

The dependence of optimal cognitive functioning on sufficient and undisturbed sleep has been demonstrated by sleep deprivation studies (Killgore, 2010; Reynolds and Banks, 2010). Deprivation (Pilcher and Huffcutt, 1996), reduction (Banks and Dinges, 2007) and fragmentation (Bonnet and Arand, 2003) of sleep all result in increased sleepiness, impaired performance and disturbed mood in healthy subjects. Undisturbed recovery sleep is sufficient to reverse the negative effects of acute sleep loss and the short-term, experimentally imposed sleep deprivation has no known lasting effects on cognitive functioning.

However, the translation of these experimental findings into the clinical field of sleep medicine is limited for various reasons. First, most sleep disorders are long-lasting or chronic, and thus the amount and quality of sleep in patients is influenced by time-dependent factors, which are difficult to assess. Second, sleep disorders are diverse, thus depending on very different initiating and maintaining factors. Third, according to the heterogeneity of sleep disorders, procedures for their assessment differ widely, which complicates comparisons between them. Finally, in cases where performance deficits have been consistently established – for example in patients with severe sleep apnoea – different factors have been proposed to play a role in the development of the cognitive impairment, such as multiple sleep disruptions by respiratory-induced arousals or recurrent episodes of hypoxia during sleep (Jackson et al., submitted; Matthews and Aloia, submitted).

The primary research aim of neuropsychological investigations in sleep-disordered patients is to extract the most likely factors that may cause cognitive deficits and to disentangle their interaction. A second aim is to measure the attenuation or even resolution of cognitive deficits as a result of therapeutic interventions and to identify those factors which either facilitate or prevent changes in cognitive performance.

Other chapters in this book review the extent and nature of cognitive alterations in different sleep disorders and the effect of specific interventions on cognitive functioning. In this chapter we focus on methodological aspects of studies designed to measure the effect of therapeutic interventions on impaired cognitive functions and address the following questions:

- Which factors influence cognitive performance?
- Which considerations influence the selection of tests and procedures?
- Which strategies have been used to measure cognitive deficits?
- Which study designs have been used to explore treatment effects on cognition?

Clinical studies will be used to illustrate advantages and limitations of experimental strategies that have been applied to appraise treatment effects on cognitive deficits in sleep-disordered patients.

Factors influencing cognitive performance

Cognitive performance is influenced by a wide range of different factors both in laboratory settings and in everyday life. Factors associated with cognitive performance can be classified as person specific, task specific or specific to the test environment. Within each category one can further differentiate between fluctuating (state) factors and stable (trait) factors. This is especially true for person-specific factors. Sleep disorders and associated features, such as sleepiness or fatigue, are thought to be major contributing factors to cognitive impairment, but the other factors also have to be considered and adequately controlled before a given dysfunction can be ascribed to the sleep disorder itself.

Person-specific factors

Person-specific state and trait factors with potential influence on cognitive performance can be separated by criteria of long-term predictability. Classical trait factors are age and gender (see Table 1). It is well known that many cognitive functions decline with age, independent of age-related comorbidities (Drag and Bieliauskas, 2010). Generally, information-processing and memory tasks ('cognitive mechanics') show a stronger decay with age than knowledge-based and verbal tasks ('cognitive pragmatics', Baltes, 1993). It is largely unknown how age and disordered sleep interact in their effects on cognitive functioning. For SRBD, the combined effect of age and disordered sleep on cognitive performance seems to be non-linear across the age range and is more pronounced during middle age (Alchanatis et al., 2008; Ayalon et al., 2010) than in young patients (Ayalon et al., 2010) and otherwise healthy elderly subjects (Sforza et al., 2010). Whether this is due to compensatory mechanisms in the younger ones (Ayalon et al., 2010) and resilience or protective factors in the elderly is unclear (Richards and Sawyer, 2010). Interestingly, experimental

Table 1. Factors influencing cognitive performance

Person specific	Task specific	Setting/environment
Trait factors		
Gender	Task duration	Availability of external resources
Age	Task difficulty	Training/adaptation
Education	Task complexity	Familiarity with the task
Social status	Knowledge of results	Possibilities for compensation
Ethnicity	Memory requirements	Time of assessment
Functional reserve	Cognitive domain	Time of day
Genetic profile	Self- versus experimenter-paced	Length of test battery
Age at disease onset		Order of task administration
Severity of sleep disorder		
Duration of sleep disorder		
Medical comorbidities		
Psychiatric comorbidities		
Vision/hearing/motor function		
Medication		
Trait sleepiness		
Body weight (obesity)		
State factors		
Sleepiness		
Fatigue		
Attention		
Effort/motivation		
Mood		
Time spent awake		
Prior sleep duration		

evidence also suggests that elderly, as compared to younger subjects, are less sleepy (Lowden et al., 2009) and less vulnerable to sleep deprivation (Duffy et al., 2009). Across the age range there are also gender-specific cognitive profiles, with men believed to be performing some tasks better than women, for example mental rotation, while women perform better in free verbal recall or perceptual speed (Gong et al., 2009; Kimura, 2002).

Other stable factors that can influence cognitive functioning are education, social background and ethnicity (see Table 1). Education, in particular, has a strong and pervasive influence on neuropsychological functioning and contributes to performance levels for most age groups on many kinds of tests (Lezak et al., 2004). Medical comorbidities are another important factor that can influence cognitive functioning. In sleep medicine it can be especially difficult to separate contributions by the sleep disorder from associated comorbidities. A prominent example are mood disorders that are associated with a wide range of sleep disorders including insomnia, SRBD and RLS. Since effective treatment of a sleep disorder will also have a positive influence on associated mood disturbances, it is difficult to determine the relative contributions of these factors to the improvement in cognitive functioning.

Cognitive impairment as caused by altered sleep varies substantially in magnitude between individuals. The existence of large and stable inter-individual differences in the reaction to sleep deprivation or sleep restriction has been investigated systematically by Van Dongen et al. in recent years. While some subjects are especially vulnerable to the effect of lost sleep on cognitive functioning, others are not (Van Dongen et al., 2005). For chronic sleep disturbances it remains still to be shown what role inter-individual differences play in cognitive dysfunction and in its improvement by therapy.

Genetic vulnerability may play a role in the reaction of cognitive functioning to sleep disorders, as illustrated by a study of older women with SRBD (Spira et al., 2008). It was found that subjects who are carriers of the apolipoprotein E (APOE) ε4 allele, a known risk factor for cognitive decline, have a much greater association between the apnoea-hypopnea index (AHI) and cognitive decline than subjects who are APOE ε4 negative. Genetic vulnerability factors may therefore also play a role in treatment outcomes, although this has still to be shown.

Another important question is whether a given sleep disorder is associated with structural brain changes and, if this is the case, to which extent they are reversible by therapeutic interventions. Such brain changes could be the effect either of the sleep disorder itself or of an associated feature. In subjects with SRBD, repeatedly occurring blood gas abnormalities during sleep probably induce structural nervous system cellular injury (Zimmerman and Aloia, 2006). If this is true, it would be consistent with the observation that treatment of SRBD results in only partial remission of cognitive functions (Bédard et al., 1993; Engleman and Joffe, 1999; Naëgelé et al., 1995). Others have suggested that impaired alertness is the main reason for cognitive dysfunction (Verstraeten, 2007). This view is supported by studies which did not find structural brain damage in patients with SRBD (O'Donoghue et al., 2005; Robbins et al., 2005).

Additional factors, such as the severity of the disease, are of primary interest when measuring impaired cognitive functions and their potential improvement under therapy. However, there are no simple or one-dimensional measures of severity for any of the various sleep disorders, and therefore approximative appraisals or surrogate measures have been suggested. Such measures rely on recorded sleep (polysomnography, Multiple Sleep Latency Test (MSLT), Maintenance of Wakefulness Test (MWT)), on symptom-specific physiological measures (e.g. AHI), on subjective ratings of sleepiness (e.g. Epworth Sleepiness Scale, ESS; Johns, 1991) or on disease-specific rating scales (e.g. Ullanlinna Narcolepsy Scale, Hublin et al., 1994). In patients with SRBD, different measures of disease severity correlated significantly with measures of cognitive impairment. This was shown for hypoxemia versus executive functions and vigilance (Bédard et al., 1991; Montplaisir et al., 1992), number of microarousals versus memory deficits (Daurat et al., 2008), sleep quality versus processing speed (Naismith et al., 2004) and subjective rating of sleepiness versus reaction time (Lis et al., 2008).

In primary insomniacs, the pre-therapy cognitive disposition has been studied as another person-specific factor which may influence the treatment outcome. Edinger et al. (2008b) compared patients who had relatively high levels of unhelpful sleep-related beliefs (Type 1) with patients who had less pronounced sleep-related beliefs (Type 2). After 8 weeks of treatment with cognitive behaviour therapy (CBT), Type 1 patients showed better performance in multiple subjective and objective tests, while Type 2 patients did not.

Sleepiness, as a person-specific factor, deserves a separate mentioning here, because it can be conceptualized on both a trait and a state level. For instance, the ESS assesses habitual sleepiness over an extended period. However, superimposed on the general level of sleepiness, fluctuations occur in the range of hours, due to time-of-the-day, or even more rapid minute-to-minute fluctuations due to alerting or soporific stimuli (Cluydts et al., 2002). As a consequence, substantial within-subject fluctuations of sleepiness and their effects on performance can be expected, which are not represented in the ESS score.

Sleepiness, fatigue and mood are typical state factors (see Table 1), which fluctuate in response to internal conditions and external demands, as associated with specific tasks and general environmental conditions (see below). For example, the longer a task or task battery, the more likely it will produce fatigue that in turn will affect performance. On the other hand, complex and stimulating tasks might increase the arousal level and thereby boost task performance (Scott, 1966). An outstanding question is to what extent higher order tasks such as executive functioning are influenced by basic levels of alertness, attention and arousal (cf. Verstraeten and Cluydts, 2004). Indeed, it can be argued that performance on any complex task can never be interpreted in isolation, and should be interpreted within the context of ancillary measures of the level of sleepiness.

Task-specific factors

Task-specific factors that influence cognitive performance have been delineated in studies exploring the effect of sleep deprivation (overview in Johnson, 1982). The most influential factors are the duration of the task, with longer tasks being more sensitive to sleep deprivation, and task difficulty (Bonnet, 2005). It has been argued, but not demonstrated definitively, that the more difficult a task, the more vulnerable it will be to sleep loss (Stricker et al., 2006). Knowledge of results or feedback attenuates the effect of sleep deprivation, and self-paced tasks are more resistant against sleep loss than experimenter-paced tasks.

In the context of treatment studies, the reliability of a task is another important feature. The lower the test–retest reliability of a task, the larger the treatment effect has to be to produce a statistically significant result. Additionally, learning effects, which occur when a task is being given twice, must be considered. Test repetition may have different effects in different domains of cognitive testing. For example, it has been argued that executive functions are not in maximal use for the execution of routine, well-learned behaviours, but that they are especially called upon in novel, unfamiliar contexts where no previously established routines exist (Shallice, 1990). Therefore, the 'ideal' executive task involves a combination of novelty, effort and working memory demands (Philipps, 1997) and this poses a challenge for repeated testing.

If tests of different complexity are used, one has to control for the interaction of different perceptual and cognitive functions which are involved in task performance. If a higher order cognitive function, for example performance of an executive task, is impaired, this means that the impairment may be attributed to the targeted function itself, or to a more basic function on which the higher order cognitive function relies. Basic functions which need to be regarded in this respect are alertness, attention, arousal and vigilance (for definitions and interaction of underlying systems, see Part V, Attention, in Gazzaniga, 1995). If performance of an executive function is impaired, one should thus examine whether processing speed (e.g. in a reaction time task) is undisturbed or lowered. In the latter case, impaired performance on an executive function task cannot be interpreted unambiguously as a deficit in executive functioning since the deficit of the higher function may be due to a deficit in a lower function, for example motor speed, which results probably from sleepiness. Verstraeten and colleagues (Verstraeten, 2007; Verstraeten and Cluydts, 2004) have emphasized the need to use appropriate neuropsychological tasks and statistical models, which allow separating the contribution of simple and complex tasks when performance is impaired.

In the common case where several neuropsychological tasks are combined into a test battery, additional effects must be considered. These pertain to the duration and complexity of the test battery – factors which influence fatigue, motivation and effort of the subject (Johnson, 1982; Wilkinson, 1961). While carry-over and transfer effects between sessions have been documented for performance tasks in classical studies (Poulton and Freeman, 1966), their potential role in single sessions with different tasks is less clear. In any case, test fatigue and effects of massed practice should be regarded, especially when designing studies with sleep-disordered patients (Rieth et al., 2010).

Environmental factors and setting

Adaptation to the test situation, familiarity with tests and practice (training) are important situational factors influencing the outcome of neuropsychological testing. To illustrate this point, Fig. 1 shows results of the Trail Making Test B (TMT B) from 17 treatment studies in SRBD patients. We have selected this test because it was most frequently used in this patient group to assess cognitive functioning. The TMT B measures the time a subject needs to connect, in increasing order, alternating numbers and letters spread across a page. This test for executive functioning involves the sub-functions visual search, psychomotor speed, memory and set shifting. Figure 1 shows that in the majority of studies, test performance was faster after treatment; however, there was a threefold variability of the average time subjects needed to complete the test, ranging from 40 to 120 s in the different studies. Severity of the breathing disorder or length of treatment does not fully account for this variability. This suggests that the studies differed in test material, instructions or other aspects of test performance, which resulted in remarkably different test completion times. The data illustrate that uncontrolled factors of the setting will strongly influence results of neuropsychological performance testing. If cognitive performance is measured in patients with sleep disorders, factors of the setting should be standardized as carefully as when performing physiological tests, such as the MSLT (Standards of Practice Committee of the American Academy of Sleep Medicine, 2005).

Environmental factors that influence cognitive functioning include the presence or absence of noise, ambient temperature, lightning conditions and others. Many of these factors can be subsumed under the heading of distracting factors. They clearly differ between a laboratory setting with standardized conditions and everyday life conditions. A problem arising from the differences between laboratory and field settings concerns the predictive value of cognitive test results for everyday functioning (Marcotte et al., 2010). Memorizing a shopping list in the lab may be fundamentally different from memorizing such a list at home in the face of various distractors. As a consequence, ecological validity of the task and the test situation has to be considered before results can be meaningfully generalized (Chaytor and Schmitter-Edgecombe, 2003).

The measurement of cognitive deficits in patients with sleep disturbances

Test selection

An essential feature of a neuropsychological test is its sensitivity to detect cognitive deficits. If it is intended to measure a clearly defined function, such as verbal memory, validated tests for this function are available and can be applied. However, the selection of adequate tests is more difficult if it is not known which functions are disturbed, and this is the normal case if one examines cognitive deficits in patients with sleep disturbances. The situation is further complicated by the fact that in the majority of cases a suspected impairment will not be caused by a definite brain lesion or a degenerative disorder, but will rather result from a functional disturbance, which may be fluctuating, depending on internal and external conditions. If the sleep disturbance is associated

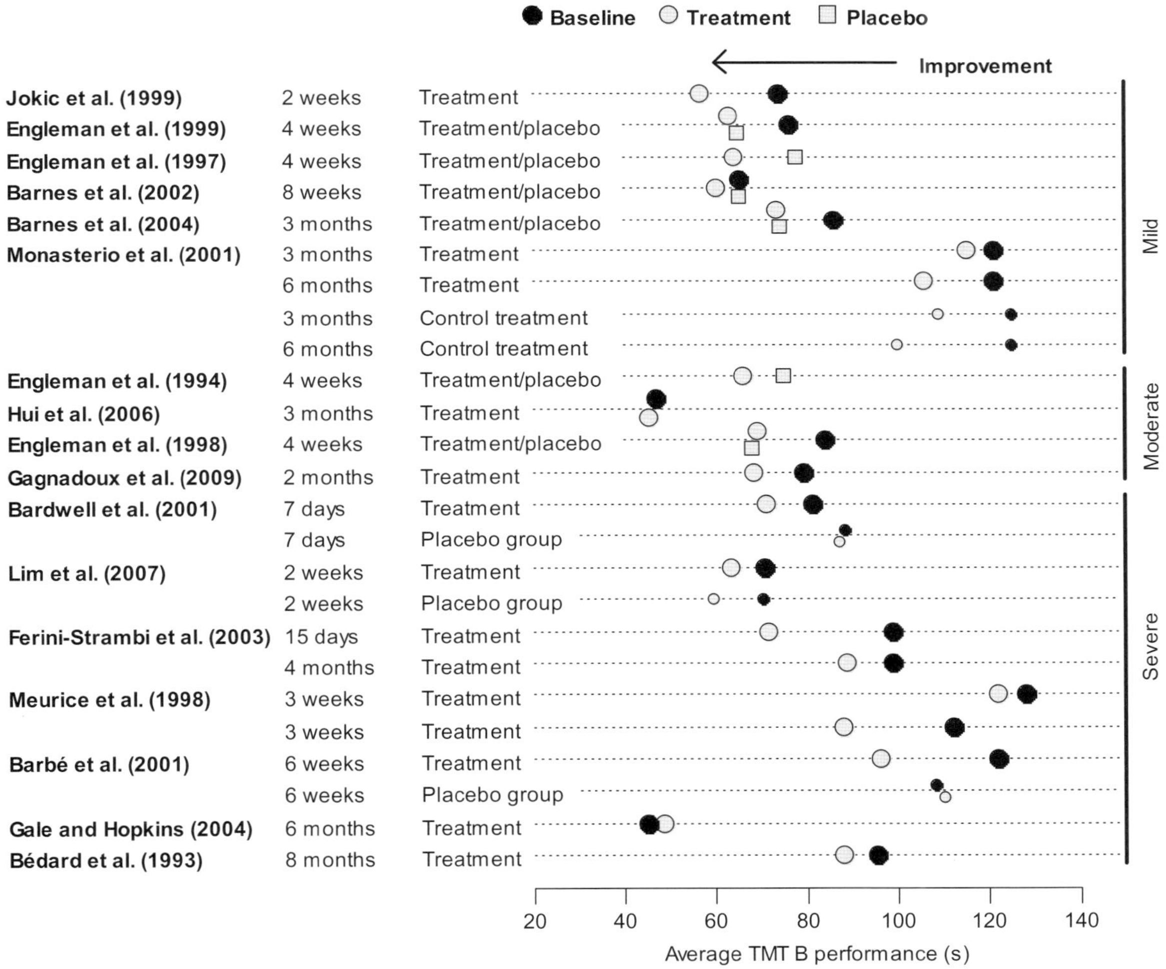

Fig. 1. Group-average performance in the Trail Making Test B (TMT B) in 17 studies with positive airway pressure (PAP) treatment in patients with sleep-related breathing disorders (SRBD). Column 1 gives the study reference and column 2 study duration. In the third column treatment refers to PAP treatment, treatment/placebo signifies cross-over studies where the same group received both PAP and placebo, and placebo group refers to parallel-group studies. Control treatment consisted of weight reduction and avoidance of alcohol. Severity of SRBD (right border) was classified as mild (apnoea-hypopnea index, AHI: 5–20), moderate (AHI: 21–50) or severe (AHI: >50). Changes within control or placebo groups are denoted by smaller symbols.

with pronounced sleepiness, as for example in severe cases of narcolepsy or SRBD, performance on many different tests will be impaired, because most tests have been developed and validated in subjects with normal attention. However, if sleepiness is less pronounced, or fatigue is a prevailing symptom, as for example in insomnia, it is more difficult to select sensitive tests to detect potential cognitive deficits. The reason for this is that sleepiness has a direct negative impact on basic attentional functions such as sustained attention which in turn contribute critically to task performance for a wide variety of tests, while the effect of fatigue on such functions is less clear. As a result of this complex situation, a multitude of different tests and protocols have been used. In a review of 57 studies describing cognitive functioning in patients with sleep disorders, we counted 170 different tasks that had been employed, most of them in only one study (Fulda and Schulz, 2001). Based on the known interdependence of the different tasks, they can be clustered into specific cognitive dimensions, for example Lezak's taxonomy of neuropsychological functions (Lezak et al., 2004).

One strategy to avoid test heterogeneity, which impedes replicability, would be to use a standard battery of neuropsychological tests covering the most essential neurocognitive functions, such as attention, memory, construction or executive functions. This would allow comparing results across studies. Such a test battery has been proposed for SRBD (Décary et al., 2000). The basic principle of this strategy is to get *point estimates* for different cognitive functions by a single measurement. If a sample, which is representative for a diagnostic group, has point estimates that are either significantly lower than norm values or lower than the scores of a sample of control subjects, the measured function would be assumed to be impaired in the patient group. The use of a standard battery thus allows identifying a pattern of impaired and unimpaired cognitive functions for a given diagnostic category.

A main weakness of this procedure is that the different tests are not independent estimates of different cognitive functions if they are performed with the same sample of subjects. In this case, any uncontrolled internal or external factors may exert similar effects on all tasks, that is the error terms of the different task measurements are not independent. To overcome this weakness, a replication for the battery of tests with a new sample would be needed before a firm statement on specific cognitive deficits can be made.

An alternative strategy is to measure performance under increasing cognitive demand, that is to systematically vary the mental load which is needed to solve a task successfully. Such an experimental strategy probably provides a more sensitive measure of cognitive deficits in sleep-disordered patients than a number of one-trial performances on different tasks. Altena et al. (2008a) followed such a strategy when they compared performance on a simple and a complex vigilance task. The simple task (110 asterisks sequentially appearing on a computer screen on the same location but with variable and random time intervals) differed from the complex task (either the target letter p or the distractor letter d appearing in the middle of the screen) in specific parameters. Subjects were instructed to respond as accurately and as quickly as possible to the targets while ignoring distractors. The authors compared the performance of a group of insomniac patients with matched controls before and after a 6-week multi-component treatment phase. Before therapy, insomniac patients performed faster than controls on the simple task and slower on the complex task. After therapy 'normal performance' was restored, that is compared to baseline, patients' reaction times became slower on the simple task and faster on the complex task with the effect that reaction times were now more similar to those of controls. However, regression to the mean in the post-therapy test session remains as an alternative explanation of the results.

Using tasks with an increasing cognitive demand is a promising strategy to assess cognitive impairment in patients with sleep disorders. This was also shown by Edinger et al. (2008a) who found significant differences between insomniac patients and control subjects in a complex and highly demanding switching attention test but not in a simple reaction time test, or a continuous performance test.

A further parameter that may increase sensitivity of a task to detect cognitive impairment is test duration, or time-on-task. One example is the Steer Clear, a simple computerized driving simulation task that measures sustained attention, which was used to compare the performance of patients with sleep apnoea, narcolepsy and healthy controls (Findley et al., 1999). Interestingly, the groups differed not only in the mean level of performance but also in intra-individual variability over time. Time-on-task decrement was low in control subjects, intermediate in sleep apnoea patients and significantly higher in narcoleptic patients. These examples show that systematic variations of task parameters, such as difficulty of the task and task duration, are effective means to increase sensitivity of a test to recognize performance deficits in patients with sleep disturbances and also to differentiate between various diagnostic groups.

Imaging techniques, such as functional magnetic resonance imaging (fMRI), offer additional tools to recognize group differences in either task-related activation of certain brain areas or activation by compensatory processes (Desseilles et al., 2008). However, studies such as the one by Altena et al. (2008b) show how complex the relationship between cognitive test results and fMRI can be. In the pre-treatment test situation insomniac patients performed significantly better on a letter and on a category fluency task, while the fMRI showed hypoactivation of medial and inferior prefrontal cortical areas, which are assumed to be critically involved in task performance. Insomniac patients were then separated into a group which received non-pharmacological, behavioural treatment and a waiting-list group. After 6 weeks task performance was improved in both groups, probably due to training; however, the treatment by time interaction was only near-significant for letter fluency and not for category fluency. At the same time, prefrontal hypoactivation had recovered in the therapy group but not in the waiting-list condition. The results show that (i) brain activation, as measured by imaging techniques, has no simple predictive value for performance in cognitive tasks and (ii) imaging-measured brain activity and task performance may react differently to treatment.

Single versus repeated measurement of cognitive functions

The vast majority of sleep disorders studies have relied on a single test performance at a pre-defined time of day. However, the few studies that have assessed cognitive performance repeatedly during the day show that groups not only differ in the level but also in the temporal pattern of performance (Schneider et al., 2004). While most studies with single measurements did not find significant differences between insomniac patients and control subjects (Fulda and Schulz, 2001), studies with frequently repeated tasks during 10 h (Schneider et al., 2004) or during 24 h of a modified constant routine protocol (Varkevisser and Kerkhof, 2005) or just four or five times a day (Edinger et al., 2008a; Mendelson et al., 1984; Murphy and Campbell, 1996) showed significant performance differences between insomniacs and controls in some tasks. At the moment it is an open question whether the knowledge that performance will be evaluated repeatedly over a longer period of time had an influence on the motivation, effort, or strategy with which insomniac patients performed the tasks. In any case, one can hypothesize that repeated measurements will be more sensitive than single measurements to detect group differences and treatment effects.

Study design and sampling strategies

A wide range of study designs are available to study the effect of an intervention on cognitive functioning. The randomized controlled trial remains the gold standard of intervention research, but in sleep research this design is not always feasible for practical or ethical reasons and alternative study designs have been used. Any choice of a study design comes with its own costs and potential limitations to the interpretation or generalization of the findings and this will be detailed in the following.

The American Academy of Sleep Medicine (AASM) has classified the level of evidence regarding intervention studies into five grades with the highest level of evidence (level I) given to randomized well-designed trials with low alpha (type I) and beta (type II) errors (see below) (e.g. Morgenthaler et al., 2006). The lowest level of evidence is given to case series, that is observational studies with no control group. The reason for this grading is that without a control group alternative explanations for a change in cognitive functioning cannot be ruled out. Major alternative explanations are simple time effects, that is performance gets better on its own, practice effects due to repeated testing, regression to the mean or other unspecific factors such as doctor's contact.

An example for evidence level V is the longitudinal study of Borak et al. (1996), who compared the performance of 20 patients with severe SRBD at baseline, after 3 and 12 months of CPAP treatment. They found that visual and spatial memory was improved after 3 months, whereas speed of work improved after 12 months of treatment. While cognitive performance improved under treatment, emotional status did not. The study design, however, does not allow ruling out that, besides CPAP, some of the factors just mentioned have contributed to the outcome.

Level IV and level III evidence are non-randomized studies that compare performance of a group of treated patients to a similar group of patients who did not receive the intervention either in the past (historically controlled, level IV) or at the same time as the intervention group (concurrently controlled, level III). An example for level IV evidence is a study by Vignola et al. (2000) who compared cognitive performance of elderly insomniacs with prolonged use of benzodiazepines to that of elderly insomniacs without medication and a group of good sleepers. The research question was whether elderly insomniac patients with benzodiazepine use show cognitive impairment in comparison to unmedicated patients. While both insomnia groups performed worse than good sleeping controls on a composite measure of attention and concentration, they did not differ from each other. The main concern here is the comparability of the two insomnia groups. There may be other unknown or unmeasured processes besides medication, which could be responsible for the outcome. It can be suspected that only patients that tolerated benzodiazepines fairly well would continue to use them for a prolonged period of time while subjects that experienced adverse effects would have discontinued drug use on their own. Thus, a selection bias must be considered in this type of study. Level III to V studies, which are subsumed under the heading of non-randomized studies, are useful to generate research hypotheses and guide selection of cognitive tasks and test procedures, while they do not give reliable evidence on the effects of treatment on cognition.

Level II and I evidence are randomized controlled studies, that is a group of patients is randomized to receive active treatment or an appropriate control condition. The quality of the randomization process is judged according to the concealment of treatment allocation schedule and the generation of the allocation sequence. Schulz et al. (1995) have empirically shown that studies with inadequately concealed treatment allocation are subject to be associated with bias, since they yield larger estimated treatment effects than adequately controlled studies. Equally important is the choice of an appropriate control condition to ensure that neither the experimenter and personnel conducting the study nor the patient is aware whether the actual condition is active treatment or sham treatment. This seems to be simple in case of drug treatment, where the placebo pills can be made undistinguishable in appearance (and taste) from the active pill. However, it is more difficult to control blinding when the active treatment has frequent side effects. Dopamine agonists, for example which are used to treat RLS, frequently give rise to nausea, especially in the beginning of treatment. Such prominent, unwanted effects obviously endanger the blinding of treatment. For that reason, domperidone, an antiemetic drug, has been used as an adjunct in treatment studies with dopaminergic drugs (Trenkwalder et al., 2004).

The search for an adequate control condition is also essential in studies where patients with obstructive sleep apnoea are treated with nasal CPAP. In this case oral placebos have been used (Engleman et al., 1997) or sham CPAP, that is CPAP with sub-therapeutic pressure, which is an established control condition (Montserrat et al., 2001; Rodway et al., 2010). In the case of oral placebos in treatment of SRBD, treatment allocation may be non-detectable for the patient, but is clearly recognizable for the experimenter. For behavioural, cognitive or multimodal treatments it can be particularly difficult to design adequate control conditions (Steinmark and Borkovec, 1974; Woolfolk and McNulty, 1983). In many studies waiting-list control groups were employed, where subjects are informed that they have been scheduled for treatment but should wait until a free place in a treatment group is available. However, waiting-list control groups are subject to implicit counter-demand characteristics. As the patient knows that he or she is not being treated actually, he or she does not expect improvement.

If the treatment conditions have been decided, the next step is to choose an adequate study design to compare the treatment conditions. In a cross-over design, a group of subjects receives both active and control treatment, one after the other, and with a sequence that is randomized between subjects. While a cross-over design, as compared with a parallel-group design, needs only half the number of subjects or less to get the same statistical power, it needs adequate control to avoid potential carry-over from one treatment to the other. A wash-out phase of suitable length between successive treatment phases is common practice in drug trials; however, this procedure increases total study duration. In addition, order effects must be considered in cross-over trials, that is the order in which active and control treatment are administered may affect the outcome. Cross-over designs also tend to suffer from greater attrition, because subjects have to be longer under study restrictions.

An alternative is the parallel-group design. Parallel-group designs rely on the randomized allocation of patients to a treatment and a control group. Given an adequate group size, randomization can be expected to result in roughly equivalent groups. In smaller studies, however, randomization could also yield groups that substantially differ in size or baseline characteristics. In this case, block randomization with random allocation in blocks is an alternative. The basic idea of block randomization is to divide potential patients into blocks and implement the experimental design within each block or homogeneous subgroup. Block building can be based on the number of subjects, for example each 10 consecutive patients, or important baseline characteristics such as disease severity. This method ensures equal treatment allocation within each block.

Finally, in designing a study, the statistical parameters alpha and beta should be considered. The alpha error is the probability that the null hypothesis is rejected when in fact it is true. It can be thought of as the false positive error, and the acceptable alpha level is generally set at 5% or less. An inflation of the alpha error occurs when non-independent multiple (e.g. post hoc) tests are conducted within the same sample. One way to control this in clinical trials is to adjust the alpha error inversely proportional to the number of non-independent tests. Another strategy is to formulate primary and secondary outcomes a priori, and to employ a hierarchical testing structure whereby secondary outcomes are only analysed if the primary outcome shows a significant effect.

The beta error, which is often referred to as statistical power (one minus beta), is the probability that the null hypothesis is not rejected given that the alternative hypothesis is actually true. It can be thought of as the false negative error, and the acceptable beta level is generally set at 20% or less (i.e. the a priori statistical power of the study is typically required to be at least 80%). The beta error depends directly on the size of the effect and the number of subjects. Small effect sizes will need larger groups before the effect will become statistically significant, while large effects will be significant also when comparing small groups. Trials that are statistically underpowered because they were performed with too few subjects may lead to the wrong conclusion that a treatment had no effect (i.e. a beta error), when in fact the treatment effect was not large enough to be detected. A realistic estimate of the expected size of the treatment effect, based on knowledge from prior studies, is therefore highly advisable to compute the sample size when planning a study (a so-called power calculation).

Treatment studies of SRBD in adults: designs and results

A survey of published studies in the area of SRBD suggests that a wide variety of different designs and comparisons have been employed, and the numerous factors implemented are compiled in Table 2. The multifaceted designs have to be considered when comparing the effect of treatment on cognitive performance between studies.

The most evidence on the effect of treatment on cognitive functioning has accumulated for the positive airway pressure (PAP) treatment of obstructive sleep apnoea, where more than 50 studies are available. For cognitive functioning by far the most frequent comparison is made between baseline assessment in untreated patients and following subsequent PAP treatment of variable length. In only a minority of studies has PAP treatment been compared to a control condition such as sham CPAP (Barbé et al., 2001; Bardwell et al., 2001; Henke et al., 2001; Marshall et al., 2005), oral placebo (Barnes et al., 2002, 2004; Engleman et al., 1994, 1997, 1998, 1999; Lim et al., 2007) or conservative treatment (most often weight reduction and avoidance of alcohol; see Engleman et al., 1993; Lojander et al., 1999; Monasterio et al., 2001). Several studies compared PAP treatment with another active treatment such as theophylline (Saletu et al., 1999), oxygen (Lim et al., 2007), positional treatment (Jokic et al., 1999), surgery (Conradt et al., 1998) or oral devices (Barnes et al., 2004; Hoekema et al., 2007; Gagnadoux et al., 2009). In a few studies, one PAP treatment was compared to another PAP treatment (Bakker et al., 2010; Marshall et al., 2008; Meurice et al., 1998; Senn et al., 2003) or to withdrawal of treatment (Kribbs et al., 1993; Turkington et al., 2004). Finally, an increasing number of studies have

Table 2. Features of study design and sampling in treatment studies in SRBD

A: Sort of comparison	
1	Treatment versus no treatment (baseline, withdrawal of treatment)
2	Treatment versus control condition (or control group)
3	Treatment versus pseudo-treatment (oral placebo, sham CPAP, other)
4	Two active treatments (CPAP, positional treatment, oral appliance, surgery, other)
5	Within treatment (baseline, acute, short term, long term, withdrawal)
B: Comparators	
1	Sham CPAP
2	Oral placebo
3	Conventional treatment (weight reduction etc.)
4	Positional training
5	Oral appliances
6	ENT operation (UPPP, others)
7	Add-on treatment (oxygen, modafinil, others)
C: Treatment duration	
1	Acute (1 night to 1 week)
2	Short term (2 weeks to 6 months)
3	Long term (>6 months)
4	Withdrawal
D: SRBD (OSAS) severity	
1	Mild
2	Moderate
3	Severe
E: Compliance with treatment	
1	Low compliance
2	High compliance
F: Other effects controlled in some studies	
1	Learning effects
2	Carry-over effects
3	Effects of pre-morbid intelligence

compared PAP treatment to PAP treatment with an add-on medication with stimulants, to reduce residual sleepiness after PAP treatment, which is a known clinical problem in a subgroup of SRBD patients (Bittencourt et al., 2008; Hirshkowitz et al., 2007; Kingshott et al., 2001; Roth et al., 2006, 2008; Williams et al., 2008, 2010).

Several studies compared performance of patient groups in the treated and the untreated state (Castronovo et al., 2009; Ferini-Strambi et al., 2003; Feuerstein et al., 1997; Hoekema et al., 2007; Kotterba et al., 1998; Orth et al., 2002; Randerath et al., 2000; Saunamäki et al., 2009; Thomas et al., 2005; Tonon et al., 2007), or against a healthy control group. However, in only three studies was the control group tested more than once (George et al., 1997; Mazza et al., 2006; Muñoz et al., 2000) as a control for learning effects (Engleman et al., 1994, 1997, 1998, 1999) or carry-over effects (Engleman et al., 1994). Finally, several studies have drawn attention to the effect of PAP use on cognitive functioning by comparing compliant versus non-compliant patients (Aloia et al., 2001, 2003; Engleman et al., 1999; Felver-Gant et al., 2007; Kingshott et al., 2000; Zimmerman et al., 2006).

Overall, cognitive functioning in SRBD is improved in some but not all tasks following CPAP treatment, and results are described in detail by Matthews and Aloia (submitted). All in all, out of over 50 treatment studies, only 14 compared CPAP treatment to either a placebo condition or conservative treatment, and these studies have documented learning effects or other systematic changes in cognitive measures, unrelated to CPAP treatment per se. This necessitates caution when interpreting results. Placebo-controlled studies that included cognitive outcomes have only been conducted for shorter periods of time, the longest study being 3 months (Barnes et al., 2004). When CPAP was compared to conservative treatment, consisting of weight reduction and reduction of alcohol consumption, no differences in cognitive tests were seen after periods of 3–12 months in patients with mild (Monasterio et al., 2001), moderate (Lojander et al., 1999) or severe (Engleman et al., 1993) SRBD. This was the case despite the fact that, at the end of the studies, CPAP treatment had effectively reduced sleep-related breathing whereas conservative treatment had not (Lojander et al., 1999; Monasterio et al., 2001).

Treatment studies of SRBD in children: designs and results

In children, SRBD is associated with deficits of attention and alertness (Beebe, 2006; Halbower and Mahone, 2006). Adenotonsillectomy is a standard treatment of childhood SRBD with a success rate of 60–80% (Friedman et al., 2009; Lipton and Gozal, 2003). Assessment of cognitive functions in treatment studies with children is a difficult task since cognitive functions change rapidly during development in children.

From 12 studies with cognitive task performance before and after AT, only 5 had a control group, either healthy non-scoring children (Friedman et al., 2003; Hogan et al., 2008; Kohler et al., 2009) or children scheduled for unrelated surgery (Ali et al., 1996; Chervin et al., 2006). None of the studies was placebo-controlled, presumably for ethical reasons and practicability. Follow-up periods ranged from 5 to 12 months in control group studies and from 2 to 9 months in studies without a control group (Table 3). Similar to treatment studies in adults, also in children a multitude of different tasks have been employed, with limited convergence between studies. Improvement from baseline to post-surgery performance was most consistently found for attention (Ali et al., 1996; Avior et al., 2004; Chervin et al., 2006; Galland et al., 2006; Guilleminault et al., 1982; Hogan et al., 2008; Li et al., 2006; Owens et al., 2000). In addition, improvement has been reported for memory (Kohler et al., 2009), reasoning (Friedman et al., 2003), verbal fluency (Owens et al., 2000) and sensorimotor function (Kohler et al., 2009; Owens et al., 2000). In studies with a control group, some improvement was also seen in the controls (Friedman et al., 2003; Kohler et al., 2009).

Table 3. Studies assessing cognitive tasks performance in children with sleep-disordered breathing before and after adenotonsillectomy (AT)

Study (follow-up duration)	Subjects	Cognitive tests	Significant changes pre–post	Significant changes compared to control group
Studies with control group				
Kohler et al. (2009) (6 months)	44 children with SDB, 3–13 years, versus 48 non-snoring control children	Stanford Binet Intelligence Scale (15 tasks, 18 scores); NEPSY (13 tasks, 17 scores)	Both groups: verbal working memory, sensorimotor function, memory for names and faces	Visual spatial performance
Chervin et al. (2006) (1 year)	78 children scheduled for AT, 5–13 years, versus 27 children scheduled for unrelated surgery	Cognitive attention index (3 tasks, 1 score)	Cognitive attention index improved only in children scheduled for AT	Cognitive attention index
Friedman et al. (2003) (6–10 months)	27 children with OSAS, 5–9 years, versus 14 healthy control	K-ABC intelligence scales (6 tasks, 9 scores)	OSAS: Gestalt closure, triangles, word order, matrix analogies, spatial memory, sequential processing scale, simultaneous processing scale, mental processing composite Control: simultaneous processing scale, mental processing composite	Gestalt closure, word order, simultaneous processing scale, mental processing composite
Ali et al. (1996) (3–6 months)	12 children with moderate SDB, 5–12 years, versus 11 children with history of snoring and sleep disturbances but without SDB (oximetry) versus 10 children referred for unrelated surgery	Continuous performance task (CPT) (2 scores); Matching Familiar Figures Test (MFFT) (2 scores)	SDB and snorers: CPT number of hits	SDB and snorers: CPT number of hits
Hogan et al. (2008) (1 year)	19 children with mild SDB, 3–7 years, versus 14 control children	(Only tests that showed significant pre-operative differences); WPPSI-III (2 tasks, 1 score); neuropsychological test battery, visual attention (1 task, 1 score)	SDB: processing speed index, visual attention	

(continued)

Table 3 (continued)

Study (follow-up duration)	Subjects	Cognitive tests	Significant changes pre–post	Significant changes compared to control group
Studies without control group				
Guilleminault et al. (1982) (3 months)	5 children with heavy snoring but no sleep apnoea, 11–14 years	Wilkinson addition test (WAT), 5 times/day (1 score)	WAT number of problems solved	
Li et al. (2006) (6 months)	40 children with SDB, 5–12 years	TOVA (1 task, 6 scores)	TOVA ADHS score, response time	
Owens et al. (2000) (6–12 months)	8 of 18 children with mild to moderate OSAS, ~8 years	2 h test battery (10 tasks, 13 scores): WISC III IQ; Peabody picture test; cancellation tests (2 tasks, 4 scores); verbal fluency; WISC III digit span; WRAML memory; Hooper visual organization; visual motor integration; finger tapping (2 scores)	Verbal fluency; finger tapping, non-dominant hand	
Montgomery-Downs et al. (2005) (~7 months)	19 children with OSAS, ~4 years (control group tested only once)	Differential Ability Scales (DAS) (7 tasks, 1 score); NEPSY (3 tasks, 3 scores)	DAS global score	
Avior et al. (2004) (2 months)	19 children with OSAS, 5–14 years	TOVA (1 task, 1 score)	TOVA score	
Galland et al. (2006) (3 months)	39 of 61 children scheduled for AT, 6–11 years (PSG showed AHI > 1.5 in 43 children)	Visual Conners' Continuous Performance Test (VCPT) II (1 task, 11 scores); Auditory Continuous Performance Test (1 task, 1 score)	VCPT: % commissions detectability	

ADHS: attention deficit hyperactivity syndrome; AHI: apnoea-hypopnoea index; AT: adenotonsillectomy; CPT: Continuous Performance Test; DAS: Differential Ability Scale; K-ABC: Kaufman Assessment Battery for Children; MFFT: Matching Familiar Figures Test; NEPSY: Neuropsychological Developmental Assessment; OSAS: obstructive sleep apnoea syndrome; SDB: sleep-disordered breathing; TOVA: Test of Variables of Attention; VCPT: Visual Conners' Continuous Performance Test; WAT: Wilkinson Addition Test; WISC: Wechsler Intelligence Scale for Children; WPPSI: Wechser PreSchool and Primary Scale of Intelligence; WRAML: Wide Range Assessment of Memory and Learning.

How treatment acts on cognitive functioning in patients with sleep disorders

There are direct and indirect ways of how treatment may act on cognitive performance. The two main direct routes are (i) by restoring and consolidating nighttime sleep and (ii) by reducing daytime sleepiness and fatigue. In addition, there are indirect ways to improve cognitive performance, for example by enhancing mood and well-being and by attenuating undesirable symptoms such as pain or stress, or comorbid disorders such as depression.

Consolidation of sleep

Improving night sleep is the primary aim of any treatment in any patient suffering from a sleep disorder. Since it is known from experimental studies that sleep curtailment and sleep fragmentation result in impaired performance (Pilcher and Huffcutt, 1996), it would be safe to hypothesize that consolidation of sleep will alleviate cognitive deficits in patients with disturbed sleep. For patients with daytime sleepiness, therapeutic improvement of sleep is thought to reduce daytime sleepiness, which in turn is expected to improve cognitive functioning (but see below).

For insomnia, convincing evidence from empirical studies that treatment improves cognitive deficits is still lacking. In addition, for insomnia there are only a handful of studies showing cognitive deficits before treatment. The case of insomnia is even more complicated by the fact that drugs, which are used for treatment, can negatively affect performance. Benzodiazepines, for instance, are associated with hangover and thus may induce next-day performance deficits in both healthy subjects and insomniac patients (Johnson and Chernik, 1982). Benzodiazepines, but also non-benzodiazepines such as zopiclone or zaleplon, and sedative antidepressants can be associated with impaired driving performance (Verster et al., 2004). Moderating factors of these effects are age, gender, time of administration, length of treatment and large inter-individual differences. For non-pharmacological treatments of chronic insomnia, evidence for improved performance in cognitive tasks is presently insufficient (e.g. Morin et al., 1999, but see Altena et al., 2008a).

Reducing sleepiness

Hypersomnias and SRBD are consistently associated with increased daytime sleepiness and decreased vigilance and attention. Adequate treatment of these disorders reduces sleepiness (Giles et al., 2006; Keam and Walker, 2007; Marshall et al., 2006), and thus supposedly increases vigilance and attention. Taking SRBD as an example, from the eight placebo-controlled studies that have assessed both objective sleepiness (MWT or MSLT) and cognitive performance, five were conducted in patients with milder forms of SRBD and none found significant differences between CPAP and placebo treatment, most likely due to ceiling effects (Barnes et al., 2002, 2004; Engleman et al., 1997, 1999; Marshall et al., 2005). Two of the five studies employed a 30 or 60 min version of the Steer Clear task and found no difference between placebo and CPAP treatment (Engleman et al., 1997, 1999), while one (Barnes et al., 2004) of three other studies (Barnes et al., 2002; Marshall et al., 2005) using the Psychomotor Vigilance Test (PVT) reported improved performance with CPAP treatment. Interestingly, the one study (Barnes et al., 2004) that found a difference in the PVT was also the longest (3 months), and by far the largest study with more than 100 participants, which suggests that the size of the treatment effect is so small that the other studies may have been underpowered. On the other hand, in case of very small effects, the clinical significance of treatment-induced changes may be questioned.

Changes in other cognitive measures, such as short-term attention or verbal fluency, were occasionally reported in some of the studies in mild SRBD patients (Barnes et al., 2002, 2004; Engleman et al., 1997, 1999). Two further studies in moderate SRBD found that CPAP was superior to placebo in reducing objective daytime sleepiness measured with the MSLT (Engleman et al., 1994, 1998). Both studies used very similar protocols, but in only one of them corresponding treatment effects were observed in cognitive measures (Engleman et al., 1994). In a final study (Barbé et al., 2001), severe SRBD patients were selected for the absence of daytime sleepiness and consequently objective sleepiness was not apparent at baseline and did not change with treatment. Accordingly, in the cognitive performance measures only 1 out of 12 measures showed a slight superiority of CPAP over placebo.

Taken together, the question whether reduction of daytime sleepiness is a prerequisite for improvement in cognitive functioning in SRBD cannot be answered with certainty. In milder cases with no daytime sleepiness, therapeutic changes in cognitive functioning appear inconsistent. In moderately affected patients, the limited evidence suggests reduction of daytime sleepiness as maybe a necessary but not sufficient condition for improvement of cognitive functioning, whereas controlled studies in severely affected patients with daytime sleepiness are lacking.

Concluding remarks

It has been shown that experimentally shortened or disturbed sleep results in impaired daytime performance in otherwise normal sleeping persons. The relationship between sleep and performance is less clear in persons suffering from sleep disorders. It is even more difficult to firmly conclude from available studies how cognitive deficits are reduced by treatment. We have discussed some of the critical points such as task selection, study designs and control of intervening factors. In the interpretation of cognitive improvements, learning effects, order effects and other systematic biases must be considered, and such effects invalidate uncontrolled studies in the field. Interpretations of a lack of improvement must take into account the sensitivity of the tasks, treatment efficacy (e.g. the presence of residual sleepiness) and treatment duration. Finally, the database is presently too small to decide with certainty by which way treatment affects cognitive performance. Reduction of daytime sleepiness may be a primary candidate for treating cognitive impairment in many sleep disorders. Ways to adapt research strategies of cognitive neuroscience to the needs of sleep medicine present a challenge for future research.

References

Alchanatis, M., Zias, N., Deligiorgis, N., Liappas, I., Chroneou, A., & Soldatos, C., et al., (2008). Comparison of cognitive performance among different age groups in patients with obstructive sleep apnea. *Sleep & Breathing*, *12*, 17–24.

Ali, N. J., Pitson, D., & Stradling, J. R. (1996). Sleep disordered breathing: Effects of adenotonsillectomy on behaviour and psychological functioning. *European Journal of Pediatrics*, *155*, 56–62.

Aloia, M. S., Di Dio, L., Ilniczky, N., Perlis, M. L., Greenblatt, D. W., & Giles, D. E. (2001). Improving compliance with nasal CPAP and vigilance in older adults with OAHS. *Sleep & Breathing*, *5*, 13–21.

Aloia, M. S., Ilniczky, N., Di Dio, P., Perlis, M. L., Greenblatt, D. W., & Giles, D. E. (2003). Neuropsychological changes and treatment compliance in older adults with sleep apnea. *Journal of Psychosomatic Research*, *54*, 71–76.

Altena, E., Van Der Werf, Y., Strijers, R. L. M., & Van Someren, E. J. W. (2008a). Sleep loss affects vigilance: Effects of chronic insomnia and sleep therapy. *Journal of Sleep Research*, *17*, 335–343.

Altena, E., Van Der Werf, Y. D., Sanz-Arigita, E. J., Voorn, T. A., Rombouts, S. A. R. B., & Kuijer, J. P. A., et al., (2008b). Prefrontal hypoactivation and recovery in insomnia. *Sleep*, *31*, 1271–1276.

Avior, G., Fishman, G., Leor, A., Sivan, Y., Kaysar, N., & Derowe, A. (2004). The effect of tonsillectomy and adenoidectomy on inattention and impulsivity as measured by the Test of Variables of Attention (TOVA) in children with obstructive sleep apnea syndrome. *Otolaryngology - Head and Neck Surgery*, *131*, 367–371.

Ayalon, L., Ancoli-Israel, S., & Drummond, S. P. (2010). Obstructive sleep apnea and age: A double-insult to brain function? *American Journal of Respiratory and Critical Care Medicine,*, *182*, 413–419.

Bakker, J., Campbell, A., & Neill, A. (2010). Randomized controlled trial comparing flexible and continuous positive airway pressure delivery: Effects on compliance, objective and subjective sleepiness and vigilance. *Sleep*, *33*, 523–529.

Baltes, P. B. (1993). The aging mind: Potential and limits. *The Gerontologist*, *33*, 580–594.

Banks, S., & Dinges, D. F. (2007). Behavioral and physiological consequences of sleep restriction. *Journal of Clinical Sleep Medicine*, *3*, 519–528.

Barbé, F., Mayoralas, L. R., Duran, J., Masa, J. F., Maimó, A., & Montserrat, J. M., et al., (2001). Treatment with continuous positive airway pressure is not effective in patients with sleep apnea but no daytime sleepiness. A randomized, controlled trial. *Annals of Internal Medicine*, *134*, 1015–1023.

Bardwell, W. A., Ancoli-Israel, S., Berry, C. C., & Dimsdale, J. E. (2001). Neuropsychological effects of one-week continuous positive airway pressure treatment in patients with obstructive sleep apnea: A placebo-controlled study. *Psychosomatic Medicine*, *63*, 579–584.

Barnes, M., Houston, D., Worsnop, C. J., Neill, A. M., Mykytyn, I. J., & Kay, A., et al., (2002). A randomized controlled trial of continuous positive airway pressure in mild obstructive sleep apnea. *American Journal of Respiratory and Critical Care Medicine*, *165*, 773–780.

Barnes, M., McEvoy, R. D., Banks, S., Tarquinio, N., Murray, C. G., & Vowles, N., et al., (2004). Efficacy of positive airway pressure and oral appliance in mild to moderate obstructive sleep apnea. *American Journal of Respiratory and Critical Care Medicine*, *170*, 656–664.

Bédard, M. A., Montplaisir, J., Malo, J., Richer, F., & Rouleau, I. (1993). Persistent neuropsychological deficits and vigilance impairment in sleep apnea syndrome after treatment with continuous positive airways pressure (CPAP). *Journal of Clinical and Experimental Neuropsychology*, *15*, 330–341.

Bédard, M., Montplaisir, J., Richer, F., Rouleau, I., & Malo, J. (1991). Obstructive sleep apnea syndrome: Pathogenesis of neuropsychological deficits. *Journal of Clinical and Experimental Neuropsychology*, *13*, 950.

Beebe, D. W. (2006). Neurobehavioral morbidity associated with disordered breathing during sleep in children: A comprehensive review. *Sleep*, *29*, 1115–1134.

Bittencourt, L. R. A., Lucchesi, L. M., Rueda, A. D., Garbuio, S. A., Palombini, L. O., & Guilleminault, C., et al., (2008). Placebo and modafinil effect on sleepiness in obstructive sleep apnea. *Progress in Neuro-Psychopharmacology & Biological Psychiatry*, *32*, 552–559.

Bonnet, M. H. (2005). Acute sleep deprivation. In: Kryger, M. H., Roth, T., Dement, W. C. (Eds.), *Principles and Practice of Sleep Medicine, 4th ed. Elsevier Saunders, Philadelphia, pp. 51–66.*

Bonnet, M. H., & Arand, D. L. (2003). Clinical effects of sleep fragmentation versus sleep deprivation. *Sleep Medicine Reviews*, *7*, 297–310.

Borak, J., Cieslicki, J. K., Koziej, M., Matuszweski, A., & Zielinski, J. (1996). Effects of CPAP treatment on psychological status in patients with severe obstructive sleep apnoea. *Journal of Sleep Research*, *5*, 123–127.

Castronovo, V., Canessa, N., Strambi, L. F., Aloia, M. S., Consonni, M., & Marelli, S., et al., (2009). Brain activation changes before and after PAP treatment in obstructive sleep apnea. *Sleep*, *32*, 1161–1172.

Chaytor, N., & Schmitter-Edgecombe, M. (2003). The ecological validity of neuropsychological tests: A review of the literature on everyday cognitive skills. *Neuropsychological Review*, *13*, 181–197.

Chervin, R. D., Ruzicka, D. L., Giordani, B. J., Weatherly, R. A., Dillon, J. E., & Hodges, E. K., et al., (2006). Sleep-disordered breathing, behavior, and cognition in children before and after adenotonsillectomy. *Pediatrics*, *117*, e769–e778.

Cluydts, R., De Valck, E., Verstraeten, E., & Theys, P. (2002). Daytime sleepiness and its evaluation. *Sleep Medicine Reviews*, *6*, 83–96.

Conradt, R., Hochban, W., Heitmann, J., Brandenburg, U., Cassel, W., & Penzel, T., et al., (1998). Sleep fragmentation and daytime vigilance in patients with OSA treated by surgical maxillomandibular advancement compared to CPAP therapy. *Journal of Sleep Research*, *7*, 217–223.

Daurat, A., Foret, J., Bret-Dibat, J., Fureix, C., & Tiberge, M. (2008). Spatial and temporal memories are affected by sleep fragmentation in obstructive sleep apnea syndrome. *Journal of Clinical and Experimental Neuropsychology*, *30*, 91–101.

Décary, A., Rouleau, I., & Montplaisir, J. (2000). Cognitive deficits associated with sleep apnea syndrome: A proposed neuropsychological test battery. *Sleep*, *23*, 369–381.

Desseilles, M., Dang-Vu, T., Schabus, M., Sterpenich, V., Maquet, P., & Schwartz, S. (2008). Neuroimaging insights into the pathophysiology of sleep disorders. *Sleep*, *31*, 777–794.

Drag, L. L., & Bieliauskas, L. A. (2010). Contemporary review 2009: Cognitive aging. *Journal of Geriatric Psychiatry and Neurology*, *23*, 75–93.

Duffy, J. F., Willson, H. J., Wang, W., & Czeisler, C. A. (2009). Healthy older adults better tolerate sleep deprivation than young adults. *Journal of the American Geriatrics Society*, *57*, 1245–1251.

Edinger, J. D., Means, M. K., Carney, C. E., & Krystal, A. D. (2008a). Psychomotor performance deficits and their relation to prior nights' sleep among individuals with primary insomnia. *Sleep*, *31*, 599–607.

Edinger, J. D., Carney, C. E., & Wohlgemuth, W. K. (2008b). Pretherapy cognitive dispositions and treatment outcome in cognitive behavior therapy for insomnia. *Behavior Therapy*, *39*, 406–416.

Engleman, H., & Joffe, D. (1999). Neuropsychological function in obstructive sleep apnoea. *Sleep Medicine Reviews*, *3*, 59–78.

Engleman, H. M., Cheshire, K. E., Deary, I. J., & Douglas, N. J. (1993). Daytime sleepiness, cognitive performance and mood after continuous positive airway pressure for the sleep apnoea/hypopnoea syndrome. *Thorax*, *48*, 911–914.

Engleman, H. M., Kingshott, R. N., Wraith, P. K., Mackay, T. W., Deary, I. J., & Douglas, N. J. (1999). Randomized placebo-controlled crossover trial of continuous positive airway pressure for mild sleep apnea/hypopnea syndrome. *American Journal of Respiratory and Critical Care Medicine*, *159*, 461–467.

Engleman, H. M., Martin, S. E., Deary, I. J., & Douglas, N. J. (1997). Effect of CPAP therapy on daytime function in patients with mild sleep apnoea/hypopnoea syndrome. *Thorax*, *52*, 114–119.

Engleman, H. M., Martin, S. E., Douglas, N. J., & Deary, I. J. (1994). Effect of continuous positive airway pressure treatment on daytime function in sleep apnoea/hypopnoea syndrome. *The Lancet*, *343*, 572–575.

Engleman, H., Martin, S., Kingshott, R., Mackay, T., Deary, I., & Douglas, N. (1998). Randomised placebo controlled trial of daytime function after continuous positive airway pressure (CPAP) therapy for the sleep apnoea/hypopnoea syndrome. *Thorax*, *53*, 341–345.

Felver-Gant, J. C., Bruce, A. S., Zimmerman, M., Sweet, L. H., Millman, R. P., & Aloia, M. S. (2007). Working memory in obstructive sleep apnea. *Journal of Clinical Sleep Medicine*, *3*, 589–594.

Ferini-Strambi, L., Baietto, C., Di Gioia, M. R., Castaldi, P., Castronovo, C., & Zucconi, M., et al., (2003). Cognitive dysfunction in patients with obstructive sleep apnea (OSA): Partial reversibility after continuous positive airway pressure (CPAP). *Brain Research Bulletin*, *61*, 87–92.

Feuerstein, C., Naëgelé, B., Pépin, J. L., & Lévy, P. (1997). Frontal lobe-related cognitive functions in patients with sleep apnea syndrome before and after treatment. *Acta Neurologica Belgica*, *97*, 96–107.

Findley, L. J., Suratt, P. M., & Dinges, D. F. (1999). Time-on-task decrements in "steer clear" performance of patients with sleep apnea and narcolepsy. *Sleep*, *22*, 804–809.

Friedman, B. C., Hendeles-Amitai, A., Kozminsky, E., Leiberman, A., Friger, M., & Tarasiuk, A., et al., (2003). Adenotonsillectomy improves neurocognitive function in children with obstructive sleep apnea syndrome. *Sleep*, *26*, 999–1005.

Friedman, M., Wilson, M., Lin, H. C., & Chang, H. W. (2009). Updated systematic review of tonsillectomy and adenoidectomy for treatment of pediatric obstructive sleep apnea/hypopnea syndrome. *Otolaryngology - Head and Neck Surgery*, *140*, 800–808.

Fulda, S., & Schulz, H. (2001). Cognitive dysfunction in sleep disorders. *Sleep Medicine Reviews*, *5*, 423–445.

Gagnadoux, F., Fleury, B., Vielle, B., Pételle, B., Meslier, N., & N'Guyen, X. L., et al., (2009). Titrated mandibular advancement versus positive airway pressure for sleep apnoea. *The European Respiratory Journal*, *34*, 914–920.

Gale, S. D., & Hopkins, R. O. (2004). Effects of hypoxia on the brain: Neuroimaging and neuropsychological findings following carbon monoxide poisoning and obstructive sleep apnea. *Journal of the International Neuropsychological Society*, *10*, 60–71.

Galland, B. C., Dawes, P. J., Tripp, E. G., & Taylor, B. J. (2006). Changes in behavior and attentional capacity after adenotonsillectomy. *Pediatric Research*, *59*, 711–716.

Gazzaniga, M. S. (Ed.), 1995. *The cognitive neurosciences*. The MIT Press, Cambridge.

George, C. F., Boudreau, A. C., & Smiley, A. (1997). Effects of nasal CPAP on simulated driving performance in patients with obstructive sleep apnoea. *Thorax*, *52*, 648–653.

Giles, T. L., Lasserson, T. J., Smith, B. H., White, J., Wright, J., & Cates, C. J. (2006). Continuous positive airways pressure for obstructive sleep apnoea in adults. *Cochrane Database of Systematic Reviews*, *3*, CD001106.

Gong, G., Rosa-Neto, P., Carbonell, F., Chen, Z. J., He, Y., & Evans, A. C. (2009). Age- and gender-related differences in the cortical anatomical network. *The Journal of Neuroscience*, *29*, 15684–15693.

Guilleminault, C., Winkle, R., Korobkin, R., & Simmons, B. (1982). Children and nocturnal snoring: Evaluation of the effects of sleep related respiratory resistive load and daytime functioning. *European Journal of Pediatrics*, *139*, 165–171.

Halbower, A. C., & Mahone, E. M. (2006). Neuropsychological morbidity linked to childhood sleep-disordered breathing. *Sleep Medicine Reviews*, *10*, 97–107.

Henke, K. G., Grady, J. J., & Kuna, S. T. (2001). Effect of nasal continuous positive airway pressure on neuropsychological function in sleep apnea-hypopnea syndrome. A randomized, placebo-controlled trial. *American Journal of Respiratory and Critical Care Medicine*, *163*, 911–917.

Hirshkowitz, M., Black, J. E., Wesnes, K., Niebler, G., Arora, S., & Roth, T. (2007). Adjunct armodafinil improves wakefulness and memory in obstructive sleep apnea/hypopnea syndrome. *Respiratory Medicine*, *101*, 616–627.

Hoekema, A., Stegenga, B., Bakker, M., Brouwer, W. H., de Bont, L. G. M., & Wijkstra, P. J., et al., (2007). Simulated driving in obstructive sleep apnoea-hypopnoea; effects of oral appliances and continuous positive airway pressure. *Sleep & Breathing*, *11*, 129–138.

Hogan, A. M., Hill, C. M., Harrison, D., & Kirkham, F. J. (2008). Cerebral blood flow velocity and cognition in children before and after adenotonsillectomy. *Pediatrics*, *122*, 75–82.

Hublin, C., Kaprio, J., Partinen, M., Koskenvuo, M., & Heikkilä, K. (1994). The Ullanlinna Narcolepsy Scale: Validation of a measure of symptoms in the narcoleptic syndrome. *Journal of Sleep Research*, *3*, 52–59.

Hui, D. S. C., Ko, F. W. S., Chan, J. K. W., To, K. W., Fok, J. P. C., & Ngai, J. C., et al., (2006). Sleep-disordered breathing and continuous positive airway pressure compliance in a group of commercial bus drivers in Hong Kong. *Respirology*, *11*, 723–730.

Jackson, M., Howard, M. & Barnes, M. (2011). Cognitive and daytime functioning in sleep-related breathing disorders. In G. Kerkhof & H. V. Dongen (Eds.), *Human sleep and cognition, Vol. 2*, Elsevier, submitted.

Johns, M. W. (1991). A new method for measuring daytime sleepiness: The Epworth sleepiness scale. *Sleep*, *14*, 540–545.

Johnson, L. C. (1982). Sleep deprivation and performance. In: Monk, T. H. (Ed.), *Biological rhythms, sleep and performance*. Wiley, Chichester, pp. 111–141.

Johnson, L. C., & Chernik, D. A. (1982). Sedative-hypnotics and human performance. *Psychopharmacology*, *76*, 101–113.

Jokic, R., Klimaszewski, A., Crossley, M., Sridhar, G., & Fitzpatrick, M. F. (1999). Positional treatment vs. continuous positive airway pressure in patients with positional obstructive sleep apnea syndrome. *Chest*, *115*, 771–781.

Keam, S., & Walker, M. C. (2007). Therapies for narcolepsy with or without cataplexy: Evidence-based review. *Current Opinion in Neurology*, *20*, 699–703.

Killgore, W. D. S. (2010). Effects of sleep deprivation on cognition. Kerkhof, G., Van Dongen, H. (Eds.), *Human sleep and cognition, progress in brain research. Vol. 185*, Elsevier, Amsterdam.

Kimura, D. (2002). Sex hormones influence human cognitive pattern. *Neuroendocrinology Letters, 23*(Suppl. 4); 67–77.

Kingshott, R. N., Vennelle, M., Coleman, E. L., Engleman, H. M., Mackay, T. W., & Douglas, N. J. (2001). Randomized, double-blind, placebo-controlled crossover trial of modafinil in the treatment of residual excessive daytime sleepiness in the sleep apnea/hypopnea syndrome. *American Journal of Respiratory and Critical Care Medicine, 163*, 918–923.

Kingshott, R. N., Vennelle, M., Hoy, C. J., Engleman, H. M., Deary, I. J., & Douglas, N. J. (2000). Predictors of improvements in daytime function outcomes with CPAP therapy. *American Journal of Respiratory and Critical Care Medicine, 161*, 866–871.

Kohler, M. J., Lushington, K., van den Heuvel, C. J., Martin, J., Pamula, Y., & Kennedy, D. (2009). Adenotonsillectomy and neurocognitive deficits in children with sleep disordered breathing. *PLoS ONE, 4*, e7343.

Kotterba, S., Rasche, K., Widdig, W., Duscha, C., Blombach, S., & Schultze-Werninghaus, G., et al., (1998). Neuropsychological investigations and event-related potentials in obstructive sleep apnea syndrome before and during CAP-therapy. *Journal of the Neurological Sciences, 159*, 45–50.

Kribbs, N. B., Pack, A. I., Kline, L. R., Getsy, J. E., Schuett, J. S., & Henry, J. N., et al., (1993). Effects of one night without nasal CPAP treatment on sleep and sleepiness in patients with obstructive sleep apnea. *The American Review of Respiratory Disease, 147*, 1162–1168.

Léger, D., & Bayon, V. (2010). Societal costs of insomnia. *Sleep Medicine Reviews*, 14(6):379-89.

Lezak, M. D., Howieson, D. B., Loring, D. W., Hannay, H. J., & Fischer, J. S. (2004). *Neuropsychological assessment, 4th ed. Oxford University Press, Oxford.*

Li, H. -Y., Huang, Y. -S., Chen, N. -H., Fang, T. -J., & Lee, L. -A. (2006). Impact of adenotonsillectomy on behavior in children with sleep-disordered breathing. *The Laryngoscope, 116*, 1142–1147.

Lim, W., Bardwell, W. A., Loredo, J. S., Kim, E., Ancoli-Israel, S., & Morgan, E. E., et al., (2007). Neuropsychological effects of 2-week continuous positive airway pressure treatment and supplemental oxygen in patients with obstructive sleep apnea: A randomized placebo-controlled study. *Journal of Clinical Sleep Medicine, 3*, 380–386.

Lipton, A. J., & Gozal, D. (2003). Treatment of obstructive sleep apnea in children: Do we really know how? *Sleep Medicine Reviews, 7*, 61–80.

Lis, S., Krieger, S., Hennig, D., Röder, C., Kirsch, P., & Seeger, W., et al., (2008). Executive functions and cognitive subprocesses in patients with obstructive sleep apnoea. *Journal of Sleep Research, 17*, 271–280.

Lojander, J., Kajaste, S., Maasilta, P., & Partinen, M. (1999). Cognitive function and treatment of obstructive sleep apnea syndrome. *Journal of Sleep Research, 8*, 71–76.

Lowden, A., Anund, A., Kecklund, G., Peters, B., & Åkerstedt, T. (2009). Wakefulness in young and elderly subjects driving at night in a car simulator. *Accident Analysis & Prevention, 41*, 1001–1007.

Marcotte, T., Scott, J., Kamat, R., & Heaton, R. (2010). Neuropsychology and the prediction of everyday functioning. In: Marcotte, T., Grant, I. (Eds.), *Neuropsychology of everyday functioning*. Guilford Press, New York, pp. 5–38.

Marshall, N. S., Barnes, M., Travier, N., Campbell, A. J., Pierce, R. J., & McEvoy, R. D., et al., (2006). Continuous positive airway pressure reduces daytime sleepiness in mild to moderate obstructive sleep apnoea: A meta-analysis. *Thorax, 61*, 430–434.

Marshall, N. S., Neill, A. M., & Campbell, A. J. (2008). Randomised trial of compliance with flexible (C-Flex) and standard continuous positive airway pressure for severe obstructive sleep apnea. *Sleep & Breathing, 12*, 393–396.

Marshall, N. S., Neill, A., Campbell, A., & Sheppard, D. (2005). Randomised controlled crossover trial of humidified continuous positive airway pressure in mild obstructive sleep apnoea. *Thorax, 60*, 427–432.

Matthews, E. & Aloia, M. (2011). Cognitive recovery following positive airway pressure (PAP) in sleep apnea. In G. Kerkhof & H. V. Dongen (Eds.), *Human sleep and cognition, Vol. 2*, Elsevier, submitted.

Mazza, S., Pépin, J., Naëgelé, B., Rauch, E., Deschaux, C., & Ficheux, P., et al., (2006). Driving ability in sleep apnoea patients before and after CPAP treatment: Evaluation on a road safety platform. *The European Respiratory Journal, 28*, 1020–1028.

Mendelson, W. B., Garnett, D., Gillin, J. C., & Weingartner, H. (1984). The experience of insomnia and daytime and nighttime functioning. *Psychiatry Research, 12*, 235–250.

Meurice, J. C., Paquereau, J., Denjean, A., Patte, F., & Series, F. (1998). Influence of correction of flow limitation on continuous positive airway pressure efficiency in sleep apnoea/hypopnoea syndrome. *The European Respiratory Journal, 11*, 1121–1127.

Monasterio, C., Vidal, S., Duran, J., Ferrer, M., Carmona, C., & Barbé, F., et al., (2001). Effectiveness of continuous positive airway pressure in mild sleep apnea-hypopnea syndrome. *American Journal of Respiratory and Critical Care Medicine, 164*, 939–943.

Montgomery-Downs, H. E., Crabtree, V. M., & Gozal, D. (2005). Cognition, sleep and respiration in at-risk children treated for obstructive sleep apnoea. *European Respiratory Journal, 25*, 336–342.

Montplaisir, J., Bédard, M. A., Richer, F., & Rouleau, I. (1992). Neurobehavioral manifestations in obstructive sleep apnea syndrome before and after treatment with continuous positive airway pressure. *Sleep, 15*, S17–S19.

Montserrat, J. M., Ferrer, M., Hernandez, L., Farré, R., Vilagut, G., & Navajas, D., et al., (2001). Effectiveness of CPAP treatment in daytime function in sleep apnea syndrome: A randomized controlled study with an optimized placebo. *American Journal of Respiratory and Critical Care Medicine*, *164*, 608–613.

Morgenthaler, T., Kramer, M., Alessi, C., Friedman, L., Boehlecke, B., & Brown, T., et al., (2006). Practice parameters for the psychological and behavioral treatment of insomnia: An update. An American Academy of Sleep Medicine report. *Sleep*, *29*, 1415–1419.

Morin, C. M., Hauri, P. J., Espie, C. A., Spielman, A. J., Buysse, D. J., & Bootzin, R. R. (1999). Nonpharmacologic treatment of chronic insomnia. An American Academy of Sleep Medicine review. *Sleep*, *22*, 1134–1156.

Muñoz, A., Mayoralas, L. R., Barbé, F., Pericás, J., & Agusti, A. G. (2000). Long-term effects of CPAP on daytime functioning in patients with sleep apnoea syndrome. *The European Respiratory Journal*, *15*, 676–681.

Murphy, P. J., & Campbell, S. S. (1996). Enhanced performance in elderly subjects following bright light treatment of sleep maintenance insomnia. *Journal of Sleep Research*, *5*, 165–172.

Naëgelé, B., Thouvard, V., Pépin, J. L., Lévy, P., Bonnet, C., & Perret, J. E., et al., (1995). Deficits of cognitive executive functions in patients with sleep apnea syndrome. *Sleep*, *18*, 43–52.

Naismith, S., Winter, V., Gotsopoulos, H., Hickie, I., & Cistulli, P. (2004). Neurobehavioral functioning in obstructive sleep apnea: Differential effects of sleep quality, hypoxemia and subjective sleepiness. *Journal of Clinical and Experimental Neuropsychology*, *26*, 43–54.

O'Donoghue, F. J., Briellmann, R. S., Rochford, P. D., Abbott, D. F., Pell, G. S., & Chan, C. H. P., et al., (2005). Cerebral structural changes in severe obstructive sleep apnea. *American Journal of Respiratory and Critical Care Medicine*, *171*, 1185–1190.

Orth, M., Leidag, M., Kotterba, S., Widdig, W., de Zeeuw, J., & Walther, J. W., et al., (2002). Abschätzung des Unfallrisikos bei obstruktivem Schlafapnoe-Syndrom (OSAS) durch Fahrsimulation [Estimation of accident risk in obstructive sleep apnea syndrome (OSAS) by driving simulation]. *Pneumologie*, *56*, 13–18.

Owens, J., Spirito, A., Marcotte, A., McGuinn, M., & Berkelhammer, L. (2000). Neuropsychological and behavioral correlates of obstructive sleep apnea syndrome in children: A preliminary study. *Sleep & Breathing*, *4*, 67–78.

Philip, P. (2005). Sleepiness of occupational drivers. *Industrial Health*, *43*, 30–33.

Philipps, L. (1997). Do "frontal tests" measure executive function? Issues of assessment and evidence from fluency test. In: Rabitt, D. (Ed.), *Methodology of frontal and executive function*. Psychology Press, East Sussex, pp. 7–35.

Pilcher, J. J., & Huffcutt, A. I. (1996). Effects of sleep deprivation on performance: A meta-analysis. *Sleep*, *19*, 318–326.

Poulton, B. C., & Freeman, P. R. (1966). Unwanted asymmetrical transfer effects with balanced experimental designs. *Psychological Bulletin*, *66*, 1–8.

Randerath, W. J., Gerdesmeyer, C., Siller, K., Gil, G., Sanner, B., & Rühle, K. H. (2000). A test for the determination of sustained attention in patients with obstructive sleep apnea syndrome. *Respiration*, *67*, 526–532.

Reynolds, A. C., & Banks, S. (2010). Sleep deprivation, chronic sleep restriction and sleep disruption. Kerkhof, G., Van Dongen, H. (Eds.), *Human sleep and cognition, progress in brain research. Vol. 185*, Elsevier, Amsterdam.

Richards, K., & Sawyer, A. M. (2010). What we don't know about sleep-related breathing disorders in the elderly. *Sleep*, *33*, 423–425.

Rieth, C. A., Cai, D. J., McDevitt, E. A., & Mednick, S. C. (2010). The role of sleep and practice in implicit and explicit motor learning. *Behavioral Brain Research*, *214*(2); 470–474.

Robbins, J., Redline, S., Ervin, A., Walsleben, J. A., Ding, J., & Nieto, F. J. (2005). Associations of sleep-disordered breathing and cerebral changes on MRI. *Journal of Clinical Sleep Medicine*, *1*, 159–165.

Rodway, G. W., Weaver, T. E., Mancini, C., Cater, J., Maislin, G., & Staley, B., et al., (2010). Evaluation of sham-CPAP as a placebo in CPAP intervention studies. *Sleep*, *33*, 260–266.

Roth, T., Rippon, G. A., & Arora, S. (2008). Armodafinil improves wakefulness and long-term episodic memory in nCPAP-adherent patients with excessive sleepiness associated with obstructive sleep apnea. *Sleep & Breathing*, *12*, 53–62.

Roth, T., White, D., Schmidt-Nowara, W., Wesnes, K. A., Niebler, G., & Arora, S., et al., (2006). Effects of armodafinil in the treatment of residual excessive sleepiness associated with obstructive sleep apnea/hypopnea syndrome: A 12-week, multicenter, double-blind, randomized, placebo-controlled study in nCPAP-adherent adults. *Clinical Therapeutics*, *28*, 689–706.

Saletu, B., Oberndorfer, S., Anderer, P., Gruber, G., Divos, H., & Lachner, A., et al., (1999). Efficiency of continuous positive airway pressure versus theophylline therapy in sleep apnea: Comparative sleep laboratory studies on objective and subjective sleep and awakening quality. *Neuropsychobiology*, *39*, 151–159.

Saunamäki, T., Jehkonen, M., Huupponen, E., Polo, O., & Himanen, S. (2009). Visual dysfunction and computational sleep depth changes in obstructive sleep apnea syndrome. *Clinical EEG and Neuroscience*, *40*, 162–167.

Schneider, C., Fulda, S., & Schulz, H. (2004). Daytime variation in performance and tiredness/sleepiness ratings in patients with insomnia, narcolepsy, sleep apnea and normal controls. *Journal of Sleep Research*, *13*, 373–383.

Schulz, K. F., Chalmers, I., Hayes, R. J., & Altman, D. G. (1995). Empirical evidence of bias. Dimensions of methodological quality associated with estimates of treatment effects in controlled trials. *The Journal of the American Medical Association*, *273*, 408–412.

Scott Jr., W. E. (1966). Activation theory and task design. *Organizational Behavior and Human Performance*, *1*, 3–30.

Senn, O., Brack, T., Matthews, F., Russi, E. W., & Bloch, K. E. (2003). Randomized short-term trial of two autoCPAP devices versus fixed continuous positive airway pressure for the treatment of sleep apnea. *American Journal of Respiratory and Critical Care Medicine*, *168*, 1506–1511.

Sforza, E., Roche, F., Thomas-Anterion, C., Kerleroux, J., Beauchet, O., & Celle, S., et al., (2010). Cognitive function and sleep related breathing disorders in a healthy elderly population: The SYNAPSE study. *Sleep*, *33*, 515–521.

Shallice, T. (1990). *From neuropsychology to mental structure.* Cambridge University Press, Cambridge.

Standards of Practice Committee of the American Academy of Sleep Medicine (2005). Practice parameters for clinical use of the multiple sleep latency test and the maintenance of wakefulness test. *Sleep*, *28*, 113–121.

Spira, A. P., Blackwell, T., Stone, K. L., Redline, S., Cauley, J. A., & Ancoli-Israel, S., et al., (2008). Sleep-disordered breathing and cognition in older women. *Journal of the American Geriatrics Society*, *56*, 45–50.

Steinmark, S. W., & Borkovec, T. D. (1974). Active and placebo treatment effects on moderate insomnia under counterdemand and positive demand instructions. *Journal of Abnormal Psychology*, *83*, 157–163.

Stricker, J. L., Brown, G. G., Wetherell, L. A., & Drummond, S. P. (2006). The impact of sleep deprivation and task difficulty on networks of fMRI brain response. *Journal of the International Neuropsychological Society*, *12*, 591–597.

Szentkirályi, A., Madarász, C. Z., & Novák, M. (2009). Sleep disorders: Impact on daytime functioning and quality of life. *Expert Review of Pharmacoeconomics & Outcomes Research*, *9*, 49–64.

Thomas, R. J., Rosen, B. R., Stern, C. E., Weiss, J. W., & Kwong, K. K. (2005). Functional imaging of working memory in obstructive sleep-disordered breathing. *Journal of Applied Physiology*, *98*, 2226–2234.

Tonon, C., Vetrugno, R., Lodi, R., Gallassi, R., Provini, F., & Iotti, S., et al., (2007). Proton magnetic resonance spectroscopy study of brain metabolism in obstructive sleep apnoea syndrome before and after continuous positive airway pressure treatment. *Sleep*, *30*, 305–311.

Trenkwalder, C., Hundemer, H., Lledo, A., Swieca, J., Polo, O., & Wetter, T., et al., (2004). Efficacy of pergolide in treatment of restless legs syndrome: The PEARLS Study. *Neurology*, *62*, 1391–1397.

Turkington, P., Sircar, M., Saralaya, D., & Elliott, M. (2004). Time course of changes in driving simulator performance with and without treatment in patients with sleep apnoea hypopnoea syndrome. *Thorax*, *59*, 56–59.

Van Dongen, H. P. A., Vitellaro, K. M., & Dinges, D. F. (2005). Individual differences in adult human sleep and wakefulness: Leitmotif for a research agenda. *Sleep*, *28*, 479–496.

Varkevisser, M., & Kerkhof, G. A. (2005). Chronic insomnia and performance in a 24-h constant routine study. *Journal of Sleep Research*, *14*, 49–59.

Verster, J. C., Veldhuijzen, D. S., & Volkerts, E. R. (2004). Residual effects of sleep medication on driving ability. *Sleep Medicine Reviews*, *8*, 309–325.

Verstraeten, E. (2007). Neurocognitive effects of obstructive sleep apnea syndrome. *Current Neurology and Neuroscience Reports*, *7*, 161–166.

Verstraeten, E., & Cluydts, R. (2004). Executive control of attention in sleep apnea patients: Theoretical concepts and methodological considerations. *Sleep Medicine Reviews*, *8*, 257–267.

Vignola, A., Lamoureux, C., Bastien, C. H., & Morin, C. M. (2000). Effects of chronic insomnia and use of benzodiazepines on daytime performance in older adults. *The Journals of Gerontology. Series B, Psychological Sciences and Social Sciences*, *55*, P54–P62.

Wilkinson, R. T. (1961). Interaction of lack of sleep with knowledge of results, repeated testing, and individual differences. *Journal of Experimental Psychology*, *63*, 263–271.

Williams, S. C., Marshall, N. S., Kennerson, M., Rogers, N. L., Liu, P. Y., & Grunstein, R. R. (2010). Modafinil effects during acute CPAP withdrawal: A randomized crossover double-blind placebo-controlled trial. *American Journal of Respiratory and Critical Care Medicine*, *181*, 825–831.

Williams, S. C., Rogers, N. L., Marshall, N. S., Leung, S., Starmer, G. A., & Grunstein, R. R. (2008). The effect of modafinil following acute CPAP withdrawal: A preliminary study. *Sleep & Breathing*, *12*, 359–364.

Woolfolk, R., & McNulty, T. (1983). Relaxation treatment for insomnia: A component analysis. *Journal of Consulting and Clinical Psychology*, *51*, 495–503.

Zimmerman, M. E., & Aloia, M. S. (2006). A review of neuroimaging in obstructive sleep apnea. *Journal of Clinical Sleep Medicine*, *2*, 461–471.

Zimmerman, M. E., Arnedt, J. T., Stanchina, M., Millman, R. P., & Aloia, M. S. (2006). Normalization of memory performance and positive airway pressure adherence in memory-impaired patients with obstructive sleep apnea. *Chest*, *130*, 1772–1778.

G. A. Kerkhof and H. P. A. Van Dongen (Eds.)
Progress in Brain Research, Vol. 185
ISSN: 0079-6123

CHAPTER 6

Total sleep deprivation, chronic sleep restriction and sleep disruption

Amy C. Reynolds[†] and Siobhan Banks[†,*]

[†]*Centre for Sleep Research, University of South Australia, Adelaide, SA, Australia*

Abstract: Sleep loss may result from total sleep deprivation (such as a shift worker might experience), chronic sleep restriction (due to work, medical conditions or lifestyle) or sleep disruption (which is common in sleep disorders such as sleep apnea or restless legs syndrome). Total sleep deprivation has been widely researched, and its effects have been well described. Chronic sleep restriction and sleep disruption (also known as sleep fragmentation) have received less experimental attention. Recently, there has been increasing interest in sleep restriction and disruption as it has been recognized that they have a similar impact on cognitive functioning as a period of total sleep deprivation. Sleep loss causes impairments in cognitive performance and simulated driving and induces sleepiness, fatigue and mood changes. This review examines recent research on the effects of sleep deprivation, restriction and disruption on cognition and neurophysiologic functioning in healthy adults, and contrasts the similarities and differences between these three modalities of sleep loss.

Keywords: Total sleep deprivation; chronic sleep restriction; sleep disruption; sleep fragmentation; performance; cognition; neurophysiologic

Common forms of sleep loss are total sleep deprivation, chronic sleep restriction (also sometimes referred to as partial sleep deprivation) and sleep fragmentation or disruption. Total sleep deprivation is the elimination of sleep for a period of time (at least one night) to significantly prolong wakefulness. Sleep restriction is a reduction in sleep time below an individual's usual baseline or the amount of sleep needed on a regular basis to maintain optimal performance. This is probably the

* Corresponding author.
Tel.: (+) 61 88302 2657; Fax: (+) 61 88302 6623.
E-mail: siobhan.banks@unisa.edu.au

DOI:10.1016/B978-0-444-53702-7.00006-3

most frequently experienced form of sleep loss in everyday life (Banks and Dinges, 2007). Sleep disruption is the interruption or fragmentation of sleep, commonly seen in sleep disorders such as sleep apnea where frequent arousals disrupt the normal dynamics of sleep. Sleep disruption is associated with an increase in awakenings and, typically, a reduction of deep sleep, and can contribute to daytime sleepiness (Stepanski, 2002).

This review examines the effects of experimental sleep deprivation, sleep restriction and sleep disruption on normal, healthy, adult populations with a particular focus on neurocognitive consequences.

Basal sleep need

A variety of factors determine the amount of sleep an individual habitually obtains, such as genetic, environmental and societal factors. Sleep needs can be described as habitual sleep duration in the absence of pre-existing sleep debt (Dinges et al., 2005). Given this definition, basal need for sleep appears to be between 7.5 and 8.5 h per day in healthy adult humans. This is based on a study in which any prior sleepiness was removed through many nights of extended sleep that stabilized at a mean of 8.17 h (Wehr et al., 1993). A similar sleep need (8.16 h per night) was found statistically in a study investigating chronic sleep restriction (Van Dongen et al., 2003).

Total sleep deprivation

The first published investigations of the effect of total sleep deprivation on cognition date back to the late 19th century (Patrick and Gilbert, 1896). The early experiments used lengthy periods of sleep deprivation (e.g. 90 h) and found that memory and reaction time were significantly affected. These studies initiated a new area of research and since then many hundreds of more detailed and systematic studies have been conducted. To date, total sleep deprivation is still the most common laboratory-based manipulation of sleep and many individuals regularly experience it as part of shift work (e.g. truck drivers, nurses, anaesthesiologists, airline pilots etc.). Accurately determining the effects of sleep deprivation on cognitive functioning is important for these safety sensitive jobs.

Cognitive effects of total sleep deprivation

The cognitive deficits associated with total sleep deprivation have been well described by many studies (for review, see Durmer and Dinges, 2005). While the majority of cognitive performance measures show decrements with total sleep deprivation, some are considered more sensitive than others. The psychomotor vigilance test (PVT; Dinges and Powell, 1985) is one of the most sensitive cognitive assays to sleep loss. It is an objective measure of vigilant attention and reliably demonstrates changes in reaction time with changes in sleep opportunity. It is considered sensitive enough to demonstrate the effects of even small changes in prior sleep and wakefulness, and it is used in a large number of studies. These studies have continuously shown a deleterious effect of total sleep deprivation on vigilant attention (Doran et al., 2001; Van Dongen et al., 2004). Other cognitive domains aside from attention have also been found to deteriorate with total sleep deprivation. These include constructive thinking (Killgore et al., 2008), spatial working memory (Heuer et al., 2005), cognitive throughput (Van Dongen et al., 2003) and verbal memory (Horne and Reyner, 1999). Total sleep deprivation can result in task perseveration with reduced creative thinking (Harrison and Horne, 1999) and an inability to perceive the likelihood of making errors (Harrison and Horne, 2000).

Cognitive responses become unpredictable with total sleep deprivation and this variability is thought to reflect state instability (Doran et al., 2001). State instability refers to moment-to-moment shifts in the relationship between wake maintenance and sleep initiation (Doran et al., 2001). Individuals begin to show state instability when the biological mechanisms responsible for initiating sleep start to interfere with cognitive performance. This makes performance more variable and increasingly reliant on deliberate effort to stay awake. The consequences of state instability can be seen with increasing errors of omission (when subjects fail to respond to a stimulus), and errors of commission (when subjects respond when not required) (Doran et al., 2001; Durmer and Dinges, 2005).

Advances in technology have recently enabled researchers to observe brain changes associated with sleep deprivation. With functional magnetic resonance imaging (fMRI) the effect of sleep deprivation on specific brain regions responsible for certain cognitive task can be investigated (Drummond and Brown, 2001). Studies have shown that neural activity in a number of different brain regions is altered following a period of total sleep deprivation. When wakefulness is extended beyond 35 h (i.e. one night of total sleep deprivation), activation during working memory tasks shifts from temporal to parietal regions (Drummond and Brown, 2001). This shift has been interpreted as a compensatory mechanism to protect working memory. Other studies have observed activation decreases in the frontal regions of the brain following total sleep deprivation, which have been associated with reduced working memory, planning and inhibition (Muzur et al., 2002). There is considerable support for the hypothesis that the frontal region is important for high-level cognitive functioning (Foucher et al., 2004) and that changes in activation in this region are associated with reduced performance.

Impact of total sleep deprivation on the electroencephalogram

Electroencephalography (EEG) measures the electrical activity of the brain using electrodes placed on the scalp. It has often been used to investigate the effects of sleep deprivation on neurocognitive functioning. EEG patterns can be described by amplitude and frequency and traditionally, EEG frequencies are divided into several frequency bands: delta (1–4 Hz), theta (4–8 Hz), alpha (8–12 Hz), beta (12–30 Hz) and gamma (30–90 Hz). During sleep, particular changes occur within these bands in relationship to the various sleep stages (Rechtschaffen and Kales, 1968). For instance, slow-wave sleep (sleep stages 3 and 4) is characterized by strong delta activity, whereas rapid eye movement (REM) sleep is signified by theta activity. During recovery sleep periods following total sleep deprivation, the amount of slow-wave sleep in the sleep EEG is enhanced above baseline levels (Banks et al., 2010; Borbely et al., 1981). During extended periods without sleep, an increase in theta activity is generally seen in the waking EEG (Finelli et al., 2000), which may be evidence that that sleep is intruding upon wakefulness.

Event-related potentials (ERPs), which are EEG patterns aligned to a specific stimulus (usually the onset of a tone or visual cue), allow for analysis of cortical processing related to a specific brain activity. Certain components of ERPs have been found to reflect specific forms of information processing, related to sensory, motor and/or cognitive functions (Ford and Pfefferbaum, 1991). In total sleep deprivation research, two ERP components, N100 (sometimes called N1) and P300 (sometimes called P3) have been the main focus of investigation.

N1 represents a negative polarity deflection in the EEG waveform about 100 ms after stimulus presentation. It has been found to be associated with the processing of auditory and visual stimuli in the primary sensory areas (Rennie et al., 2002). N1 is thought to be important for attentional processing because patients with frontal lesions exhibit a reduction in N1 amplitude as well as a reduction in attentional capacities (Knight et al., 1995). A reduction in N1 amplitude can also be seen during total sleep deprivation for auditory responses (Boonstra et al., 2005), and visual- (Corsi-Cabrera et al., 1999) and motor-evoked potentials (Boonstra et al., 2005).

P3 appears as a positive deflection of the electroencephalograph voltage at the frontal scalp around 300 ms post-stimulus. P3 is associated with frontal lobe functioning and can be elicited by presenting the subject with a visual or auditory stimulus that is either unexpected or highly relevant for the task at hand (Pritchard, 1981). Following sleep deprivation, the onset of P3 is delayed and its amplitude reduced (Morris et al., 1992). It seems that the amplitude reductions of N1 and P3 after sleep deprivation are related to changes in attention and thus to changes in sensory processing (Lee et al., 2003).

Effect of total sleep deprivation on objective sleepiness

Sleep propensity, or the drive for sleep, is increased by total sleep deprivation. An increased sleep propensity is associated with a reduction in the time taken to fall asleep (i.e. sleep latency), which can be objectively recorded and is widely used as a measure of sleepiness in clinical settings. The multiple sleep latency test (MSLT; Carskadon and Dement, 1982) and the maintenance of wakefulness test (MWT; Mitler et al., 1982) are used to physiologically evaluate sleep propensity by measuring sleep latency. Brain activity is measured using EEG during both tests to determine the point at which subjects fall asleep.

During the MSLT, subjects are requested to lie down and try to fall asleep for a period of about 20 min. This is repeated several times a day. The MWT differs from the MSLT in that subjects are instructed to remain seated in an upright position and attempt to stay awake. The duration of each session of the MWT is usually set to 40 min, although variations exist. Both of these tests are sensitive to sleep deprivation, where time taken to fall asleep is inversely related to duration of time awake (Banks and Dinges, 2005; Carskadon and Dement, 1982).

Sleep propensity is also reflected in physiological intrusions upon wakefulness such as sleep attacks (i.e. involuntary naps), slow eyelid closures, slow rolling eye movements and intrusive daydreaming while engaged in cognitive work (Dinges and Kribbs, 1991; Kleitman, 1963).

Effect of total sleep deprivation on subjective sleepiness

A number of subjective measures are affected by a period of total sleep deprivation, including fatigue, sleepiness and mood. Early studies reported increased ‘desire to go to sleep’ and the need for subjects to ‘close their eyes’ during sleep deprivation (Patrick and Gilbert, 1896). Indeed, virtually all total sleep deprivation studies have observed alterations in subjective feelings of sleepiness and/or fatigue (see Durmer and Dinges, 2005, for a comprehensive review). Generally, self reported mood is also affected by sleep deprivation. In the majority of sleep deprivation studies, there is an increase in negative mood states, with reports of fatigue and confusion as well as reduced energy and enthusiasm (Pilcher and Huffcutt, 1996). While it is probable that there are also threshold changes in anxiety and frustration with total sleep deprivation, investigating these aspects of mood in laboratory settings can be difficult as researchers actively work to keep subjects happy and motivated.

Age effects on cognitive performance during total sleep deprivation

Several studies have suggested that older individuals perform better during total sleep deprivation than their younger counterparts (Duffy et al., 2009). Older individuals have been found to have faster reaction times and feel less sleepy, even after controlling for baseline differences prior to sleep loss. Additionally, their performance is more consistent overall (Duffy et al., 2009). Reduced habitual sleep duration in older adults has been suggested as the reason for this difference. This implies that when older individuals experience total sleep deprivation, the impact is not as great on them as it is for younger adults (Duffy et al., 2009). An alternative hypothesis is that the neurobiological mechanisms responsible for sleep initiation are reduced in older adults – specifically the region of the hypothalamus known as the ventrolateral preoptic nucleus, involved in enabling this transition, is impaired with age. This possibly would be associated with a more stable wake state during total sleep deprivation, and thus results in less cognitive deficits (Fuller et al., 2006).

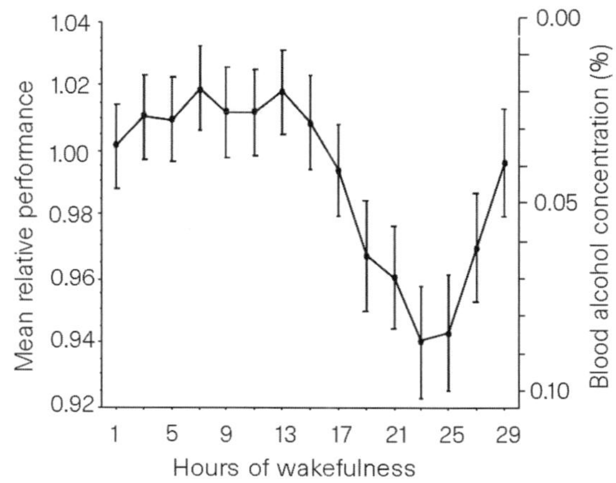

Fig. 1. Performance in a sustained wakefulness condition expressed as mean performance relative to baseline and the percentage blood alcohol concentration equivalent. Error bars ± s.e.m. are shown. After 17 h of sustained wakefulness (03:00) cognitive psychomotor performance decreased to a level equivalent to the performance impairment observed at a blood alcohol concentration of 0.05%. After 24 h of sustained wakefulness (08:00) cognitive psychomotor performance decreased to a level equivalent to the performance deficit observed at a blood alcohol concentration of roughly 0.10%. Reproduced with permission from Dawson and Reid (1997).

Total sleep deprivation, accidents and alcohol

The implications of sleep loss outside the laboratory are far-reaching. One real-world example is the demonstrated link between total sleep deprivation and accidents, particularly in regards to traffic and work place incidents. An increased number of accidents occur with extended wakefulness and this is of particular concern in safety sensitive industries such as medicine (Landrigan et al., 2004) and aviation (Caldwell et al., 2009).

A number of studies have compared a night of total sleep deprivation with effects of alcohol intoxication and found that impaired performance is on a par across both conditions (Dawson and Reid, 1997; Fairclough and Graham, 1999). In a seminal study by Dawson and Reid (1997), it was found that after 17 h of wakefulness, performance on a cognitive task was equivalent to a blood alcohol concentration of 0.05% (see Fig. 1). They also found that performance at 8 a.m. after staying awake all night was equivalent to performance with blood alcohol content 0.10%. Comparisons such as these are important to help the wider community appreciate the impact even a modest amount of sleep loss can have on safety.

Several studies have also investigated the separate and combined effects of alcohol and total sleep deprivation on driving performance. These have generally found that steering deviation is more affected when alcohol and sleep deprivation are combined than during conditions of alcohol or total sleep deprivation alone, even if the amounts of alcohol consumed are low (Arnedt et al., 2001; Fairclough and Graham, 1999; Horne et al., 2003). This suggests that the combined effects of moderate total sleep deprivation and legal amounts of alcohol consumption can significantly increase risk of driving accidents.

Sleep restriction

Sleep restriction, also known as partial sleep deprivation, occurs when sleep is reduced below an individual's usual baseline or the amount of sleep needed on a regular basis to maintain optimal performance. It is a common phenomenon, as sleep time is affected by a multitude of factors including social responsibilities, work requirements and medical illnesses. A number of different approaches to understanding the mechanisms behind sleep restriction and its effects on cognitive functioning have been explored. These include restricted time in bed in a laboratory setting (Hartley, 1974), and specifically targeting different sleep stages and restricting sleep accordingly (Ferrara et al., 1999).

The past 15 years have seen an increased focus on ensuring methodological integrity in sleep restriction protocols to determine whether these insignificant findings were accurate. Where many older studies were conducted outside of the laboratory, more recent studies have been run in tightly controlled laboratory environments (e.g. Banks et al., 2010; Van Dongen et al., 2003).

Impact of chronic sleep restriction on hippocampus and implications for cognitive performance

The hippocampal region of the brain is important for cognitive function. Damage to the hippocampus makes forming new memories difficult and often also affects memories formed before the damage. It was once thought that damage to the hippocampus was permanent but recent research in rats has established that new neurons are regularly generated in this area of the adult brain. While the exact function of these new cells is unknown it is thought that they are involved in learning and memory processes and the regulation of mood. Several studies have investigated the effect of sleep loss on the development of these neurons (for a review, see Meerlo et al., 2009). Disruption of sleep for one night appears to have little effect on the rate of cell production (van der Borght et al., 2006) but chronic sleep restriction or disruption of sleep has cumulative effects that lead to a reduction of neuronal development (Roman et al., 2005). Additionally, sleep restriction interferes with the normal increase in neurogenesis that occurs with hippocampus-dependent learning tasks (e.g. spatial learning) (Hairston et al., 2005). It is hypothesized that decreases in cell production are related to the decreases in REM sleep commonly seen in total sleep deprivation and sleep restriction (Guzman-Marin et al., 2005). The mechanisms by which sleep loss affects aspects of neurogenesis are largely unknown, but it has been proposed that adverse effects of sleep loss may be mediated by stress and glucocorticoids (Mirescu et al., 2006). While most of the current research on adult neurogenesis has been conducted in rats, this new data raises the possibility that chronically restricted or disturbed sleep associated with lifestyle, stress or diseases may affect the production of new neurons in the adult human brain as well. Magnetic resonance imaging studies in humans have confirmed the role of sleep in hippocampal function and the formation of memory (Peigneux et al., 2004) but more research is needed to examine if sleep impacts neurogenesis in humans and what the direct implications may be for cognitive function.

Cognitive effects of sleep restriction

Controlled experiments on healthy adults have found clear evidence that cognitive performance functions such as attention, working memory and cognitive throughput deteriorate systematically across days when sleep duration is chronically restricted (Banks et al., 2010; Belenky et al., 2003; Van Dongen et al., 2003). Subjects experiencing less than 7 h of sleep a night for five or more consecutive nights showed cumulative effects of sleep restriction on their daytime performance as measured by the psychomotor vigilance task (Banks et al., 2010; Belenky et al., 2003; Van Dongen et al., 2003). Specifically, decreased mean response speed (Belenky et al., 2003) and increased cognitive lapses (Banks et al., 2010; Van Dongen et al., 2003) were evident. The cumulative effect of reducing sleep time on daytime performance in the study by Van Dongen et al. (2003) is demonstrated in Fig. 2 panel A.

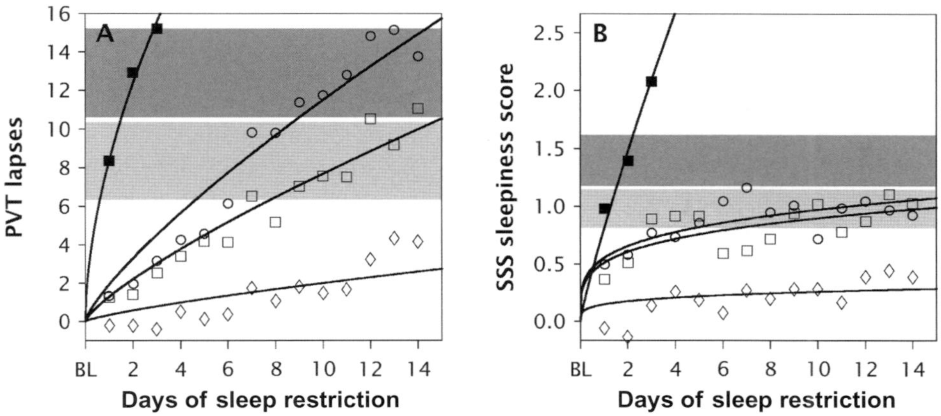

Fig. 2. Performance and subjective sleepiness responses to varying doses of daily sleep. Each panel displays group averages for subjects in either 8 h (◇), 6 h (□) or 4 h (○) chronic sleep restriction conditions across 14 days, and in a total sleep deprivation condition (■) across 3 days. Subjects were tested every 2 h each day; data points represent the daily average (07:30–23:30) expressed relative to baseline (BL). Panel A shows psychomotor vigilance task (PVT) performance lapses (reaction times ≥500 ms) and panel B shows Stanford Sleepiness Scale (SSS) self-ratings. Upward corresponds to worse performance on the PVT and greater sleepiness on the SSS. The mean ± s.e.m. ranges of performance and sleepiness for 1 and 2 days of total sleep deprivation are shown as light and dark grey bands, respectively, allowing comparison of the total sleep deprivation condition and the chronic sleep restriction conditions. It is clear that subjective ratings of sleepiness (Panel B) do not track actual PVT performance (Panel A). This suggests that once sleep restriction is chronic, subjects cannot introspect with regard to their actual sleepiness levels. Reproduced with permission from Van Dongen et al. (2003).

In another, classic study, Carskadon and Dement (1981) restricted sleep to 5 h per night for seven consecutive nights. They found MSLT scores were significantly reduced after the second restriction night and continued a declining trend from baseline values of 17 min to about 7 min after the last night of sleep reduction. These studies suggest that when the sleep period is regularly restricted to approximately 7 h or less, the healthy adults develop sleepiness and cognitive impairments that accumulate across days.

Impairment as a result of sleep restriction is not limited to findings on laboratory performance tasks. It has also been found that as little as one night of sleep restriction to 5 h can significantly impair simulated driving performance. Participants in a study by Banks et al. (2004) showed increased crashes following this short period of restricted sleep. This effect is not isolated to short-term sleep restriction, as these results are also seen in laboratory studies of chronic sleep restriction regardless of the daytime or nighttime nature of the sleep opportunity (Dorrian et al., 2003).

The cause of altered cognitive functioning when sleep is restricted is not well defined. However, it has been postulated that the inhibitory neuromodulator adenosine and its dynamically regulated receptor may be responsible (Van Dongen et al., 2010). Adenosine is a by-product of brain metabolism and it is implicated in sleep promotion and suppression of arousal with increasing daytime wakefulness. The density of the adenosine receptor appears to be increased following sleep loss (Elmenhorst et al., 2007), possibly resulting in heightened sensitivity to further sleep loss. This mechanism could be responsible for the cumulative decreases in cognitive performance observed in sleep-restricted individuals (Porkka-Heiskanen et al., 1997) by progressively increasing sleepiness across days of sleep restriction.

Subjective sleepiness, mood and sleep restriction

When sleep is restricted to less than 6 h per night for a number of days, individuals tend to report only moderate sleepiness even though their cognitive function is considerably impaired (Van Dongen et al., 2003). Therefore, while subjects show increasing deficits in performance, they seem less able to accurately report their sleepiness (see Fig. 2). Sleep restriction also affects mood (Dinges et al., 1997) and sociability (Haack and Mullington, 2005) and has been found to exacerbate psychosomatic symptoms including feelings of muscular pain, nausea, headache and generalized body pain (Haack and Mullington, 2005). As such, sleep restriction may degrade long-term well being.

Sleep disruption

Sleep disruption is the least researched form of sleep loss. However, a number of studies have shown that disrupted sleep has significant consequences for cognitive functioning (for review, see Bonnet and Arand, 2003). The effects of sleep disruption are particularly pertinent for populations who experience fragmented sleep opportunities as a result of occupational demands, environmental disturbance or certain medical conditions. Further research in this area is particularly important, as studies have shown that if significantly disturbed, even a normal duration of sleep can result in reduced alertness and impaired cognition.

Disrupting sleep by changing its architecture

By their very nature, sleep disruption or fragmentation studies change the structure and duration of sleep. Exactly how sleep is disrupted is methodologically important, as various techniques may differentially impact cognitive performance the next day (Bonnet, 1985). In a number of studies, a specific sleep stage was targeted for experimental fragmentation (e.g. slow-wave sleep, or REM sleep). In other experimental manipulations, sleep was fragmented to mimic a sleep disorder or disruptive environmental situation (Basner et al., 2006; Martin et al., 1996). In such studies, subjects may be awakened with tones in order to produce the fragmentation. While this produces a standardized event leading to easily recognized breaks in sleep continuity, it typically causes more changes in sleep architecture as compared to a transient EEG arousals and tends to result in greater cognitive deterioration (Magee et al., 1987). Many forced awakenings can also lead to an accumulation of stage 1 sleep and wakefulness (Levine et al., 1987), altering not only the sleep architecture but also total sleep time (Philip et al., 1994).

Sleepiness, cognition and mood following sleep disruption

Sleep disruption shortens subsequent sleep latency (as measured by the MSLT) (Roehrs et al., 1994) in a manner that is proportional to the frequency of sleep fragmentation (see Fig. 3, Bonnet and Arand, 2003). It appears that a reduction of total time is not needed to increase objective sleepiness as measured by sleep latency (Wesensten et al., 1999).

With regard to cognitive functioning, most of the sleep disruption literature has focused on the cognitive domain of vigilant attention (as measured by the previously described PVT) and found that it is deleteriously affected by slow-wave sleep fragmentation (Bonnet and Arand, 2003). Other types of cognitive performance affected by sleep disruption include working memory and cognitive speed. While PVT performance is impaired following a night of sleep disruption, older individuals perform better than younger individuals (Bonnet, 1989a), suggesting that they are more tolerant to its effects, perhaps for the reasons mentioned above in the section on total sleep deprivation and age.

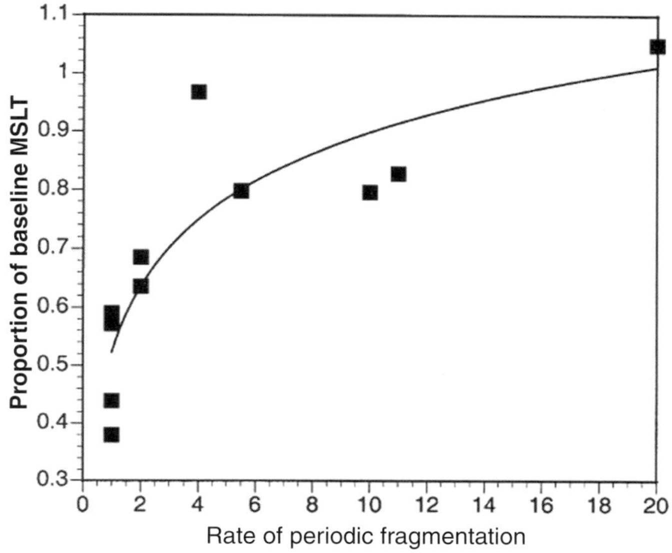

Fig. 3. MSLT sleep latency after sleep fragmentation expressed as a proportion of baseline MSLT sleep latency as observed in several sleep fragmentation studies, plotted as a function of rate of sleep fragmentation during the night. Objectively defined sleepiness increases as the rate of fragmentation is increased, where rate of fragmentation is defined as the interval, in minutes, between the onset of sleep and the sleep disturbance. Data shown are from Bonnet (1986a), Stepanski et al. (1987), Bonnet (1989b) and Roehrs et al. (1994). Reproduced with permission from Bonnet and Arand (2003).

In a study of anaesthetists (Murray and Dodds, 2003), sleep disruption due to on-call work was found to have a significant effect on steering error during a simulated driving task. Another study of medical officers found that mood was not affected by sleep disruption (Deary and Tait, 1987), but subsequent more carefully controlled studies have found that subjective measures of mood and sleepiness are negatively impacted after a night of sleep fragmentation (Martin et al., 1996).

Some people experience sleep disruption because they live close to a busy highway or an airport. Nocturnal noise, particularly aircraft landings and take-offs, fragments sleep and interferes with the duration of specific sleep stages, such as deep sleep (Basner et al., 2006). Studies have shown that attention and memory are both affected by nocturnal aircraft noise (Elmenhorst et al., 2010), but exactly which changes in sleep structure account for these daytime performance impairments remains unclear and needs further examination.

A comparison between sleep deprivation, restriction and disruption

Total sleep deprivation, sleep restriction and sleep disruption all adversely affect cognitive functioning. While sleep disruption has received less systematic investigation than total sleep deprivation and sleep restriction, it has been found to result in a reduction in cognitive functioning on par with total sleep deprivation (Bonnet and Arand, 2003; Wesensten et al., 1999). Similarly, cognitive deficits can accumulate over multiple days of sleep restriction to levels comparable to one or two nights of total sleep deprivation.

Comparison of sleep restriction and total sleep deprivation

The cognitive effects of sleep restriction and total sleep deprivation have been directly compared in several studies. In one such study by Van Dongen et al. (2003), performance decrements that had accumulated over 14 nights of sleep restriction at 4 h sleep per night were found to be similar to 2 nights of total sleep deprivation. One of the key differences, however, between total sleep deprivation and sleep restriction was in self-reported sleepiness and mood (see Fig. 2). While studies of total sleep deprivation have found increased self-reported fatigue and sleepiness in parallel with impaired cognitive performance, individuals experiencing chronic sleep restriction lack the ability to accurately introspect their level of impairment. Instead, ratings of sleepiness and mood tend to plateau after several days while cognitive performance continues to deteriorate. So even though sleep restriction, on a chronic basis, produces similar cognitive deficits to total sleep deprivation, the introspective process is different between the two types of sleep loss. This has potential implications for risk taking and safety (Van Dongen and Hursh, 2010), as individuals may be more inclined to drive, for example while significantly impaired.

Comparison between sleep disruption and sleep deprivation

The effects of sleep disruption are essentially indistinguishable from the effects of total sleep deprivation when the disruption is severe, resulting in comparable alertness and performance deficits. For example, Bonnet (1986b) found that next day MSLT mean sleep latency results were not significantly different between a group whose sleep had been fragmented every minute and a group totally deprived of sleep for 64 h. Levine et al. (1987) also directly compared the effects of sleep disruption and total sleep deprivation on objective sleepiness (MSLT) and found that they produced similar results, which demonstrates that the continuity as well as the overall quantity of sleep is important for performance. Healthy older participants have been found to be less cognitively impaired (when compared to younger individuals) during both total sleep deprivation (Duffy et al., 2009) and sleep restriction studies (Stenuit and Kerkhofs, 2005), suggesting that the mediating effect of age on cognitive performance (discussed above) is not altered by the type of sleep loss sustained.

Decrements in cognitive performance during total sleep deprivation and sleep disruption have both been compared to performance after alcohol consumption. Studies have found that cognitive function (driving performance, vigilance and response speed) after 21 h of total sleep deprivation (Williamson and Feyer, 2000) or a night of sleep disruption (Powell et al., 1999) is comparable to performing with a blood alcohol level of 0.08%. This illustrates that both types of sleep loss are equally potent.

Conclusion

Limiting or disrupting sleep opportunities in normal, healthy subjects has significant negative effects on cognitive performance, sleepiness and neurophysiologic functioning. These findings are highly relevant in modern society, with sleep loss increasingly common in the general population. The ramifications of reduced or disrupted sleep opportunities may extend beyond cognitive effects into general safety, health and well being.

Abbreviations

EEG	electroencephalography
ERPs	event-related potentials
N1	negative polarity ERP with a peak of 100 ms
P3	positive polarity ERP with a peak of 300 ms

PVT psychomotor vigilance test
fMRI functional magnetic resonance imaging
MSLT multiple sleep latency test
MWT maintenance of wakefulness test
REM rapid eye movement

Acknowledgements

Siobhan Banks is supported by a University of South Australia Research Fellowship for Women in Science. Amy Reynolds is supported by a University of South Australia Postgraduate Award.

References

Arnedt, J. T., Wilde, G. J., Munt, P. W., & MacLean, A. W. (2001). How do prolonged wakefulness and alcohol compare in the decrements they produce on a simulated driving task? *Accident Analysis and Prevention*, *33*, 337–344.

Banks, S., & Dinges, D. F. (2005). Is the maintenance of wakefulness test sensitive to varying amounts of recovery sleep after chronic sleep restriction? *Sleep*, *28*, A136.

Banks, S., & Dinges, D. F. (2007). Behavioral and physiological consequences of sleep restriction. *Journal of Clinical Sleep Medicine*, *3*, 519–528.

Banks, S., Catcheside, P., Lack, L., Grunstein, R. R., & McEvoy, R. D. (2004). Low levels of alcohol impair driving simulator performance and reduce perception of crash risk in partially sleep deprived subjects. *Sleep*, *27*, 1063–1067.

Banks, S., Van Dongen, H. P. A., Maislin, G., & Dinges, D. F. (2010). Neurobehavioral dynamics following chronic sleep restriction: Dose-response effects of one night for recovery. *Sleep*, *33*, 1013–1026.

Basner, M., Samel, A., & Isermann, U. (2006). Aircraft noise effects on sleep: Application of the results of a large polysomnographic field study. *Journal of the Acoustical Society of America*, *119*, 2772–2784.

Belenky, G., Wesensten, N. J., Thorne, D. R., Thomas, M. L., Sing, H. C., & Redmond, D. P., et al., (2003). Patterns of performance degradation and restoration during sleep restriction and subsequent recovery: A sleep dose-response study. *Journal of Sleep Research*, *12*, 1–12.

Bonnet, M. H. (1985). Effect of sleep disruption on sleep, performance, and mood. *Sleep*, *8*, 11–19.

Bonnet, M. H. (1986a). Performance and sleepiness as a function of frequency and placement of sleep disruption. *Psychophysiology*, *23*, 263–271.

Bonnet, M. H. (1986b). Performance and sleepiness following moderate sleep disruption and slow wave sleep deprivation. *Physiology & Behavior*, *37*, 915–918.

Bonnet, M. H. (1989a). The effect of sleep fragmentation on sleep and performance in younger and older subjects. *Neurobiology of Aging*, *10*, 21–25.

Bonnet, M. H. (1989b). Infrequent periodic sleep disruption: Effects on sleep, performance and mood. *Physiology & Behavior*, *45*, 1049–1055.

Bonnet, M. H., & Arand, D. L. (2003). Clinical effects of sleep fragmentation versus sleep deprivation. *Sleep Medicine Reviews*, *7*, 297–310.

Boonstra, T. W., Daffertshofer, A., & Beek, P. J. (2005). Effects of sleep deprivation on event-related fields and alpha activity during rhythmic force production. *Neuroscience Letters*, *388*, 27–32.

Borbely, A. A., Baumann, F., Brandeis, D., Strauch, I., & Lehmann, D. (1981). Sleep deprivation: Effect on sleep stages and EEG power density in man. *Electroencephalography and Clinical Neurophysiology*, *51*, 483–495.

Caldwell, J. A., Mallis, M. M., Caldwell, J. L., Paul, M. A., Miller, J. C., & Neri, D. F. (2009). Fatigue countermeasures in aviation. *Aviation, Space, and Environmental Medicine*, *80*, 29–59.

Carskadon, M. A., & Dement, W. C. (1981). Cumulative effects of sleep restriction on daytime sleepiness. *Psychophysiology*, *18*, 107–113.

Carskadon, M. A., & Dement, W. C. (1982). The multiple sleep latency test: What does it measure? *Sleep*, *5*(Suppl 2); S67–S72.

Corsi-Cabrera, M., Arce, C., Del Rio-Portilla, I. Y., Perez-Garci, E., & Guevara, M. A. (1999). Amplitude reduction in visual event-related potentials as a function of sleep deprivation. *Sleep*, *22*, 181–189.

Dawson, D., & Reid, K. (1997). Fatigue, alcohol and performance impairment. *Nature*, *388*, 235.

Deary, I. J., & Tait, R. (1987). Effects of sleep disruption on cognitive performance and mood in medical house officers. *British Medical Journal (Clinical Research Edition)*, *295*, 1513–1516.

Dinges, D. F., & Kribbs, N. B. (1991). Performing while sleepy: Effects of experimentally induced sleepiness. In: Monk, T. H. (Ed.), *Sleep, sleepiness and performance*. Wiley, Winchester, England, pp. 97–128.

Dinges, D. F., & Powell, J. W. (1985). Microcomputer analyses of performance on a portable, simple visual RT task during sustained operations. *Behavior Research Methods, Instruments, & Computers*, *17*, 3.

Dinges, D. F., Pack, F., Williams, K., Gillen, K. A., Powell, J. W., & Ott, G. E., et al., (1997). Cumulative sleepiness, mood disturbance, and psychomotor vigilance performance decrements during a week of sleep restricted to 4–5 h per night. *Sleep*, *20*, 267–277.

Dinges, D. F., Rogers, N., & Baynard, M. (2005). Chronic sleep deprivation. In: Kryger, M. H., Roth, T., Dement, W. C.

(Eds.), *Principles and practices of sleep medicine*. Elsevier Saunders, Philadelphia, PA.

Doran, S. M., Van Dongen, H. P., & Dinges, D. F. (2001). Sustained attention performance during sleep deprivation: Evidence of state instability. *Archives Italiennes de Biologie (Pisa)*, *139*, 253–267.

Dorrian, J., Dinges, D. F., Rider, R. L., Price, N. J., & Rogers, N. (2003). Simulated driving performance during chronic partial sleep deprivation. *Sleep*, *26*, A182–A183.

Drummond, S. P., & Brown, G. G. (2001). The effects of total sleep deprivation on cerebral responses to cognitive performance. *Neuropsychopharmacology*, *25*, S68–S73.

Duffy, J. F., Willson, H. J., Wang, W., & Czeisler, C. A. (2009). Healthy older adults better tolerate sleep deprivation than young adults. *Journal of the American Geriatrics Society*, *57*, 1245–1251.

Durmer, J. S., & Dinges, D. F. (2005). Neurocognitive consequences of sleep deprivation. *Seminars in Neurology*, *25*, 117–129.

Elmenhorst, E. M., Elmenhorst, D., Wenzel, J., Quehl, J., Mueller, U., & Maass, H., et al., (2010). Effects of nocturnal aircraft noise on cognitive performance in the following morning: Dose-response relationships in laboratory and field. *International Archives of Occupational and Environmental Health*, *83*, 743–751.

Elmenhorst, D., Meyer, P. T., Winz, O. H., Matusch, A., Ermert, J., & Coenen, H. H., et al., (2007). Sleep deprivation increases A1 adenosine receptor binding in the human brain: A positron emission tomography study. *The Journal of Neuroscience*, *27*(9); 2410–2415.

Fairclough, S. H., & Graham, R. (1999). Impairment of driving performance caused by sleep deprivation or alcohol: A comparative study. *Human Factors*, *41*, 118–128.

Ferrara, M., De Gennaro, L., & Bertini, M. (1999). The effects of slow-wave sleep (SWS) deprivation and time of night on behavioral performance upon awakening. *Physiology & Behavior*, *68*, 55–61.

Finelli, L. A., Baumann, H., Borbely, A. A., & Achermann, P. (2000). Dual electroencephalogram markers of human sleep homeostasis: Correlation between theta activity in waking and slow-wave activity in sleep. *Neuroscience*, *101*, 523–529.

Ford, J. M., & Pfefferbaum, A. (1991). Event-related potentials and eyeblink responses in automatic and controlled processing: Effects of age. *Electroencephalography and Clinical Neurophysiology*, *78*, 361–377.

Foucher, J. R., Otzenberger, H., & Gounot, D. (2004). Where arousal meets attention: A simultaneous fMRI and EEG recording study. *Neuroimage*, *22*, 688–697.

Fuller, P. M., Gooley, J. J., & Saper, C. B. (2006). Neurobiology of the sleep-wake cycle: Sleep architecture, circadian regulation, and regulatory feedback. *Journal of Biological Rhythms*, *21*, 482–493.

Guzman-Marin, R., Suntsova, N., Methippara, M., Greiffenstein, R., Szymusiak, R., & McGinty, D. (2005). Sleep deprivation suppresses neurogenesis in the adult hippocampus of rats. *European Journal of Neuroscience*, *22*, 2111–2116.

Haack, M., & Mullington, J. M. (2005). Sustained sleep restriction reduces emotional and physical well-being. *Pain*, *119*, 56–64.

Hairston, I. S., Little, M. T., Scanlon, M. D., Barakat, M. T., Palmer, T. D., & Sapolsky, R. M., et al., (2005). Sleep restriction suppresses neurogenesis induced by hippocampus-dependent learning. *Journal of Neurophysiology*, *94*, 4224–4233.

Harrison, Y., & Horne, J. A. (1999). One night of sleep loss impairs innovative thinking and flexible decision making. *Organizational Behavior and Human Decision Processes*, *78*, 128–145.

Harrison, Y., & Horne, J. A. (2000). The impact of sleep deprivation on decision making: A review. *Journal of Experimental Psychology Applied*, *6*, 236–249.

Hartley, L. R. (1974). A comparison of continuous and distributed reduced sleep schedules. *Quarterly Journal of Experimental Psychology*, *26*, 8–14.

Heuer, H., Kohlisch, O., & Klein, W. (2005). The effects of total sleep deprivation on the generation of random sequences of key-presses, numbers and nouns. *Quarterly Journal of Experimental Psychology A*, *58*, 275–307.

Horne, J., & Reyner, L. (1999). Vehicle accidents related to sleep: A review. *Occupational and Environmental Medicine*, *56*, 289–294.

Horne, J. A., Reyner, L. A., & Barrett, P. R. (2003). Driving impairment due to sleepiness is exacerbated by low alcohol intake. *Occupational and Environmental Medicine*, *60*, 689–692.

Killgore, W. D., Kahn-Greene, E. T., Lipizzi, E. L., Newman, R. A., Kamimori, G. H., & Balkin, T. J. (2008). Sleep deprivation reduces perceived emotional intelligence and constructive thinking skills. *Sleep Medicine*, *9*, 517–526.

Kleitman, N. (1963). *Sleep and wakefulness*. University of Chicago Press, Chicago, IL.

Knight, R. T., Grabowecky, M. F., & Scabini, D. (1995). Role of human prefrontal cortex in attention control. *Advanced Neurology*, *66*, 21–34 discussion 34-26.

Landrigan, C. P., Rothschild, J. M., Cronin, J. W., Kaushal, R., Burdick, E., & Katz, J. T., et al., (2004). Effect of reducing interns' work hours on serious medical errors in intensive care units. *The New England Journal of Medicine*, *351*, 1838–1848.

Lee, H. J., Kim, L., & Suh, K. Y. (2003). Cognitive deterioration and changes of P300 during total sleep deprivation. *Psychiatry and Clinical Neurosciences*, *57*, 490–496.

Levine, B., Roehrs, T., Stepanski, E., Zorick, F., & Roth, T. (1987). Fragmenting sleep diminishes its recuperative value. *Sleep*, *10*, 590–599.

Magee, J., Harsh, J., & Badia, P. (1987). Effects of experimentally-induced sleep fragmentation on sleep and sleepiness. *Psychophysiology*, *24*, 528–534.

Martin, S. E., Engleman, H. M., Deary, I. J., & Douglas, N. J. (1996). The effect of sleep fragmentation on daytime function. *American Journal of Respiratory and Critical Care Medicine*, *153*, 1328–1332.

Meerlo, P., Mistlberger, R. E., Jacobs, B. L., Heller, H. C., & McGinty, D. (2009). New neurons in the adult brain: The role of sleep and consequences of sleep loss. *Sleep Medicine Reviews*, *13*, 187–194.

Mirescu, C., Peters, J. D., Noiman, L., & Gould, E. (2006). Sleep deprivation inhibits adult neurogenesis in the hippocampus by elevating glucocorticoids. *Proceedings of the National Academy of Sciences of the United States of America*, *103*, 19170–19175.

Mitler, M. M., Gujavarty, K. S., & Browman, C. P. (1982). Maintenance of wakefulness test: A polysomnographic technique for evaluation treatment efficacy in patients with excessive somnolence. *Electroencephalography and Clinical Neurophysiology*, *53*, 658–661.

Morris, A. M., So, Y., Lee, K. A., Lash, A. A., & Becker, C. E. (1992). The P300 event-related potential. The effects of sleep deprivation. *Journal of Occupational Medicine*, *34*, 1143–1152.

Muecke, S. (2005). Effects of rotating night shifts: Literature review. *Journal of Advanced Nursing*, *50*(4); 433–439.

Murray, D., & Dodds, C. (2003). The effect of sleep disruption on performance of anaesthetists–a pilot study. *Anaesthesia*, *58*, 520–525.

Muzur, A., Pace-Schott, E. F., & Hobson, J. A. (2002). The prefrontal cortex in sleep. *Trends in Cognitive Sciences*, *6*, 475–481.

Patrick, G. T. W., & Gilbert, J. A. (1896). On the effects of loss of sleep. *Psychological Review*, *3*, 469–483.

Peigneux, P., Laureys, S., Fuchs, S., Collette, F., Perrin, F., & Reggers, J., et al., (2004). Are spatial memories strengthened in the human hippocampus during slow wave sleep? *Neuron*, *44*, 535–545.

Philip, P., Stoohs, R., & Guilleminault, C. (1994). Sleep fragmentation in normals: A model for sleepiness associated with upper airway resistance syndrome. *Sleep*, *17*, 242–247.

Pilcher, J. J., & Huffcutt, A. I. (1996). Effects of sleep deprivation on performance: A meta-analysis. *Sleep*, *19*, 318–326.

Porkka-Heiskanen, T., Strecker, R. E., Thakkar, M., Bjorkum, A. A., Greene, R. W., & McCarley, R. W. (1997). Adenosine: A mediator of the sleep-inducing effects of prolonged wakefulness. *Science*, *276*, 1265–1268.

Powell, N. B., Riley, R. W., Schechtman, K. B., Blumen, M. B., Dinges, D. F., & Guilleminault, C. (1999). A comparative model: Reaction time performance in sleep-disordered breathing versus alcohol-impaired controls. *Laryngoscope*, *109*, 1648–1654.

Pritchard, W. S. (1981). Psychophysiology of P300. *Psychological Bulletin*, *89*, 506–540.

Rechtschaffen, A., & Kales, A. (1968). *A manual of standardized terminology, techniques and scoring system for sleep stages of human subjects.* Public Health Service, U.S. Government Printing Office, Washington, DC.

Rennie, C. J., Robinson, P. A., & Wright, J. J. (2002). Unified neurophysical model of EEG spectra and evoked potentials. *Biological Cybernetics*, *86*, 457–471.

Roehrs, T., Merlotti, L., Petrucelli, N., Stepanski, E., & Roth, T. (1994). Experimental sleep fragmentation. *Sleep*, *17*, 438–443.

Roman, V., Van der Borght, K., Leemburg, S. A., Van der Zee, E. A., & Meerlo, P. (2005). Sleep restriction by forced activity reduces hippocampal cell proliferation. *Brain Research*, *1065*, 53–59.

Stenuit, P., & Kerkhofs, M. (2005). Age modulates the effects of sleep restriction in women. *Sleep*, *28*, 1283–1288.

Stepanski, E., Lamphere, J., Roehrs, T., Zorick, F., & Roth, T. (1987). Experimental sleep fragmentation in normal subjects. *International Journal of Neuroscience*, *33*, 207–214.

Stepanski, E. J. (2002). The effect of sleep fragmentation on daytime function. *Sleep*, *25*, 268–276.

van der Borght, K., Ferrari, F., Klauke, K., Roman, V., Havekes, R., & Sgoifo, A., et al., (2006). Hippocampal cell proliferation across the day: Increase by running wheel activity, but no effect of sleep and wakefulness. *Behavioural Brain Research*, *167*, 36–41.

Van Dongen, H. P. A., & Hursh, S. R. (2010). Fatigue, performance, errors and accidents. In: Kryger, M. H., Roth, T., Dement, W. C. (Eds.), *Principles and practice of sleep medicine, 5th ed.* Elsevier Saunders, Philadelphia.

Van Dongen, H. P., Baynard, M. D., Maislin, G., & Dinges, D. F. (2004). Systematic interindividual differences in neurobehavioral impairment from sleep loss: Evidence of trait-like differential vulnerability. *Sleep*, *27*, 423–433.

Van Dongen, H. P. A., Belenky, G., & Krueger, J. M. (2010). Investigating the temporal dynamics and underlying mechanisms of cognitive fatigue. In: Ackerman, P. L. (Ed.), *Cognitive fatigue*. American Psychological Association, Washington, DC, pp. 127–147.

Van Dongen, H. P. A., Maislin, G., Mullington, J. M., & Dinges, D. F. (2003). The cumulative cost of additional wakefulness: Dose-response effects on neurobehavioral functions and sleep physiology from chronic sleep restriction and total sleep deprivation. *Sleep*, *26*, 117–126.

Wehr, T. A., Moul, D. E., Barbato, G., Giesen, H. A., Seidel, J. A., & Barker, C., et al., (1993). Conservation of photoperiod-responsive mechanisms in humans. *American Journal of Physiology*, *265*, R846–857.

Wesensten, N. J., Balkin, T. J., & Belenky, G. (1999). Does sleep fragmentation impact recuperation? A review and reanalysis. *Journal of Sleep Research*, *8*, 237–245.

Williamson, A. M., & Feyer, A. M. (2000). Moderate sleep deprivation produces impairments in cognitive and motor performance equivalent to legally prescribed levels of alcohol intoxication. *Occupational and Environmental Medicine*, *57*, 649–655.

G. A. Kerkhof and H. P. A. Van Dongen (Eds.)
Progress in Brain Research, Vol. 185
ISSN: 0079-6123

CHAPTER 7

Effects of sleep deprivation on cognition

William D.S. Killgore*

Neuroimaging Center, McLean Hospital, Harvard Medical School, Belmont, MA, USA

Abstract: Sleep deprivation is commonplace in modern society, but its far-reaching effects on cognitive performance are only beginning to be understood from a scientific perspective. While there is broad consensus that insufficient sleep leads to a general slowing of response speed and increased variability in performance, particularly for simple measures of alertness, attention and vigilance, there is much less agreement about the effects of sleep deprivation on many higher level cognitive capacities, including perception, memory and executive functions. Central to this debate has been the question of whether sleep deprivation affects nearly all cognitive capacities in a global manner through degraded alertness and attention, or whether sleep loss specifically impairs some aspects of cognition more than others. Neuroimaging evidence has implicated the prefrontal cortex as a brain region that may be particularly susceptible to the effects of sleep loss, but perplexingly, executive function tasks that putatively measure prefrontal functioning have yielded inconsistent findings within the context of sleep deprivation. Whereas many convergent and rule-based reasoning, decision making and planning tasks are relatively unaffected by sleep loss, more creative, divergent and innovative aspects of cognition do appear to be degraded by lack of sleep. Emerging evidence suggests that some aspects of higher level cognitive capacities remain degraded by sleep deprivation despite restoration of alertness and vigilance with stimulant countermeasures, suggesting that sleep loss may affect specific cognitive systems above and beyond the effects produced by global cognitive declines or impaired attentional processes. Finally, the role of emotion as a critical facet of cognition has received increasing attention in recent years and mounting evidence suggests that sleep deprivation may particularly affect cognitive systems that rely on emotional data. Thus, the extent to which sleep deprivation affects a particular cognitive process may depend on several factors, including the magnitude of global decline in general alertness and attention, the degree to which the specific cognitive function depends on emotion-processing networks, and the extent to which that cognitive process can draw upon associated cortical regions for compensatory support.

Keywords: Sleep deprivation; cognition; attention; vigilance; perception; emotion; executive function; decision making

* Corresponding author.
Tel.: +(617) 855-3166; Fax: +(617) 855-2770.
E-mail: killgore@mclean.harvard.edu

DOI:10.1016/B978-0-444-53702-7.00007-5

Introduction

Most of us will spend approximately one-third of our lives asleep. Despite the large proportion of our existence that it consumes, there remains little scientific consensus regarding the actual function that sleep provides. Scientific debate aside, even most non-experts would agree that without adequate sleep, nearly every aspect of waking life becomes more effortful, laboured and emotionally less fulfilling. Nothing seems to bring as much clarity to the function of sleep as spending a night without it. When deprived of sufficient sleep, most of us feel sleepy and physically drained, our mood is noticeably flattened if not somewhat dour, and our thinking feels sluggish and unfocused. Even to the non-expert, sleep has obvious importance for sustaining normal functioning at several levels, including basic alertness, emotional experience and a host of complex cognitive processes.

Despite common wisdom that sleep is important for sustaining performance, in the daily bustle of life, sleep is sometimes considered to be something of a minor nuisance – a perfunctory part of the daily routine, akin to bathing, oral hygiene and waste elimination. To the casual observer, sleep appears to be a state of unproductive dormancy – time that might seem wasted and better devoted to more productive, lucrative or entertaining pursuits. When work, school or social demands encroach, people often trade sleep for additional time to devote to such activities. Furthermore, insufficient sleep is often the norm among many professions, such as medical residents, military personnel and shift-workers. Thus, scientific study of the effects of sleep deprivation can provide unique insights, not only regarding the nature and function of sleep but also of practical importance for enhancing the health and well being of workers who must perform optimally despite periods with little to no sleep.

The present chapter presents a selective review of the effects of sleep deprivation on a number of cognitive processes. Because human cognition is complex and higher order capacities often build upon more elementary cognitive functions, the chapter will begin with a discussion of the effects of sleep loss on simple alertness, vigilance and attention, the foundation for other aspects of waking cognition. We will then focus on the consequences of sleep deprivation on various aspects of sensory perception, emotion and long-term memory processes. Finally, we will discuss the effects of sleep deprivation on several of the most complex cognitive processes, including mental flexibility, planning and sequencing, abstract concept formation and decision making. Many other cognitive capacities (e.g. language) would also be appropriate for a discussion of this type, but due to space limitations such coverage is beyond the scope of this chapter.

Alertness, vigilance and simple attention

Without some degree of alertness and attention, it is virtually impossible to engage in complex cognitive processing. These basic capacities serve as the foundation for higher level cognition. Interestingly, alertness and vigilance also appear to be the cognitive capacities most consistently and dramatically impacted by insufficient sleep (Lim and Dinges, 2008, 2010). During a normal day, alertness remains relatively stable throughout typical waking hours in a healthy rested person. With sufficient sleep, even circadian (i.e. near-24-h) fluctuations in alertness and more rapid variations (e.g. the post lunch dip) during normal waking hours are trivial and difficult to detect without extremely sensitive tests. Nevertheless, when the envelope of continuous wakefulness is pushed beyond about 16 h, most individuals begin to show a substantial slowing of reaction time (RT) and worsening of performance accuracy on tests of psychomotor vigilance (Goel et al., 2009), declines that continue to worsen as wakefulness is sustained throughout the night into the early morning hours.

Psychomotor vigilance performance

The most commonly used metric for evaluating alertness and vigilance during sleep loss is the Psychomotor Vigilance Test (PVT) (Dinges and Powell, 1985), a 10-min simple RT test that repeatedly presents a visual cue at pseudo-random intervals ranging from 2 to 10 s. At each cue presentation, the subject simply presses a button as quickly as possible to register a response, clear the stimulus and start the next trial. The PVT is exquisitely sensitive to the slowing of RT and increased attentional lapses that occur during periods of total sleep deprivation (Doran et al., 2001) or chronic sleep restriction (Dinges et al., 1997). The PVT has become the 'gold standard' for assessment of the effects of sleep deprivation on cognition because it is highly reliable, sensitive to prolonged wakefulness and circadian influences, and shows very little effect of learning (Dinges et al., 1997; Van Dongen et al., 2003), making it ideal for repeated administrations over the course of a lengthy study.

A recent review by Lim and Dinges (2008) outlined several general conclusions about the effects of sleep deprivation on vigilance performance as measured by the PVT. First, they note that sleep deprivation leads to a general slowing of response times, which includes a worsening of average RT for all trials, as well as slowing of the fastest 10% of responses during the task. The latter point is important, as it suggests that sleep loss adversely affects even the best performances, not just the typical responses. Measures of response speed are extremely sensitive to sleep loss, as demonstrated by Doran et al. (2001). They measured PVT performance every 2 h in two groups over an 88-h period of sleep deprivation. One group remained awake for the entire period, while the other group received a 2-h nap once every 12 h. In comparison to the group receiving only a short nap twice a day, those who remained awake the entire time showed significant slowing of response times, greater variability in performance and increased errors of omission and commission (Doran et al., 2001).

Total sleep deprivation is not necessary in order to observe decrements in psychomotor vigilance response speed, however. In fact, restricting sleep by only a couple of hours per night (e.g. 6 h per night) can lead to significant slowing of response times that, if prolonged for up 2 weeks, can reach impairment levels that are comparable to about two nights of total sleep deprivation (Van Dongen et al., 2003). Chronic sleep restriction to about 5 h per night appears to produce even greater decrements in psychomotor vigilance performance, but these declines eventually level off at a substantially reduced level; further restriction to less than about 4 h nightly appears to lead to continued degradation in vigilance performance (Belenky et al., 2003; Van Dongen et al., 2003).

The second conclusion about psychomotor vigilance suggested in the review by Lim and Dinges is that sleep deprivation leads to an increase in the number and duration of attentional lapses (i.e. periods during which the subject fails to respond to the cue, usually defined as a response of 500 ms or longer) as well as an increase in errors of commission or false alarms (i.e. responses when no cue has been presented or incorrect responses). Some have suggested that longer lapses may actually represent 'microsleeps', or brief periods where sleep-like brain activity may momentarily interrupt ongoing wakefulness (Peiris et al., 2008; Poudel et al., 2009). There is evidence that the number of lapses at any particular time point is correlated with the duration of those lapses, suggesting that this index is particularly useful as a measure of sleepiness (Lim and Dinges, 2008).

It is also true that the ability to sustain psychomotor vigilance also decreases with the duration of the task (Lim and Dinges, 2008). This is known as the 'time-on-task effect' (i.e. the progressive worsening of performance with sustained focus on a cognitive task) and is greatly exacerbated during sleep deprivation. In fact, during even a single night of sleep loss, decrements in performance on a boring monotonous task can be seen within only a few minutes (Gillberg and Akerstedt, 1998). The time on task effect appears to be strongly affected by motivation and some evidence suggests that its effects can be mitigated by incentives or rewards (Steyvers and Gaillard, 1993). The standard version of the PVT lasts 10-min, which appears to be ample duration to induce time-on-task effects in sleep-deprived individuals. However, shorter variants of the PVT have been used successfully to show performance decrements during sleep loss. For instance, a series of studies from the Walter Reed Army Institute of Research used a shorter 5-min variant of the PVT to examine the effectiveness of stimulant countermeasures such as caffeine, dextroamphetamine and modafinil at sustaining alertness and vigilance during prolonged sleep deprivation (Killgore et al., 2008b; Wesensten et al., 2005). Even a 5-min variant of the PVT appears to be of sufficient duration to elicit significant effects of sleep deprivation and is sensitive to the effects of stimulant countermeasures. These studies showed that with sufficient dosage, speed of responding could be temporarily restored to near baseline levels by these commonly used psychostimulants, even after two to three nights of total sleep deprivation (Killgore et al., 2008b; Wesensten et al., 2005).

Finally, psychomotor vigilance performance is highly sensitive to the magnitude of homeostatic sleep pressure (i.e. the biological drive for sleep), which accumulates with longer durations of wakefulness, as well as the normal diurnal fluctuations in alertness that occur throughout the day. These latter observations comprise the two-process model (Borbely, 1982), which posits that sleep propensity and alertness are regulated by the combined interaction of two biological processes involving a homeostatic drive for sleep that accumulates over time awake (process S) and an oscillating circadian process that modulates the level of alertness (process C) (see Fig. 1). Thus, the longer an individual remains awake, the greater the

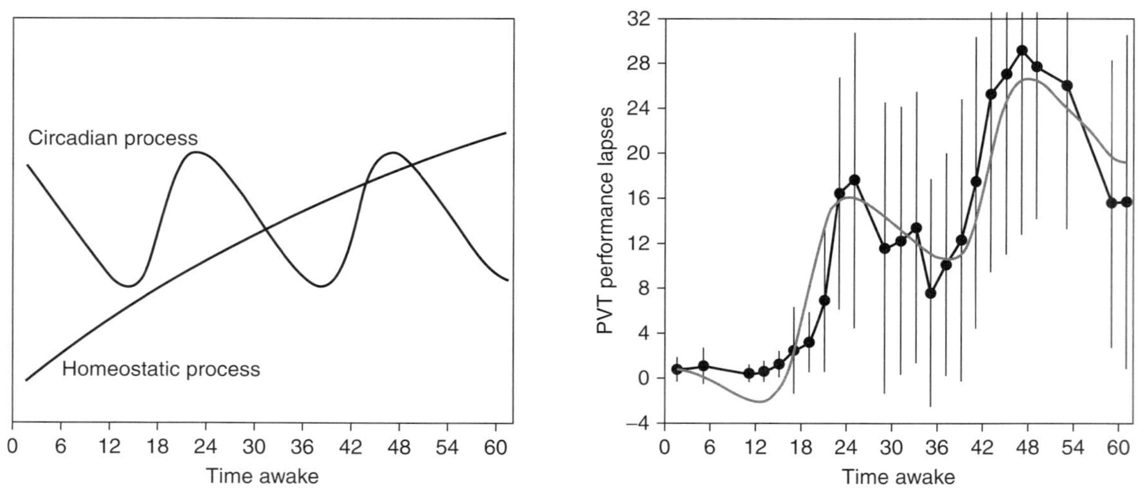

Fig. 1. Dynamic influences on cognitive performance by two key neurobiological processes: a homeostatic process and a circadian process. The left panel shows a gradual increase of the homeostatic process across 62 h of total sleep deprivation, representing the progressive build-up of pressure for sleep over time awake; and an oscillatory pattern of the circadian process with a period of (approximately) 24 h, representing the waxing and waning of pressure for wakefulness over time of day. The right panel shows the sum of these two influences as a model of performance impairment (grey curve), superimposed on actual measurements of performance during 62 h of total sleep deprivation in a laboratory (black curve). The data shown in the right panel are averages (black circles) with one standard deviation on each side (whiskers) over 12 healthy adults. Reprinted with permission from Van Dongen and Belenky (2009).

homeostatic pressure to fall asleep (S). However, this pressure will be either reduced or increased according to a 24-h sinusoidal pattern (C) throughout the day. During sleep deprivation, performance degradation will be most severe at the circadian nadir during the early morning hours (Babkoff et al., 1991).

Attention and motor tracking

A particularly compelling and practically relevant account of the decline in vigilance and attention was demonstrated by a simple but elegant study that equated hours of wakefulness with blood alcohol concentration during a visual-motor tracking task (Dawson and Reid, 1997). In that study, performance on a simple test of hand–eye tracking and coordination worsened in a linear manner during a 28-h period of overnight sleep deprivation. Moreover, performances during sleep deprivation were statistically equated with those of the same subjects at various blood alcohol concentration levels manipulated and measured on a different day. Findings showed that after 10 h of continuous wakefulness, each additional hour awake was equivalent to an increase of 0.004% blood alcohol concentration until about 26 h of wakefulness. In practical terms, by 17-h of wakefulness performance was equivalent to a blood alcohol concentration of 0.05%, while 24 h awake was roughly equivalent to performance at 0.10%, a level meeting or exceeding the legal limit for intoxication in all states in the United States. The implications are clear – on average, a person who has gone for even one single night without sleep is about as impaired on early morning hand–eye coordination as an individual drinking alcohol to the legal limit of intoxication.

Wake state instability

The longer a person remains awake, the stronger the biological pressure for sleep. During periods of intentional wakefulness, the accumulating homeostatic pressure for sleep exists in opposition to the individual's motivation to remain awake. Motivational control over the waking state is presumed to be modulated by top-down cortical control systems, most likely involving prefrontal executive regions, whereas the involuntary drive for sleep emerges from bottom-up systems involving brainstem and hypothalamic nuclei (Lim and Dinges, 2008), or possibly, from emergent properties of local neuronal assemblies as a function of prior use (Krueger et al., 2008). When sleep pressure is low, there is little tension in this system and waking alertness and vigilance performance remains stable. However, as an individual attempts to sustain wakefulness beyond about 16 h, the tension between the mounting homeostatic pressure for sleep and motivated attempts to fight off sleep becomes greater, leading to increased variability in alertness and progressively unreliable performance. This theory, known as the 'wake state instability' hypothesis (Doran et al., 2001), suggests that the hallmark of sleep deprivation is increased variability in performance due to the interaction of reciprocally inhibiting neurobiologic systems, one attempting to keep the individual awake and the other exerting pressure to fall sleep (Goel et al., 2009). This instability is often most easily observed in performance lapses (i.e. PVT reaction times longer than 500 ms), which become more frequent and longer in duration as the period of continuous wakefulness is extended (Doran et al., 2001). Eventually, lapses become so extreme in duration (e.g. 30 s or longer) that they qualitatively shift from momentary periods of inattention to what can be described as a functional sleep attack (Lim and Dinges, 2008). According to Lim and Dinges, these sleep attacks are virtually non-existent in normally rested individuals, but begin to be observed with greater frequency as the period of wakefulness is extended beyond the normal period of waking.

Neuroimaging correlates

What might be occurring in the brain during sustained attention and what occurs during a lapse? Is the process the same when a person is well rested versus sleep deprived? Early neuroimaging studies using positron emission tomography (PET) showed that sleep deprivation is associated with reduced metabolic activity within a network of brain regions important for attention, information processing and executive control, including the prefrontal cortex, anterior cingulate, thalamus, basal ganglia and cerebellum, and the magnitude of declines in activity within the thalamus, prefrontal and parietal regions is correlated with measures of alertness and cognitive performance (Thomas et al., 2000). More recently, studies capitalizing on the superior temporal resolution of functional magnetic resonance imaging (fMRI) have supported the existence of a cortical network important for sustained attention and have shown that the functioning of this network is altered during sleep deprivation. For instance, Drummond and colleagues used event-related fMRI to examine the functional brain correlates of the PVT in healthy individuals when well rested and again following 36 h of total sleep deprivation (Drummond et al., 2005). Faster responses were associated with activation within a cortical sustained attention network including prefrontal, motor and parietal cortical regions, and subcortical structures such as the basal ganglia. In contrast, slow responses were associated with greater activation of medial prefrontal regions implicated in the 'default mode network', a network of medial cortical regions that tends to be most active when external cognitive processing demands are minimized. Following sleep deprivation, slow responses were associated with even greater activation of default mode regions (Drummond et al., 2005). Because the default mode network is generally activated when subjects are awake but at rest, daydreaming, or not otherwise involved in goal-directed behaviours, the authors posit that sleep loss may result in inappropriate activation of default systems or may lead to a failure to effectively allocate resources to task-relevant brain regions when needed.

Other fMRI studies have also shown that sleep deprivation is associated with reduced activation of frontal and parietal networks and altered functioning within the thalamus. Notably, Chee et al. (2008) found that lapses following a night of sleep deprivation were different from those that occurred during rested wakefulness. While infrequent, lapses of attention do occur even in normally rested individuals, usually during boring monotonous tasks. The occurrence of these lapses is believed to originate from transient disruptions in ongoing prefrontal cortical control systems. In contrast, lapses occurring after total sleep deprivation were not only associated with attenuated activation of frontal controls systems but also showed significantly reduced activation of parietal attention regions, visual cortex and thalamus relative to lapses during the rested state (Chee et al., 2008). These findings suggest that lapses during sleep deprivation are qualitatively different from those that occur when an individual is well rested, primarily as a function of reduced visual sensory processing. Overall, neuroimaging research suggests that sleep loss alters normal functioning of the sustained attention network and leads to increased disengagement from external sensory input.

Individual differences

When it comes to the ability to sustain performance when sleep deprived, not all individuals are created equal. Some people appear to be little affected or are well able to compensate for the effects of sleep loss on alertness and vigilance, whereas others seem to be much less resistant. Moreover, these effects appear to be relatively stable within individuals across different sessions of sleep deprivation (Van Dongen et al., 2004). In their seminal study, Van Dongen and colleagues reported that 67.5% of between-session variability in PVT performance, and more than 90% of variability in subjective sleepiness ratings could be explained by systematic individual differences. These authors have proposed that consistent inter-individual differences in the susceptibility to performance impairment from sleep loss are so reliable within individuals as to reflect a trait-like phenomenon (Van Dongen et al., 2004). It has been suggested that prior sleep history, baseline cognitive functioning, standard blood and urine laboratory test findings or psychological traits such as personality do not significantly predict these individual differences (Van Dongen and Belenky, 2009), although some recent studies have reported such relationships (Killgore et al., 2007e, 2008a, 2009a). While the specific criteria that define the basis for these individual difference traits are still being debated, there is emerging evidence that variability in specific polymorphisms of human clock genes may play a prominent role in sensitivity to the effects of sleep loss, sleep pressure and circadian influences (von Schantz, 2008).

Interestingly, the effects of sleep deprivation on psychomotor vigilance appear to be moderated by the age of the individual (Duffy et al., 2009). A number of studies have shown that younger adults tend to show greater decrements in psychomotor vigilance performance, including slowing of RT, increased lapses and unintentional sleep episodes during periods of sleep deprivation, sleep restriction and forced desynchrony of sleep periods relative to older individuals (Adam et al., 2006; Duffy et al., 2009; Silva et al., 2010; Stenuit and Kerkhofs, 2005). In general, while older adults may show slightly slower baseline RT scores, they are less impaired by a night or more of sleep loss than younger adults.

Sensory perception

In contrast to the voluminous literature on the effects of sleep deprivation on alertness, vigilance and attention, surprisingly less research has focused on how lack of sleep affects sensory and perceptual processes. Some of the major findings in this realm will be discussed next.

Visuospatial perception

The effect of sleep deprivation on the ability to accurately perceive visual stimuli has been examined in several studies in recent years. Building on a large body of work in the field of cognitive neuropsychology, Manly et al. (2005) studied visuospatial attention biases in sleep-deprived individuals. It has been well established that healthy rested individuals show a consistent bias to overestimate the length of the left section of bisected horizontal lines, a finding that has been attributed to the dominance of the right cerebral hemisphere for attention and spatial processing. Interestingly, Manly and colleagues showed that relative to rested wakefulness, there was a rightward shift in attention following sleep deprivation, leading to an attenuation of the normal leftward bias. These findings raised the possibility that sleep loss may particularly impair right hemisphere (i.e. left visual field) functioning and alter normal visuospatial perception.

When lateralized perceptual findings are observed, they tend to support the notion that the right hemisphere may be more adversely affected by sleep loss than the left. However, this finding has not been supported universally. For example, evidence for a specific perceptual deficit in the left visual field was not found in a subsequent study by Kendall et al. (2006), who examined visual perception of small light flashes across a 150° horizontal visual arc during a divided attention paradigm. Rather than leading to lateralized visual perception deficits, 31–35 h of sleep deprivation was associated with a global worsening of response omissions across the entire field of visual perception. In another study, Killgore and colleagues examined the effect of 23 h of sleep deprivation on a standardized clinical neuropsychological test of visuospatial perception (Killgore et al., 2007b), the Judgement of Line Orientation Test (JLOT).

Contrary to their hypotheses, performance on the JLOT did not decline as a function of sleep loss despite highly significant impairments in PVT performance immediately following the task, suggesting that under conditions of free stimulus viewing and without time constraints, the simple visual ability to judge the relative angle of lines does not appear to be degraded meaningfully as a function of one night of sleep loss. Furthermore, there was no observed laterality effect on this task. Finally, a recent study by Roge and Gabaude (2009) showed that a single night of sleep loss was sufficient to reduce visual perceptual sensitivity on a computerized visual perception task and led to more conservative perceptual decisions in a manner that paralleled changes that occur during the aging process. Together these findings suggest that the effect of sleep deprivation on visual processes is subtle and may be easily compensated for when time constraints are not an issue and may be completely absent on less sensitive clinical measures, which are designed to measure the gross presence of neuropathology.

Using sophisticated fMRI techniques, Chee and colleagues have shown that during sleep deprivation, there is a significant decline in visual task-related activation within extrastriate regions of the occipital cortex, which are primarily involved in visual sensory processing, and this decline is particularly evident during lapses (Chee et al., 2008). A second study by the same group examined the effect of sleep deprivation on brain function during a visual memory task and a matched visual perceptual load task. Findings clearly showed that sleep deprivation was associated with reduced activation within visual processing regions of the occipital cortex, which correlated with poorer performance on both tasks (Chuah and Chee, 2008). Reduced visual processing during sleep deprivation might be due to use-dependent fatigue effects or even localized sleep within visual regions that are overly taxed during prolonged wakefulness. Alternatively, it is possible that the declines in visual processing and deactivation of visual cortex may simply emerge from weakened attention biasing signals from the prefrontal and parietal cortices. Chee and Tan (2010) recently tested these two competing hypotheses using fMRI and found greater support for the latter explanation, suggesting that the visual deficits associated with sleep deprivation are primarily due to an attenuation of normal top-down attention biasing systems rather than a primary deficit in the functioning of visual cortex.

Auditory perception

Relative to visual perception, much less is known about auditory perception during sleep deprivation. As with the studies of visual perception, the few available auditory studies also find a general decline in the latency of responses to auditory stimuli, but these may also be attributable to deficits in attention and vigilance rather than a specific deficit in auditory processing (Horne et al., 1983). One aspect of auditory perception that does appear to be affected by sleep deprivation is auditory temporal resolution – the ability to identify which of two closely paired auditory stimuli occurs first in succession. This capacity is believed to rely on the functions of the prefrontal cortex and, as such, might be particularly sensitive to sleep loss (Babkoff et al., 2005). In fact, one night of sleep deprivation was found to reduce auditory temporal resolution by over 28% (Babkoff et al., 2005), a finding which has possible implications for higher level cognitive processes such as language comprehension. At present, the effects of sleep deprivation on auditory comprehension are virtually unknown. Given the importance of auditory discrimination as well as auditory sensory perception thresholds for many dangerous work environments, this is an important yet understudied aspect of cognition during sleep deprivation.

Tactile perception/pain

At present, there are virtually no studies examining tactile sensation or perception during sleep deprivation. Whereas available evidence suggests that there is no effect of sleep deprivation on simple detection thresholds for warm and cold temperatures, there is compelling evidence to suggest that sleep deprivation is associated with a significant reduction in pain tolerance thresholds for cold and heat (Kundermann et al., 2004). A recent study showed that total sleep deprivation was associated with significant increases in ratings of spontaneous pain, including general physical discomfort, body pain, headache, muscle pain and stomach pain (Haack et al., 2009). The exact mechanisms for hyperalgesia during sleep deprivation remain to be determined (Lautenbacher et al., 2006), but it is conceivable that dysregulation of affective processing systems may contribute to this effect.

Taste perception

One very early study suggested that sleep deprivation is associated with increased sensory perceptual thresholds for sour tastes, but not for sweet or salty tastes at 24 and 48 h of total sleep deprivation (Furchtgott and Willingham, 1956). The authors pointed out that humans normally have a greater range of sensitivity to sour tastes than for salty or sweet tastes, suggesting that deficits in attention during sleep deprivation may account for the reduced sensitivity. At present, no other studies have explored this aspect of perception during sleep loss.

Olfactory perception

Olfaction is a particularly interesting sensory-perceptual modality, as it is the only sense that initially bypasses thalamic input and may provide a direct assessment of the functional integrity of the orbitofrontal cortex, a brain region that appears to be particularly affected by sleep deprivation (Thomas et al., 2000) and is critical to a number of emotional and cognitive processes (Killgore and McBride, 2006). To date, only two studies have examined the effects of sleep deprivation on the ability to accurately discriminate and identify odours. Killgore and McBride (2006) found that performance on the Smell Identification Test (SIT), a standardized measure of olfactory discrimination, declined significantly following 24 h of sleep deprivation, corresponding with declines in PVT performance. Because other aspects of complex cognition remained stable (i.e. mental flexibility and set-shifting on a temporally contiguous trail-making test), these findings were suggested to occur independently of global declines in alertness. These findings were replicated in a second independent sample following 52 h of sleep deprivation (McBride et al., 2006). Although statistically significant, odour identification declines were mild in both studies, with changes ranging between 5.2 and 6.3 percentage points on average. In contrast to the studies of odour identification, no studies have yet examined odour detection thresholds during sleep loss.

Emotional processing

Other than the well-documented declines in vigilance and attention, perhaps one of the most universally observed effects of sleep loss is altered emotional functioning. Despite a voluminous literature suggesting that mood consistently declines during sleep deprivation, there has, until recently, been very little focus on other more specific aspects of emotional processing during sleep loss, such as emotional perception, control, comprehension and expression (Walker, 2009). Interest in emotion research in general has shown a resurgence in recent years and it is now becoming clear that changes in emotional processing due to sleep loss can have profound effects on a variety of higher level cognitive processes, including memory, judgement and decision making.

Self-report measures

Anyone who has pulled an 'all nighter' or spent much time around someone who is lacking sleep is acutely aware of the general decline in mood and increased irritability and emotional volatility that rapidly ensues. For instance, even a single night of sleep deprivation leads to a significant increase in negative self-rated mood scores compared to subjects receiving a normal night of sleep (Tempesta et al., 2010). Not only do sleep-deprived individuals report worse moods on self-report inventories, they also show evidence of more frequent and amplified negative cognitions and intolerant responses to frustrating social situations. For example, when asked to provide responses to semi-projective cartoon scenarios of various types of frustrating circumstances, individuals who were sleep deprived for two nights showed significant elevation in their tendencies to redirect blame toward others for causing the hypothetical predicaments and were less willing to offer amends to bring about mutually satisfying outcomes (Kahn-Greene et al., 2006).

Not only does sleep deprivation affect emotional responses to frustrating events, it also appears to reduce self-reported coping capacities and emotional intelligence skills (Killgore et al., 2007a). Specifically, two nights of sleep deprivation were associated with a reduced tendency to think positively, decreased willingness to take effective behavioural action to solve problems, and a greater reliance on unproductive coping strategies such as superstitious and magical thinking processes. Moreover, total scores on an emotional intelligence scale declined as a function of sleep deprivation, particularly with regard to ratings of self-esteem, empathy toward others, understanding of interpersonal dynamics, impulse control, and the ability to delay gratification (Killgore et al., 2007a). Thus, sleep-deprived individuals appear to be more easily frustrated, intolerant, unforgiving, less caring, and more self-focused than when fully rested.

Sleep deprivation also appears to bring about an elevation of several dimensions of clinical mood problems and symptoms of psychopathology (Kahn-Greene et al., 2007). Relative to their baseline responses, subjects deprived of sleep for 56 h showed significant elevations on clinical scales measuring depression, anxiety, paranoia and somatic complaints (Kahn-Greene et al., 2007). In general, when sleep deprived, these healthy subjects were more likely to report increased feelings of worthlessness, inadequacy, powerlessness, failure, low self-esteem and reduced life satisfaction. Moreover, the change in scores was large enough to meet criteria for a 'clinically significant' increase in depression scores for 25% of the sample, while 17% of subjects showed clinically significant elevations on scales measuring anxiety, mania and borderline features (Kahn-Greene et al., 2007), suggesting that sleep loss has profound impacts on emotional functioning in healthy individuals.

Emotional perception

Evaluation of emotional stimuli is also affected by sleep deprivation. A recent study presented normally rested healthy subjects with a series of pleasant, neutral and unpleasant photographs and asked them to rate each of the images for emotional quality (Tempesta et al., 2010). Subjects then rated a matched set of images again following either a night of normal sleep at home or one night of total sleep deprivation in the laboratory. Interestingly, sleep loss did not alter ratings of pleasant or unpleasant images, but neutral images were rated significantly more negatively following sleep deprivation, an effect that was independent of self-rated mood. These findings suggest that sleep deprivation alters the affective perception of neutral stimuli, biasing emotional processing toward greater negativity. Perception of humour also appears to be affected by sleep loss. The ability to appreciate humour is a highly complex cognitive capacity that requires the ability to integrate contextual information with emotional processes (Killgore et al., 2006b). In one study, healthy participants were deprived of sleep for two nights and then asked to choose the 'funnier' item among pairs of verbal (news headlines) and visual (cartoons) stimuli. Sleep-deprived subjects scored approximately one standard deviation below normative data for non-sleep-deprived subjects on both types of stimuli, and this performance was not significantly different in a comparison group who received a large dose of caffeine, despite evidence of significantly higher alertness, vigilance and lower subjective sleepiness (Killgore et al., 2006b). Because caffeine led to increased alertness and vigilance performance but did not improve humour ratings above placebo, these effects do not appear to be accounted for by a general deficit in alertness.

Neural correlates

Why should sleep deprivation have such a dramatic effect on affective processing? What areas of the brain are affected by sleep loss and might account for these findings? Neuroimaging studies of the effects of sleep deprivation on brain function are beginning to clarify the processes involved. As mentioned previously, early PET studies showed significant declines in prefrontal metabolic activity during sleep deprivation, which correlated with declines in attention and cognitive processing (Thomas et al., 2000). However, the prefrontal cortex is important for more than just regulating attentional resources. Prefrontal regions also play important roles in emotional processing and personality. For instance, the more ventral and medial aspects of the prefrontal cortex appear to be important for integrating lower-order somatic, visceral and emotional inputs with higher order abstract reasoning and decision making (Damasio, 1994). The medial prefrontal cortex also has extensive inhibitory connections with primitive emotional processing areas such as the amygdala and other limbic structures (Walker, 2009). Thus, reductions in medial prefrontal metabolic activity might be expected to impair normal modulation of emotion-related amygdala responses, leading to elevations in negative affective processing.

The effect of sleep deprivation on cortico-limbic emotion regulation circuits was recently demonstrated in an fMRI study. Yoo et al. (2007a) showed emotionally evocative pictures to rested and sleep-deprived volunteers as they underwent functional brain imaging. While normally rested subjects showed the expected pattern of increased amygdala activation to the unpleasant images, those who were deprived of sleep for about 35 h showed significantly greater magnitude and spatial extent of activation within the amygdala to the same emotional images (see Fig. 2). Moreover, a functional connectivity analysis, which measures the strength of relationship among brain regions, showed that sleep deprivation was associated with significantly reduced functional connectivity between the medial prefrontal cortex and the amygdala during emotional processing relative to rested controls. This critical finding suggests that sleep deprivation weakens top-down inhibitory control over the amygdala by the prefrontal cortex, leading to dysregulation of emotional processing. These findings are concordant with emerging evidence that suggests that one critical function of sleep may be to optimize neuronal connectivity (Krueger et al., 2008). Without optimal cortico-limbic connectivity, the lower order emotional processing regions of the limbic system may be effectively 'cut-off' from the modulatory control regions of the prefrontal cortex during periods of sleep deprivation.

Learning and memory

Some of the most essential cognitive capacities to survival include the ability to acquire new information, commit such information to long-term storage, and effectively retrieve that information when needed – in other words, learning and memory. A large and growing literature suggests that sleep is critical to learning and memory, and when sleep is hindered, memory processing is correspondingly degraded (Diekelmann and Born, 2010; Goel et al., 2009; Walker and Stickgold, 2006). Sleep is hypothesized to play a number of complex and important roles in memory processing but full explication of these theories is beyond the scope of this chapter. Interested readers are referred to several excellent and comprehensive reviews (Diekelmann and Born, 2010; Walker, 2009; Walker and Stickgold, 2006). Briefly, sleep appears to be important for memory processing in two major ways. First, sleep is important before learning or encoding to prepare the brain to effectively acquire new information. Second, sleep is important following learning to facilitate the consolidation (i.e. stabilization) and integration (i.e. assimilation) of newly learned information into existing memory structures (Diekelmann and Born, 2010; Walker, 2009). While many studies of sleep processes have focused on memory consolidation, most studies of the effects of sleep deprivation on learning and memory have focused on the first issue, that is how sleep deprivation may impair the acquisition of new memories.

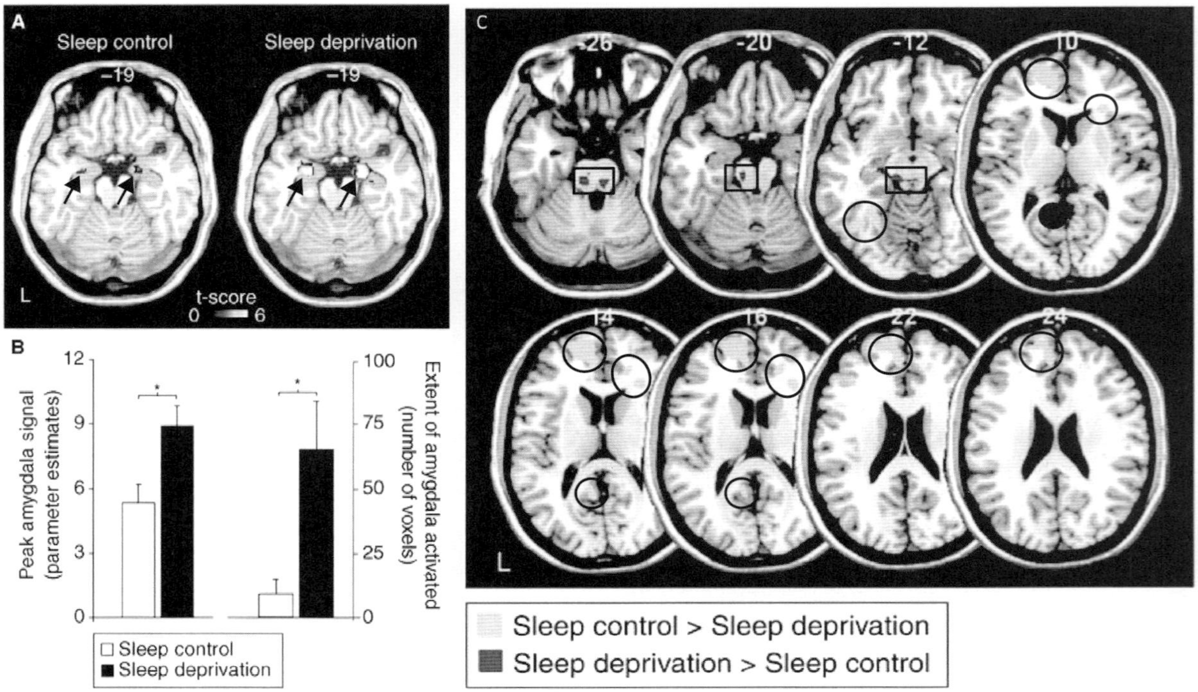

Fig. 2. Amygdala responses in rested and sleep-deprived groups. (A) Amygdala response to emotionally negative stimuli is shown for the rested and sleep-deprived conditions. (B) Corresponding differences in intensity and volumetric extent of amygdala activation are shown between the two groups (average ± s.e.m. of left and right amygdala). (C) Group level differences in amygdala functional connectivity (combined for left and right), including significantly greater connectivity in the medial-prefrontal cortex (circled areas) for the sleep-control group, yet significantly stronger connectivity with autonomic brainstem regions in the sleep-deprivation group (rectangle areas). Slice number (z-coordinate) displayed on all images. Effects are significant at $p < 0.001$; ≥ 5 contiguous voxels. Reprinted with permission from Yoo et al. (2007a). (For interpretation of the references to colour in this figure legend, the reader is referred to the web version of this book.)

Much of the work on the effects of sleep deprivation on memory has focused on declarative memory, which involves memories that are consciously accessible and either involve autobiographical memory for actual events in one's past (episodic memory) or memories for facts and general knowledge (semantic memory). These types of memory are highly dependent upon the hippocampus and medial temporal lobe structures during initial encoding. For instance, Drummond and colleagues found that 35 h of sleep deprivation resulted in significantly impaired verbal learning relative to rested wakefulness (Drummond et al., 2000). Moreover, functional neuroimaging during memory task performance revealed significantly reduced activation within temporal lobe regions during sleep deprivation relative to rested wakefulness, but increased activation within prefrontal and parietal cortices. Activation in these latter areas appeared to be compensatory in nature, as greater activation within the parietal cortex was associated with better performance on the recall test during sleep deprivation.

Similarly, in a recent study, Yoo et al. (2007b) deprived a group of healthy participants of one night of sleep and then presented them with a series of scenic photographs to encode while undergoing fMRI. A second group slept normally at home but underwent the scene-encoding procedure at the same time as the sleep-deprived subjects. Memory retention was tested for both groups after two nights of normal sleep at home. Functional imaging results showed that during encoding, the sleep-deprived group showed significantly less activation of the posterior hippocampus relative to the normally rested group. When activation associated with subsequent recall success was examined, sleep-deprived subjects showed significantly lower activation of the anterior hippocampus (Yoo et al., 2007b). These findings suggest that not only does sleep deprivation adversely affect temporal lobe regions typically involved in memory processing, other brain regions, particularly prefrontal and parietal cortices, may also be recruited to attempt to compensate for deficits and sustain performance.

Another aspect of memory, known as temporal memory, involves the ability to remember when a particular event occurred. One study examined the effect of 35 h of total sleep deprivation on these types of temporal memory judgements (Harrison and Horne, 2000a). In that study, two series of 12 facial photographs were shown, each series separated by 5 min. After a final 5-min delay, subjects were shown the previously seen faces intermixed with an equal number of new faces that served as foils. Sleep-deprived subjects were no less accurate at identifying previously seen faces than a non-sleep-deprived control group. However, they were significantly less accurate at identifying whether previously seen faces were from the distant (first) set or the more recent (second) set, and were more confident in their incorrect guesses. Because of the ordered sequencing nature of the task, the authors raised the possibility that the deficit in temporal memory suggests that sleep deprivation may also affect prefrontal executive aspects of memory organization (Harrison and Horne, 2000a).

When it comes to forming new memories, some types of material appear to be more easily remembered than others. This is especially true for emotional material. Walker and Stickgold (2006) examined the effects of sleep and sleep deprivation on memory for types of material differing in emotional valence. Participants were first deprived of sleep for 36 h or allowed to sleep normally before completing an incidental memory-encoding task. The task included words that were either emotionally positive, negative or neutral. After two additional nights of normal sleep at home, participants returned to the laboratory for a surprise recognition test. Overall, as shown in Fig. 3, sleep deprivation led to a 40% impairment in recognition scores relative to those individuals who slept normally prior to encoding. Clearly, the ability to encode the material was impaired by lack of sleep. Even more striking, however, was the effect of the pre-encoding sleep deprivation on later recognition of items from the three different emotion

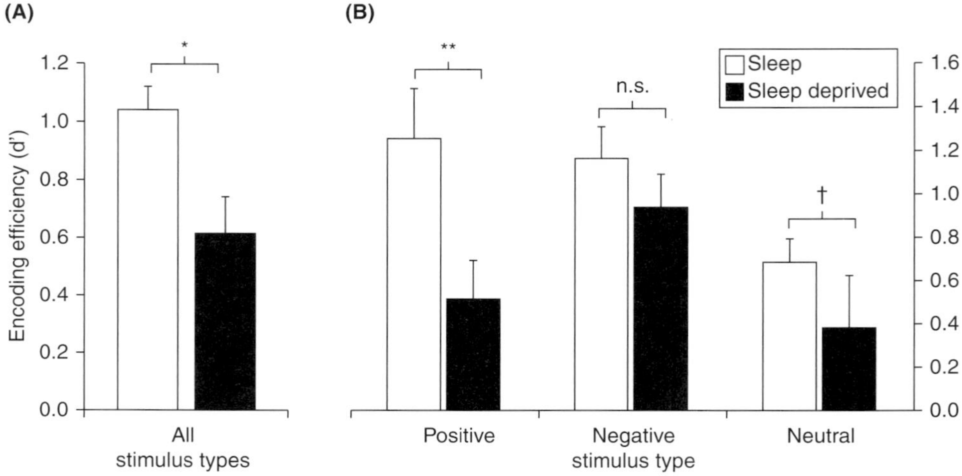

Fig. 3. Sleep deprivation and encoding of emotional and non-emotional declarative memory. Effects of 38 h of total sleep deprivation on encoding of human declarative memory (A) when combined across all emotional and non-emotional categories, (B) when separated by emotional (positive and negative valence) and non-emotional (neutral valence) categories, demonstrating a significant group (sleep, sleep deprivation) × emotion category (positive, negative and neutral) interaction. Post hoc *t*-test comparisons: †$p = 0.08$; *$p = 0.05$; **$p = 0.01$; n.s. = not significant; *d'* = *d*-prime (discrimination index). Reprinted with permission from Walker and van der Helm (2009).

categories (positive, negative and neutral). For those subjects who slept normally prior to encoding, emotional words (positive and negative) were better remembered than neutral words, consistent with prior work showing that emotional content often enhances memory. For those who were deprived of sleep, however, memory for both neutral and positive words was significantly disrupted. In fact, sleep deprivation led to a recognition deficit of 59% for positive words relative to normal sleep. Most notable, however, was the fact that retention of negative words was not significantly degraded by sleep loss. Thus, while sleep deprivation significantly impairs encoding and retention of positive and neutral stimuli, memory for negative stimuli appears to be relatively impervious to sleep loss (Walker and van der Helm, 2009). This may result in a bias favouring negative memories over neutral and positive ones when sleep deprived, which could have implications for the development and maintenance of pathological mood conditions such as depression.

In summary, sleep appears to be necessary to prepare the brain for subsequent learning. When the brain is deprived of sleep, normal hippocampal functioning becomes impaired and the formation of new memories is hindered. Interestingly, the emotional content of the to-be-remembered information is also critical. Memories for negatively valenced material appear to be more resistant to sleep loss, whereas positive and neutral memories are more susceptible to disruption by sleep deprivation.

Executive functions

The term 'executive functions' is usually used to describe a broad and loosely defined category of complex cognitive processes involved in the control and coordination of wilful action towards future goal states (Goel et al., 2009). These functions involve a host of capacities, including the ability to focus attention while ignoring irrelevant information; planning and sequencing thoughts and behaviours; updating information as contingencies change; inhibiting inappropriate thoughts or actions; forming abstract concepts; shifting mental set as appropriate; and thinking flexibly, divergently, and innovatively, just to name a few. By definition, executive functions require complex integration of information and rely on the coordinated interactions of cortical and subcortical networks within the brain. Nevertheless, of all the regions within the brain, the prefrontal cortex appears to be the linchpin for carrying out many of these highest and most complex cognitive processes.

Based on evidence from neuroimaging and cognitive studies, it has been suggested that the prefrontal cortex may be particularly vulnerable to the effects of sleep loss due to its extensive use during normal waking (Harrison et al., 2000). During the course of normal social interactions and vocational activities, the prefrontal cortex is taxed continuously as it plans, coordinates and adapts to changing demands throughout the day. Accordingly, sleep deprivation should particularly degrade complex executive functions that rely on prefrontal regions (Harrison and Horne, 2000b; Harrison et al., 2000). Interestingly, this model has received mixed support, with many studies reporting deficits on executive function tasks during sleep deprivation (Jones and Harrison, 2001), while others fail to find such effects (Pace-Schott et al., 2009; Tucker et al., 2010). The challenge now facing researchers is to clarify which types of executive function tasks are affected by sleep loss and to derive a unifying explanation of why some executive functions are degraded while others appear relatively impervious to insufficient sleep.

Working memory

One cognitive component that is universal to practically all executive function tasks is working memory (i.e. the ability to maintain and actively manipulate information in a temporary memory buffer) (Goel et al., 2009). Without the capacity to hold and manipulate information in real time, complex cognition is virtually impossible. Simply put, working memory capacity reflects the number of information units that can be sustained and juggled in the attentional spotlight at any given moment, a facility that relies heavily upon the dorsolateral regions of the prefrontal cortex (Vandewalle et al., 2009). Because the dorsolateral prefrontal cortex shows significant declines in metabolic energy consumption during sleep deprivation (Thomas et al., 2000), commensurate deficits in working memory might be expected as well.

A recent meta-analysis revealed that sleep deprivation does indeed adversely affect both accuracy and response time during working memory tasks, with effect sizes generally in the moderate range (Lim and Dinges, 2010). Impairment in working memory during sleep deprivation is associated with corresponding reductions in prefrontal activation, but may be even more susceptible to declines in other cortical regions such as the parietal cortex (Mu et al., 2005b). Some evidence suggests that the parietal cortex may play an important compensatory role during sleep deprivation (Drummond et al., 2000), and the emergence of declines in parietal functioning may be the final straw that leads to working memory impairments. Of note, Tucker et al. (2010) recently examined dissociated aspects of working memory performance during sleep deprivation, mathematically separating 'executive' from 'non-executive' components of working memory. Interestingly, that study showed that sleep loss only impaired the 'non-executive' response time aspect of the task, but not the 'executive' aspects such as working memory scanning efficiency and resistance to proactive interference. These results suggest that many studies finding working memory deficits during sleep deprivation may simply be reporting the well-established impairment of simple attention and vigilance rather than a specific deficit in the ability to manipulate cognitively held information.

Convergent thinking and logical deduction

Convergent thinking occurs when the solution to a problem can be deduced by applying established rules and logical reasoning. This type of reasoning involves solving a problem within the context of known information and narrowing down the solution based on logical inference. Harrison and Horne (2000b) reviewed an extensive literature on the effects of sleep deprivation on decision making and concluded that these processes are not significantly affected by sleep loss. Thus, complex cognitive processes, as quantified by broad intellectual functioning or IQ tests, reading comprehension, logical deduction and critical reasoning processes do not appear to be significantly degraded by even as much as two nights of sleep deprivation (Harrison and Horne, 2000b). This finding was supported by a recent meta-analysis that reported essentially no significant effect of sleep deprivation on reasoning and crystallized intelligence, including vocabulary, grammatical reasoning and nonverbal problem-solving (Lim and Dinges, 2010). Harrison and Horne (2000b) suggest that convergent thinking tasks tend to be less dependent upon prefrontal resources than other types of executive tasks, and may therefore, show little effect of sleep deprivation.

Divergent and innovative thinking

In contrast to the convergent thought processes discussed above, the ability to think laterally, innovatively and flexibly appears to be significantly impaired by sleep deprivation (Harrison and Horne, 2000b). For example, in one study, 32 h of sleep deprivation led subjects to produce less creative responses than normally rested controls, as evidenced by generation of fewer unusual or original ideas and reduced ability to shift strategy (Horne, 1988). This same study also showed that sleep deprivation reduced verbal fluency (i.e. the ability to generate novel words to a phonemic cue) and led to longer duration of planning time and more perseverations on the Tower of London Test, a measure that draws upon planning and sequencing and the ability to shift to alternative strategies. More recently, another study found that two nights of sleep deprivation led to below average performance on the number of moves taken to solve the Tower of London Task (Killgore et al., 2009b), a finding that was not improved by the administration of caffeine. Because caffeine restored psychomotor vigilance to baseline levels at roughly the same point in time, it appears that deficits in planning and sequencing may not be fully accounted for by deficits in simple attention. Similarly, Gottselig et al. (2006) examined the ability to vocally generate and maintain a continuous series of random numbers and found that sleep deprivation led to a significant increase in rule violations, response redundancy and stereotypy of responses. Furthermore, caffeine restored simple attention to the task but failed to improve more complex aspects of random number generation, suggesting that the observed executive deficits were not due simply to impaired attention and vigilance.

Harrison and Horne (1999) asked participants to play a complex marketing strategy game that required the ability to monitor ongoing events; revise plans based on new and changing information; and think flexibly, innovatively and creatively under pressure. Compared to their own performances when normally rested, sleep-deprived individuals demonstrated significantly greater rigidity of thought, perseverated on previously successful strategies that were no longer proving effective, were inefficient at updating plans in light of new data, and were unproductive at developing innovative solutions. Ultimately, the game play of the sleep-deprived group 'collapsed' and players became financially insolvent as wakefulness approached 32–36 h, whereas the performance of the same individuals when normally rested remained high as they continued to earn a profit (Harrison and Horne, 1999). While the findings of that study are provocative, the uncontrolled nature of the game makes it difficult to draw conclusions regarding the specific cognitive processes that may have been impaired by sleep loss. Nevertheless, the broad implications point to the potentially devastating effects that sleep deprivation can produce in complex real-world settings.

While the aforementioned studies suggest that sleep deprivation can severely impair divergent thinking and mental flexibility, other evidence in this regard has been less consistent. For example, the Wisconsin Card Sorting Test (WCST) is often used to identify deficits in divergent reasoning in brain-injured patients. The task assesses the ability to identify when simple rule contingencies have changed and adapt to the new rules. Damage to the prefrontal cortex frequently leads to deficits in the ability to recognize when the contingencies of this task has been switched and make appropriate behavioural adjustments. Based on findings described thus far, one might expect that sleep deprivation would lead to clear and consistent deficits on the WCST, but this is far from the case. As reviewed by Jones and Harrison (2001), a number of clinical and experimental studies of sleep-deprived individuals have found deficits on the WCST, particularly with regard to perseveration on ineffective strategies, while others have found no significant effects. It must be borne in mind, however, that tasks such as the WCST were originally developed for clinical evaluation of deficits within patients suffering from tissue lesions or other pathology of the brain. Such tasks may be well suited for detecting severe levels of brain injury, but may not demonstrate adequate sensitivity for detecting the subtle types of executive function deficits and instability of performance that may accompany sleep loss.

Another limitation of many executive function tasks used in sleep deprivation studies is that they are so complex that they rely on multiple cognitive processes (e.g. the marketing strategy game described earlier), a limitation referred to as the ‘task impurity problem’ (Tucker et al., 2010). Consequently, impairments on such tasks could be attributable to a breakdown in one or more of the other component cognitive processes and not necessarily the executive aspects of the task. For instance, when Tucker et al. (2010) separated the components contributing to performance on a phonemic verbal fluency task, they found that sleep deprivation appeared to adversely affect non-executive aspects of the task while actually leading to an improvement in the executive components. Finally, these tasks are also often fun, interesting and challenging to subjects who are participating in long boring sleep deprivation studies, and this increased novelty in itself may increase motivation and alertness long enough to temporarily improve performance. While it is clear that many divergent thinking tasks show impairment during sleep deprivation, more research is needed to identify what component processes may be affected or whether these may simply reflect a global decline in basic alertness.

Cognitive control

The ability to modulate cognitive processes, for example the ability to switch rapidly and flexibly between two different rule sets depending on the situation, is another aspect of executive functioning. A recent study examined the effect of a single night of sleep deprivation on this capacity by calculating the ‘task-switch cost’ of alternating randomly between two different cognitive tasks that rely on exactly the same visual stimuli (Couyoumdjian et al., 2010). Both tasks involved a series of single-digit numbers presented on a screen. In the first task, participants had to rapidly make a key press to indicate whether the digit was an odd or even number. In the alternate task, the same key presses had to be made to indicate if each digit was either smaller or larger than 5. On some trials, the task remained the same (i.e. trial type was repeated), while on other trials, the task shifted randomly from one rule set to another (i.e. the switch task). Compared to subjects allowed to sleep normally, sleep-deprived individuals showed deficits on the switch task, suggesting that sleep loss reduced the capacity to modify behaviour rapidly and flexibly to changing demands of the environment. Furthermore, the deficit was only observed on task-switching trials but not on repetition trials, suggesting that the effect was not due to a generalized effect of reduced alertness and attention (Couyoumdjian et al., 2010).

Another cognitive control capacity is the ability to ignore irrelevant aspects of a task and reduce cognitive interference. This process is often measured with various forms of the Stroop interference paradigm. Sagaspe et al. (2006) administered three different types of Stroop tasks to healthy subjects at several time points over a 36-h sleep deprivation period. Interestingly, no deficits were found for the standard colour-word, emotional or sleep content-specific Stroop tasks, suggesting that sleep deprivation does not reliably affect performance on these types of conflict resolution problems. One possibility for differences between the findings for the switching and interference tasks may involve the brain regions and networks involved for each. Evidence suggests that task switching often relies heavily upon the ventral regions of the brain such as the orbitofrontal cortex, whereas the Stroop paradigms often draw more heavily upon dorsal and caudal regions of the brain, such as the anterior cingulate gyrus. These regions may be differentially affected by sleep loss or differentially capable of engaging in compensatory recruitment.

Inhibitory control

The ability to inhibit inappropriate or maladaptive behaviour is another critical facet of executive functioning. This includes behaviour that might be highly adaptive or appropriate under one set of circumstances, but which may be better withheld under other circumstances. Most commonly, this capacity is measured with some variant of the 'go/no-go' paradigm, in which a participant learns to respond (i.e. 'go') to a frequently occurring stimulus but must withhold that response (i.e. 'no-go') to a less frequently occurring stimulus. This capacity appears to be modulated by predominantly right inferior lateral prefrontal cortex (Chuah et al., 2006), a region that shows decreased metabolic activity during sleep deprivation (Thomas et al., 2000), and would, therefore, be expected to show a decline in performance during periods of extended sleep loss. Drummond and colleagues studied the effects of two nights of sleep deprivation on response inhibition using a go/no-go task (Drummond et al., 2006). Subjects were significantly impaired in their ability to withhold prepotent (i.e. automatic) responses in the face of 'no-go' stimuli when tested at 23, 32 and 55 h of sleep deprivation, a capacity that returned to baseline rates following recovery sleep. Of note, the ability to respond correctly to 'go' stimuli (simple attention and response speed) was not adversely affected by sleep loss until the 55-h test session. These findings suggest that inhibitory control declined early in the course of sleep deprivation despite relatively sustained ability to attend to and respond to the stimuli (Drummond et al., 2006). These findings argue against a simple 'global decline' in basic attention as an explanation, as inhibitory processes showed deficits in the presence of intact attention to the stimuli during the first night of sleep deprivation.

Neuroimaging may also provide some insight into the neural processes involved in the changes in inhibitory capacity following sleep loss. Chuah and colleagues studied the effect of 24 h of sleep deprivation on fMRI brain activation patterns during a go/no-go task (Chuah et al., 2006). As expected, one night of sleep deprivation was associated with significant tonic reductions in task-related activation of anterior and ventrolateral prefrontal cortex. Moreover, the ability to successfully inhibit responses during sleep deprivation was associated with greater ability to recruit the right ventrolateral prefrontal cortex and right anterior insula. The authors speculate that the increased activation of these regions may reflect a compensatory response to sleep deprivation among those most able to resist its effects (Chuah et al., 2006). Thus, these data suggest that there may be an identifiable neurobiological basis for the inter-individual differences in vulnerability versus resistance to sleep deprivation discussed earlier (Mu et al., 2005a; Van Dongen, 2005).

Risk-taking, judgement and decision making

The effects of sleep deprivation on decision-making capacities are particularly complex. This complexity arises because decision making often does not rely solely upon 'cold' cognitive processes, which are purely rational and free of emotional influences. Rather, judgement and decision-making processes are often biased by, and indeed generally rely heavily upon, emotional factors that in many cases lead to more streamlined decisions. One of the most profound effects of sleep deprivation is an alteration in normal mood and emotional functioning, which may affect the assessment of risk and the types of judgements and decisions people ultimately make. This was exemplified in a study that examined the effects of 49 h of sleep deprivation on behaviour during an emotionally guided gambling task that assessed the willingness to relinquish immediate gratification to ensure long-term success (i.e. the Iowa Gambling Task – IGT) (Killgore et al., 2006a). As shown in Fig. 4, normally rested subjects gradually learned to avoid exciting high-risk decks in favour of decks providing modest but more consistent payoffs. After two

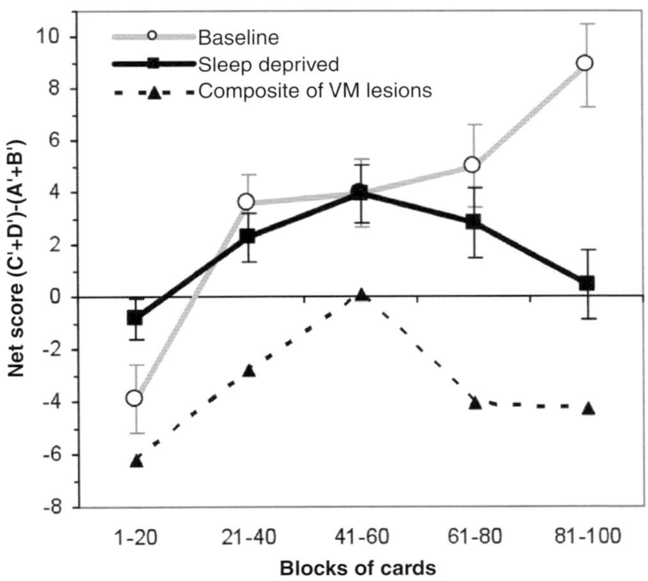

Fig. 4. Performance on the Iowa Gambling Task (IGT) at rested baseline and again following two nights of sleep deprivation. Data reflect the net score difference between the number of selections from advantageous decks (i.e. decks C' and D') minus the number of selections from disadvantageous decks (i.e. decks A' and B') for each block of 20 trials. At rested baseline (grey line with open circles), participants gradually learned to avoid disadvantageous decks and chose more frequently from advantageous decks. In contrast, following 49.5 h of sleep deprivation (black line with filled squares), the same subjects showed a significantly different pattern of performance that was best characterized by a quadratic function, demonstrating a shift in behaviour towards advantageous decks in the first half of the game followed by a reversal of behaviour towards progressively more choices from disadvantageous decks in the latter half of the game. For comparison, the figure also shows a composite line calculated by extrapolating and summarizing IGT data reported from previously published reports of patients with damage to the ventromedial prefrontal cortex (dashed line with filled triangles). Reprinted with permission from Killgore et al. (2006a).

nights of sleep loss, however, these same subjects tended to prefer riskier selections, despite the long-term losses that resulted. In fact, the pattern of performance of the sleep-deprived volunteers mirrored that typically observed among patients with lesions to the ventromedial (VM) prefrontal cortex. This same pattern was replicated in a second study that extended the period of sleep deprivation to 75 h (Killgore et al., 2007d) and was not reversed by the administration of caffeine, suggesting that the impairments are unlikely to be due simply to global deficits in alertness and vigilance. Thus, sleep deprivation may specifically impair the capacity to effectively integrate emotional cues into the decision-making process (Killgore et al., 2006a, 2007d).

The effect of sleep deprivation on risk-taking is also affected by the individual's cognitive set (i.e. whether the risk is framed in terms of gains or losses). If an outcome is presented in terms of a potential gain, sleep-deprived subjects are more likely to take risks than they would when rested, but are less likely to take risks than they ordinarily would if an outcome is framed in terms of a potential loss (McKenna et al., 2007). Recent neuroimaging findings suggest that sleep deprivation may alter expectations of gains and losses by affecting activation within reward regions of the brain. When sleep-deprived subjects made risky decisions, they showed increased activation of reward centres, consistent with an expectation of gains (Venkatraman et al., 2007). By contrast, when sleep-deprived subjects experienced losses, they show reduced activity in brain regions normally associated with aversion and punishment. In other words, sleep deprivation may alter the normal functional activity of brain networks involved in the evaluation of rewards and punishments, leading to changes in risk-related judgements that may favour unrealistic expectations of gains and underestimation of the consequences of losses.

Finally, sleep deprivation appears to have particularly salient effects on socio-emotional decisions that have implications for social exchange and morally relevant behaviour. Anderson and Dickinson (2010) presented sleep-deprived individuals with a series of 'bargaining' and 'trust' games, with actual financial consequences (Anderson and Dickinson, 2010). Thirty-six hours of sleep deprivation was associated with more aggressive social exchanges in these games, as evidenced by reduced willingness to trust an unknown partner and greater rejection of bargaining offers perceived as 'unfair', even when such rejections knowingly led to financial losses for both parties. In other words, sleep-deprived subjects preferred to reject an unfair offer outright, even if it meant earning no money for themselves from the deal, rather than accept a bargain whereby they would receive a sum of money that was significantly less than that received by the other party. These findings are consistent with the reduced empathy and increased symptoms of paranoia and feelings of persecution discussed earlier, and suggest that sleep deprivation increases the impact of emotion on decision-making processes in social situations.

Sleep deprivation also affects emotionally guided moral judgements (Killgore et al., 2007c). Killgore and colleagues presented healthy subjects with a series of moral dilemmas when they were well rested and a matched set of similar dilemmas following two nights of total sleep deprivation. For each dilemma, a difficult decision-making scenario was vividly described and a proposed solution was given for each problem. Subjects simply judged whether the proposed solution for each dilemma was 'appropriate' or 'inappropriate'. Three types of dilemmas were presented, which differed only in the emotional immediacy of the decision, ranging from benign to highly personal and emotionally intense. Interestingly, two nights of sleep deprivation had little to no effect on the speed of decision making about benign situations or even moral situations with little personal emotional involvement. However, compared to rested baseline, sleep deprivation resulted in significant slowing of decision making when the dilemma was highly emotionally charged and required direct personal involvement (see Fig. 5). Individuals were also more prone to violating their own moral positions

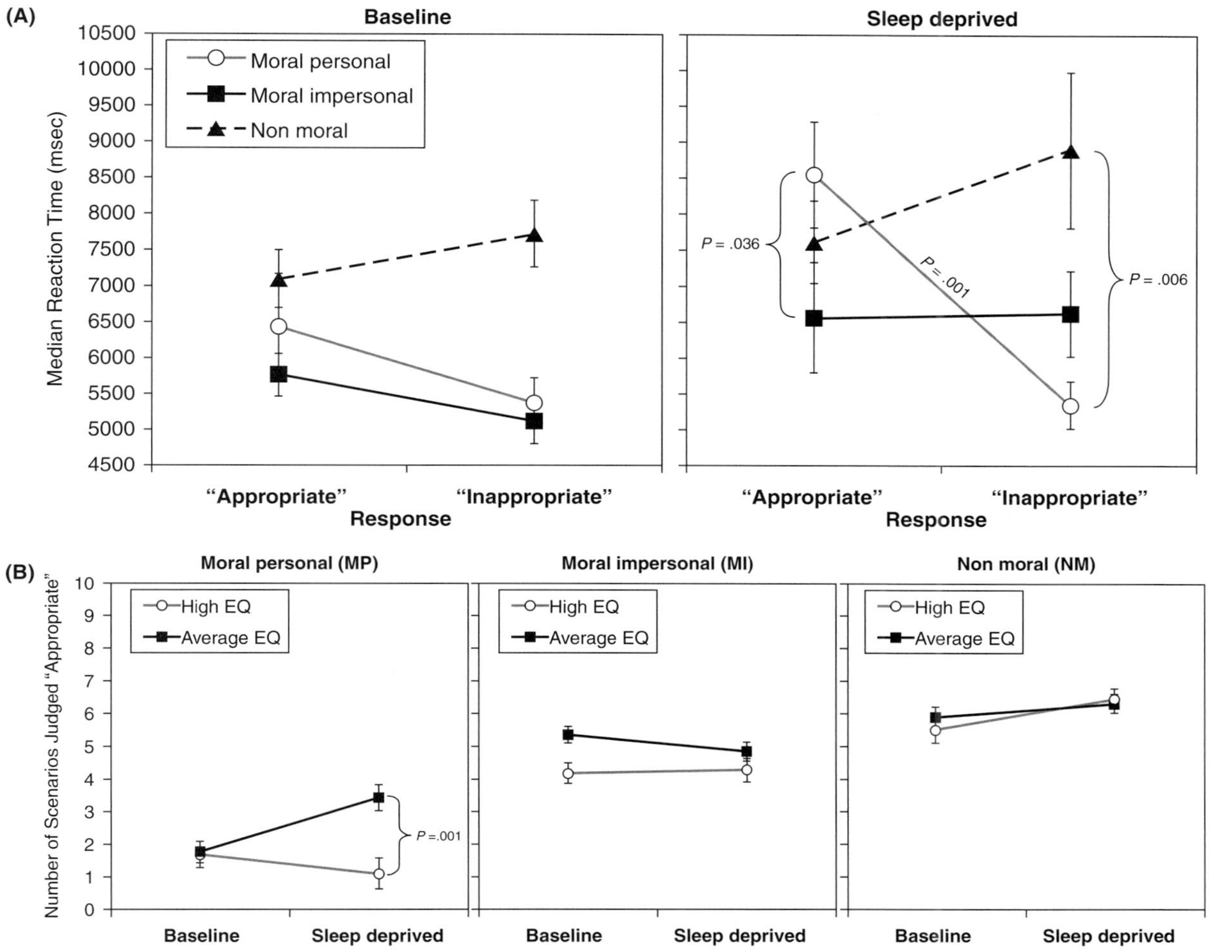

Fig. 5. Moral Personal Judgements are more affected by sleep loss than other types of judgements. (A) Median response times for moral personal, moral impersonal and non-moral dilemmas at baseline and following 53.5 h of continuous wakefulness. (B) Mean number of times various courses of action were judged as 'appropriate' for the moral personal, moral impersonal and non-moral dilemmas at baseline and following 53.5 h of sleep deprivation by individuals with high versus average (or lower) levels of Emotional Intelligence. Reprinted with permission from Killgore et al. (2007c).

when sleep deprived than when rested, and none of the findings were affected by the administration of caffeine. Again, these findings support the proposition that sleep deprivation adversely affects executive function systems, particularly those involving the ability to modulate emotional reactions and effectively integrate affective information into the decision-making process (Killgore et al., 2007c).

Conclusions

Sleep deprivation appears to have both global and specific effects on cognition, presumably due to differential susceptibility of various functionally interdependent brain systems to sleep loss or differences in the extent to which particular regions are taxed during waking. The most consistent effects of sleep deprivation include reduced attention and psychomotor vigilance and increased variability in behavioural responses, effects that are associated with altered functioning of dorsolateral prefrontal cortex and parietal regions. To the extent that cognitive processes rely on basic attention and sustained vigilance, sleep deprivation appears to have a global degrading effect. Sleep deprivation also alters normal affective processing, possibly through weakening of prefrontal inhibitory systems that allow emotional systems to run relatively unchecked, without appropriate modulation or effective integration of emotion. This affective dysregulation ultimately leads to a negative emotional bias in mood, perception and memory, reduced frustration tolerance, and difficulty using emotion to adaptively inform decision making. A number of studies have shown that many of these deficits remain even when alertness and vigilance are restored or sustained with stimulants such as caffeine, suggesting that there are specific effects of sleep loss on higher cognition beyond those accounted for by global declines in alertness and attention. Nevertheless, inconsistent findings pervade the literature on the effects of sleep deprivation on higher executive functions, and more work is necessary to identify which components of these capacities are reliably degraded by sleep loss. It is likely that any unifying explanation will view the effects of sleep deprivation as stemming from its differential influences on multiple hierarchically organized brain systems that depend to varying degrees on the reciprocal effects of cognitive control and emotional processes.

References

Adam, M., Retey, J. V., Khatami, R., & Landolt, H. P. (2006). Age-related changes in the time course of vigilant attention during 40 h without sleep in men. *Sleep*, *29*, 55–57.

Anderson, C., & Dickinson, D. L. (2010). Bargaining and trust: The effects of 36-h total sleep deprivation on socially interactive decisions. *Journal of Sleep Research*, *19*, 54–63.

Babkoff, H., Caspy, T., Mikulincer, M., & Sing, H. C. (1991). Monotonic and rhythmic influences: A challenge for sleep deprivation research. *Psychological Bulletin*, *109*, 411–428.

Babkoff, H., Zukerman, G., Fostick, L., & Ben-Artzi, E. (2005). Effect of the diurnal rhythm and 24 h of sleep deprivation on dichotic temporal order judgment. *Journal of Sleep Research*, *14*, 7–15.

Belenky, G., Wesensten, N. J., Thorne, D. R., Thomas, M. L., Sing, H. C., & Redmond, D. P., et al., (2003). Patterns of performance degradation and restoration during sleep restriction and subsequent recovery: A sleep dose-response study. *Journal of Sleep Research*, *12*, 1–12.

Borbely, A. A. (1982). A two process model of sleep regulation. *Human Neurobiology*, *1*, 195–204.

Chee, M. W., & Tan, J. C. (2010). Lapsing when sleep deprived: Neural activation characteristics of resistant and vulnerable individuals. *Neuroimage*, *51*, 835–843.

Chee, M. W., Tan, J. C., Zheng, H., Parimal, S., Weissman, D. H., & Zagorodnov, V., et al., (2008). Lapsing during sleep deprivation is associated with distributed changes in brain activation. *Journal of Neuroscience*, *28*, 5519–5528.

Chuah, L. Y., & Chee, M. W. (2008). Cholinergic augmentation modulates visual task performance in sleep-deprived young adults. *Journal of Neuroscience*, *28*, 11369–11377.

Chuah, Y. M., Venkatraman, V., Dinges, D. F., & Chee, M. W. (2006). The neural basis of interindividual variability in inhibitory efficiency after sleep deprivation. *Journal of Neuroscience*, *26*, 7156–7162.

Couyoumdjian, A., Sdoia, S., Tempesta, D., Curcio, G., Rastellini, E. L. D. E. G., & Ferrara, M. (2010). The effects of sleep and sleep deprivation on task-switching performance. *Journal of Sleep Research*, *19*, 64–70.

Damasio, A. R. (1994). *Descartes' error: Emotion, reason and the human brain.* Grosset/Putnam, New York.

Dawson, D., & Reid, K. (1997). Fatigue, alcohol and performance impairment. *Nature*, *388*, 235.

Diekelmann, S., & Born, J. (2010). The memory function of sleep. *Nature Reviews Neuroscience*, *11*, 114–126.

Dinges, D. F., & Powell, J. W. (1985). Microcomputer analyses of performance on a portable, simple, visual RT task during sustained operations. *Behavior Research Methods, Instruments, & Computers*, *17*, 652–655.

Dinges, D. F., Pack, F., Williams, K., Gillen, K. A., Powell, J. W., & Ott, G. E., et al., (1997). Cumulative sleepiness, mood disturbance, and psychomotor vigilance performance decrements during a week of sleep restricted to 4-5 h per night. *Sleep*, *20*, 267–277.

Doran, S. M., Van Dongen, H. P., & Dinges, D. F. (2001). Sustained attention performance during sleep deprivation: Evidence of state instability. *Archives Italiennes de Biologie (Pisa)*, *139*, 253–267.

Drummond, S. P., Bischoff-Grethe, A., Dinges, D. F., Ayalon, L., Mednick, S. C., & Meloy, M. J. (2005). The neural basis of the psychomotor vigilance task. *Sleep*, *28*, 1059–1068.

Drummond, S. P., Brown, G. G., Gillin, J. C., Stricker, J. L., Wong, E. C., & Buxton, R. B. (2000). Altered brain response to verbal learning following sleep deprivation. *Nature*, *403*, 655–657.

Drummond, S. P., Paulus, M. P., & Tapert, S. F. (2006). Effects of two nights sleep deprivation and two nights recovery sleep on response inhibition. *Journal of Sleep Research*, *15*, 261–265.

Duffy, J. F., Willson, H. J., Wang, W., & Czeisler, C. A. (2009). Healthy older adults better tolerate sleep deprivation than young adults. *Journal of the American Geriatric Society*, *57*, 1245–1251.

Furchtgott, E., & Willingham, W. W. (1956). The effect of sleep-deprivation upon the thresholds of taste. *American Journal of Psychology*, *69*, 111–112.

Gillberg, M., & Akerstedt, T. (1998). Sleep loss and performance: No "safe" duration of a monotonous task. *Physiology & Behavior*, *64*, 599–604.

Goel, N., Rao, H., Durmer, J. S., & Dinges, D. F. (2009). Neurocognitive consequences of sleep deprivation. *Seminars in Neurology*, *29*, 320–339.

Gottselig, J. M., Adam, M., Retey, J. V., Khatami, R., Achermann, P., & Landolt, H. P. (2006). Random number generation during sleep deprivation: Effects of caffeine on response maintenance and stereotypy. *Journal of Sleep Research*, *15*, 31–40.

Haack, M., Lee, E., Cohen, D. A., & Mullington, J. M. (2009). Activation of the prostaglandin system in response to sleep loss in healthy humans: Potential mediator of increased spontaneous pain. *Pain*, *145*, 136–141.

Harrison, Y., & Horne, J. A. (1999). One night of sleep loss impairs innovative thinking and flexible decision making. *Organizational Behavior and Human Decision Processes*, *78*, 128–145.

Harrison, Y., & Horne, J. A. (2000a). Sleep loss and temporal memory. *Quarterly Journal of Experimental Psychology A*, *53*, 271–279.

Harrison, Y., & Horne, J. A. (2000b). The impact of sleep deprivation on decision making: A review. *Journal of Experimental Psychology Applied*, *6*, 236–249.

Harrison, Y., Horne, J. A., & Rothwell, A. (2000). Prefrontal neuropsychological effects of sleep deprivation in young adults–a model for healthy aging? *Sleep*, *23*, 1067–1073.

Horne, J. A. (1988). Sleep loss and "divergent" thinking ability. *Sleep*, *11*, 528–536.

Horne, J. A., Anderson, N. R., & Wilkinson, R. T. (1983). Effects of sleep deprivation on signal detection measures of vigilance: Implications for sleep function. *Sleep*, *6*, 347–358.

Jones, K., & Harrison, Y. (2001). Frontal lobe function, sleep loss and fragmented sleep. *Sleep Medicine Reviews*, *5*, 463–475.

Kahn-Greene, E. T., Killgore, D. B., Kamimori, G. H., Balkin, T. J., & Killgore, W. D. S. (2007). The effects of sleep deprivation on symptoms of psychopathology in healthy adults. *Sleep Medicine*, *8*, 215–221.

Kahn-Greene, E. T., Lipizzi, E. L., Conrad, A. K., Kamimori, G. H., & Killgore, W. D. S. (2006). Sleep deprivation adversely affects interpersonal responses to frustration. *Personality and Individual Differences*, *41*, 1433–1443.

Kendall, A. P., Kautz, M. A., Russo, M. B., & Killgore, W. D. (2006). Effects of sleep deprivation on lateral visual attention. *International Journal of Neuroscience*, *116*, 1125–1138.

Killgore, W. D. S., & McBride, S. A. (2006). Odor identification accuracy declines following 24 h of sleep deprivation. *Journal of Sleep Research*, *15*, 111–116.

Killgore, W. D. S., Balkin, T. J., & Wesensten, N. J. (2006a). Impaired decision-making following 49 h of sleep deprivation. *Journal of Sleep Research*, *15*, 7–13.

Killgore, W. D. S., Grugle, N. L., Reichardt, R. M., Killgore, D. B., & Balkin, T. J. (2009a). Executive functions and the ability to sustain vigilance during sleep loss. *Aviation, Space, and Environmental Medicine*, *80*, 81–87.

Killgore, W. D. S., Kahn-Greene, E. T., Grugle, N. L., Killgore, D. B., & Balkin, T. J. (2009b). Sustaining executive functions during sleep deprivation: A comparison of caffeine, dextroamphetamine, and modafinil. *Sleep*, *32*, 205–216.

Killgore, W. D. S., Kahn-Greene, E. T., Lipizzi, E. L., Newman, R. A., Kamimori, G. H., & Balkin, T. J. (2007a). Sleep deprivation reduces perceived emotional intelligence and constructive thinking skills. *Sleep Medicine*, *8*, 331–343.

Killgore, W. D. S., Kendall, A. P., Richards, J. M., & McBride, S. A. (2007b). Lack of degradation in visuospatial perception of line orientation after one night of sleep loss. *Perceptual & Motor Skills*, *105*, 276–286.

Killgore, W. D. S., Killgore, D. B., Day, L. M., Li, C., Kamimori, G. H., & Balkin, T. J. (2007c). The effects of 53 h of sleep deprivation on moral judgment. *Sleep*, *30*, 345–352.

Killgore, W. D. S., Lipizzi, E. L., Kamimori, G. H., & Balkin, T. J. (2007d). Caffeine effects on risky decision-making after 75 h of sleep deprivation. *Aviation, Space, and Environmental Medicine*, *78*, 957–962.

Killgore, W. D. S., McBride, S. A., Killgore, D. B., & Balkin, T. J. (2006b). The effects of caffeine, dextroamphetamine, and modafinil on humor appreciation during sleep deprivation. *Sleep*, *29*, 841–847.

Killgore, W. D. S., McBride, S. A., Killgore, D. B., Balkin, T. J., & Kamimori, G. H. (2008a). Baseline odor identification ability predicts degradation of psychomotor vigilance during 77 h of sleep deprivation. *International Journal of Neuroscience*, *118*, 1207–1225.

Killgore, W. D. S., Richards, J. M., Killgore, D. B., Kamimori, G. H., & Balkin, T. J. (2007e). The trait of introversion-extraversion predicts vulnerability to sleep deprivation. *Journal of Sleep Research*, *16*, 354–363.

Killgore, W. D. S., Rupp, T. L., Grugle, N. L., Reichardt, R. M., Lipizzi, E. L., & Balkin, T. J. (2008b). Effects of dextroamphetamine, caffeine and modafinil on psychomotor vigilance test performance after 44 h of continuous wakefulness. *Journal of Sleep Research*, 309–321

Krueger, J. M., Rector, D. M., Roy, S., Van Dongen, H. P., Belenky, G., & Panksepp, J. (2008). Sleep as a fundamental property of neuronal assemblies. *Nature Reviews Neuroscience*, *9*, 910–919.

Kundermann, B., Spernal, J., Huber, M. T., Krieg, J. C., & Lautenbacher, S. (2004). Sleep deprivation affects thermal pain thresholds but not somatosensory thresholds in healthy volunteers. *Psychosomatic Medicine*, *66*, 932–937.

Lautenbacher, S., Kundermann, B., & Krieg, J. C. (2006). Sleep deprivation and pain perception. *Sleep Medicine Reviews*, *10*, 357–369.

Lim, J., & Dinges, D. F. (2008). Sleep deprivation and vigilant attention. *Annals of the New York Academy of Sciences*, *1129*, 305–322.

Lim, J., & Dinges, D. F. (2010). A meta-analysis of the impact of short-term sleep deprivation on cognitive variables. *Psychological Bulletin*, *136*, 375–389.

Manly, T., Dobler, V. B., Dodds, C. M., & George, M. A. (2005). Rightward shift in spatial awareness with declining alertness. *Neuropsychologia*, *43*, 1721–1728.

McBride, S. A., Balkin, T. J., Kamimori, G. H., & Killgore, W. D. S. (2006). Olfactory decrements as a function of two nights of sleep deprivation. *Journal of Sensory Studies*, *21*, 456–463.

McKenna, B. S., Dickinson, D. L., Orff, H. J., & Drummond, S. P. (2007). The effects of one night of sleep deprivation on known-risk and ambiguous-risk decisions. *Journal of Sleep Research*, *16*, 245–252.

Mu, Q., Mishory, A., Johnson, K. A., Nahas, Z., Kozel, F. A., & Yamanaka, K., et al., (2005a). Decreased brain activation during a working memory task at rested baseline is associated with vulnerability to sleep deprivation. *Sleep*, *28*, 433–446.

Mu, Q., Nahas, Z., Johnson, K. A., Yamanaka, K., Mishory, A., & Koola, J., et al., (2005b). Decreased cortical response to verbal working memory following sleep deprivation. *Sleep*, *28*, 55–67.

Pace-Schott, E. F., Hutcherson, C. A., Bemporad, B., Morgan, A., Kumar, A., & Hobson, J. A., et al., (2009). Failure to find executive function deficits following one night's total sleep deprivation in university students under naturalistic conditions. *Behavioral Sleep Medicine*, *7*, 136–163.

Peiris, M. T., Jones, R. D., Davidson, P. R., & Bones, P. J. (2008). Event-based detection of lapses of responsiveness. *Conference Proceedings – IEEE Engineering in Medicine and Biology Society*, *2008*, 4960–4963.

Poudel, G. R., Jones, R. D., Innes, C. R., Watts, R., Signal, T. L., & Bones, P. J. (2009). fMRI correlates of behavioural microsleeps during a continuous visuomotor task. *Conference Proceedings - IEEE Engineering in Medicine and Biology Society*, *2009*, 2919–2922.

Roge, J., & Gabaude, C. (2009). Deterioration of the useful visual field with age and sleep deprivation: Insight from signal detection theory. *Perceptual & Motor Skills*, *109*, 270–284.

Sagaspe, P., Sanchez-Ortuno, M., Charles, A., Taillard, J., Valtat, C., & Bioulac, B., et al., (2006). Effects of sleep deprivation on Color-Word, Emotional, and Specific Stroop interference and on self-reported anxiety. *Brain and Cognition*, *60*, 76–87.

Silva, E. J., Wang, W., Ronda, J. M., Wyatt, J. K., & Duffy, J. F. (2010). Circadian and wake-dependent influences on subjective sleepiness, cognitive throughput, and reaction time performance in older and young adults. *Sleep*, *33*, 481–490.

Stenuit, P., & Kerkhofs, M. (2005). Age modulates the effects of sleep restriction in women. *Sleep*, *28*, 1283–1288.

Steyvers, F. J., & Gaillard, A. W. (1993). The effects of sleep deprivation and incentives on human performance. *Psychology Research*, *55*, 64–70.

Tempesta, D., Couyoumdjian, A., Curcio, G., Moroni, F., Marzano, C., & De Gennaro, L., et al., (2010). Lack of sleep affects the evaluation of emotional stimuli. *Brain Research Bulletin*, *82*, 104–108.

Thomas, M., Sing, H., Belenky, G., Holcomb, H., Mayberg, H., & Dannals, R., et al., (2000). Neural basis of alertness and cognitive performance impairments during sleepiness. I. Effects of 24 h of sleep deprivation on waking human regional brain activity. *Journal of Sleep Research*, *9*, 335–352.

Tucker, A. M., Whitney, P., Belenky, G., Hinson, J. M., & Van Dongen, H. P. (2010). Effects of sleep deprivation on dissociated components of executive functioning. *Sleep*, *33*, 47–57.

Van Dongen, H. P. (2005). Brain activation patterns and individual differences in working memory impairment during sleep deprivation. *Sleep*, *28*, 386–388.

Van Dongen, H. P., & Belenky, G. (2009). Individual differences in vulnerability to sleep loss in the work environment. *Industrial Health*, *47*, 518–526.

Van Dongen, H. P., Baynard, M. D., Maislin, G., & Dinges, D. F. (2004). Systematic interindividual differences in neurobehavioral impairment from sleep loss: Evidence of trait-like differential vulnerability. *Sleep*, *27*, 423–433.

Van Dongen, H. P., Maislin, G., Mullington, J. M., & Dinges, D. F. (2003). The cumulative cost of additional wakefulness: Dose-response effects on neurobehavioral functions and sleep physiology from chronic sleep restriction and total sleep deprivation. *Sleep*, *26*, 117–126.

Vandewalle, G., Archer, S. N., Wuillaume, C., Balteau, E., Degueldre, C., & Luxen, A., et al., (2009). Functional magnetic resonance imaging-assessed brain responses during an executive task depend on interaction of sleep homeostasis, circadian phase, and PER3 genotype. *Journal of Neuroscience*, *29*, 7948–7956.

Venkatraman, V., Chuah, Y. M., Huettel, S. A., & Chee, M. W. (2007). Sleep deprivation elevates expectation of gains and attenuates response to losses following risky decisions. *Sleep*, *30*, 603–609.

von Schantz, M. (2008). Phenotypic effects of genetic variability in human clock genes on circadian and sleep parameters. *Journal of Genetics*, *87*, 513–519.

Walker, M. P. (2009). The role of sleep in cognition and emotion. *Annals of the New York Academy of Sciences*, *1156*, 168–197.

Walker, M. P., & Stickgold, R. (2006). Sleep, memory, and plasticity. *Annual Review of Psychology*, *57*, 139–166.

Walker, M. P., & van der Helm, E. (2009). Overnight therapy? The role of sleep in emotional brain processing. *Psychological Bulletin*, *135*(5); 731–748.

Wesensten, N. J., Killgore, W. D. S., & Balkin, T. J. (2005). Performance and alertness effects of caffeine, dextroamphetamine, and modafinil during sleep deprivation. *Journal of Sleep Research*, *14*, 255–266.

Yoo, S. S., Gujar, N., Hu, P., Jolesz, F. A., & Walker, M. P. (2007a). The human emotional brain without sleep–a prefrontal amygdala disconnect. *Current Biology*, *17*, R877–R878.

Yoo, S. S., Hu, P. T., Gujar, N., Jolesz, F. A., & Walker, M. P. (2007b). A deficit in the ability to form new human memories without sleep. *Nature Neuroscience*, *10*, 385–392.

G. A. Kerkhof and H. P. A. Van Dongen (Eds.)
Progress in Brain Research, Vol. 185
ISSN: 0079-6123

CHAPTER 8

Circadian rhythms and cognition

Jim Waterhouse*

Research Institute for Sport and Exercise Sciences, Liverpool John Moores University, Liverpool, UK

Abstract: Like all circadian (near-24-h) rhythms, those of cognition have endogenous and exogenous components. The origins of these components, together with effects of time awake upon cognitive performance, are described in subjects living conventionally (sleeping at night and active during the daytime). Based on these considerations, predictions can be made about changes that might be expected in the days after a time-zone transition and during night work. The relevant literature on these circumstances is then reviewed. The last section of the chapter deals with sleep-wake schedules where both regular and irregular sleeps are taken (anchor sleep).

Keywords: Cognitive performance; circadian rhythms; sleep-wake cycle; time awake; sleep loss; anchor sleep

Background

Homeostasis and rhythms

Homeostasis, keeping the internal environment within narrow limits compatible with life, is a key concept in biology. Even so, the development of methods to measure physiological and biochemical variables repeatedly and often non-invasively during the course of a 24-h period has indicated that daily rhythms are superimposed upon this stability. For example, in humans, who are normally diurnal creatures, active by day and asleep at night, core temperature is about 1–2°C higher by day than night, the excretion of excess water and waste materials by the kidneys is higher during the daytime and metabolism is mainly of glucose by day and of fats by night (Minors and Waterhouse, 1981a; Reilly et al., 1997; Waterhouse and DeCoursey, 2004a). Rhythmic changes in the body's physiology and biochemistry are ubiquitous.

These observed rhythms derive partly from our diurnal existence and the rhythmic environment in which we live; they derive also from an internal 'body clock'. One of the simplest ways to

*Corresponding author.
Tel.: (+) 44 161 432 6352.
E-mail: waterhouseathome@hotmail.com

DOI:10.1016/B978-0-444-53702-7.00008-7

illustrate the presence of this body clock is to perform a 'constant routine' (Mills et al., 1978). In this protocol, subjects are required to stay awake and sedentary or lie down for at least 24 h in an environment of constant temperature, humidity and lighting, to engage in reduced or low-level activities throughout this interval, generally reading or listening to music, and to eat identical meals at regularly spaced intervals. With such a protocol, any rhythmicity due to the individual's environment and lifestyle has been removed and any that remains must, therefore, be internal in origin.

This separation of a measured rhythm into these two components by the constant routine protocol is illustrated in Fig. 1.

The full line shows the rhythm of core temperature in a group of eight volunteers sleeping from about midnight to 08:00 h and physically and mentally active during the daytime. The rhythm shows a peak around the late afternoon and a minimum during sleep around 05:00 h. As indicated by the dashed line in Fig. 1, the rhythm of core temperature persists, but with a diminished amplitude, during the constant routine. Three general deductions can be made from these findings:

1. The rhythm observed during the constant routine must arise from within the body; it is termed the endogenous component of the rhythm and its generation is attributed to the 'body clock' (circadian pacemaker).
2. Effects due to the environment and lifestyle are present, since the two rhythms (full and dashed lines) are not identical; this difference between the two rhythms is termed the exogenous component of the rhythm.
3. In subjects living a conventional lifestyle, these two components are in phase. During the daytime, the body temperature is raised by the body clock acting in synchrony with the environment and activity; during the night, the clock, environment and inactivity all reduce core temperature.

These general concepts apply to all physiological and biochemical variables though there are differences in detail dependent upon the variable under consideration. The three main differences relate to the timing of the daily rhythm, the nature of the exogenous component and the relative strengths of

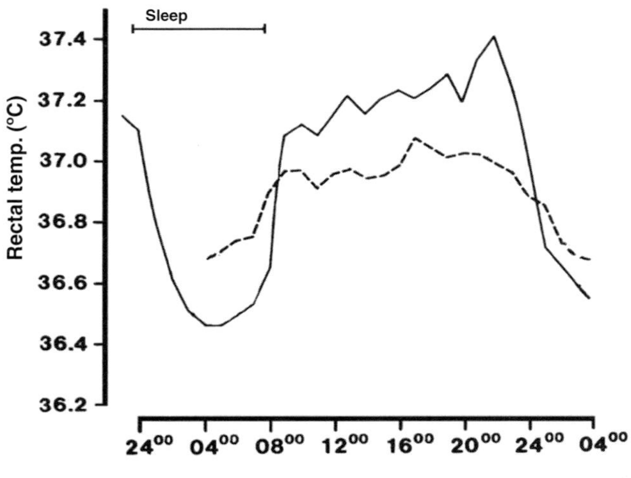

Fig. 1. Mean circadian changes in core (rectal) temperature measured hourly in eight subjects living normally and sleeping from 24:00 to 08:00 h (solid line) and then woken at 04:00 h and spending the next 24 h on a 'constant routine' (dashed line). Based on Minors and Waterhouse (1981a).

the two components of the rhythm. Some examples to illustrate these differences are as follows:

1. For variables associated with activity (cardiovascular variables and plasma adrenaline, for example), the timing is similar to that of core temperature, whereas for variables associated with growth and repair (which occur more during sleep), the phase tends to be the opposite (growth hormone and cortisol, for example).
2. The exogenous component for core temperature (as for heart rate and blood pressure) consists of increases caused by light and different types of activity (mental, physical, social and so on) during waking and decreases caused by darkness, a change in posture, sleep and inactivity during the night. For antidiuretic hormone (ADH), the exogenous influences are water intake and posture; for insulin, the exogenous influence is mainly food intake; for growth hormone, the exogenous influence is dominated by sleep onset; for melatonin, the main exogenous influence is strong light, which suppresses its secretion by the pineal gland; for cognitive performance and cognitive skills, it is the ambient conditions (light, noise and temperature, for example) under which the task is being performed. Other factors influence cognition, including time-since-waking, prior sleep loss and mood, for example, but these are not exogenous factors.
3. For many variables such as heart rate, blood pressure and growth hormone, the exogenous component of the measured rhythm is far stronger than the effect of the body clock. As a result, these rhythms always peak during the active period of the subject. By contrast, for melatonin secretion (in dim light), it is the endogenous component which is stronger; consequently, this rhythm can be used as a marker of the phase of the body clock (discussed below). In subjects living normally (i.e., without being either completely sedentary or excessively active), the two components are similar in size for core body temperature (see Fig. 1), and this variable is also often used as a clock marker.

Many experiments, including those measuring cognitive function, begin with a control phase in which ‘baseline’ measurements are taken under conditions that are controlled as closely as possible – the subject is seated and relaxed, the environmental temperature, humidity and lighting are maintained at constant values, prior activity and food/fluid intakes are standardized and so on. Even though the effects of the body clock will still be present under such circumstances, the effects of changes in the exogenous component will have been minimized by this protocol; moreover, experimental designs often fix the time of day when measurements are made, in an attempt to rule out the influence of the circadian clock altogether.

The body clock and some of its properties and roles

The body clock consists of paired suprachiasmatic nuclei (SCN) situated at the base of the hypothalamus and close to areas of the brain that exert effects throughout the body (Clayton et al., 2001; Reppert and Weaver, 2001). These effects include temperature regulation, hormone secretion and the sleep-wake and feeding cycles. When individuals are studied in time-free environments (in an underground cave, for example), the body clock and the rhythms it produces continue to be manifest. However, whereas the rhythms show a period of exactly 24 h when measured in subjects living in the 24-h world (the same as that of the solar day), this period is closer to 25 h than 24 h when measured in conditions of temporal isolation. It is for this reason that the clock and rhythms are called circadian (from Latin for about a day), and the circadian system in temporal isolation is described as ‘free running’. This period of about 25 h was originally believed to represent the intrinsic period of the body clock, but is now considered to be an overestimate of the true value due to effects of light exposure during wake times. Evidence from protocols using very dim light during the wake time or from blind subjects estimates the intrinsic period of the clock to be about 24.3 h (Shanahan and Czeisler, 2000).

Whatever its exact period, for the body clock to be of functional value, it and the rhythms it drives need to be synchronized exactly to the solar (24 h) day. This adjustment is achieved by zeitgebers (from German for time giver), occurring on a 24-h basis and resulting, directly or indirectly, from the environment. Zeitgebers adjust or re-time the body clock to the zeitgeber period. In humans, the most important zeitgeber is the light–dark cycle. Other zeitgebers, such as exercise, social factors and food intake, appear to play a minor role only when normal light–dark cycles are present. Nevertheless, under normal circumstances, all zeitgebers will act harmoniously to adjust the phase of the body clock.

When light acts upon the body clock, its effect depends on the time of presentation, and the time of the temperature minimum (normally around 05:00 h, see Fig. 1) is an important marker for this. Light presented during the 6 h after this minimum advances the body clock to an earlier time, during the 6 h before this minimum delays it to a later time and at other times exerts no significant effect upon the body clock (Khalsa et al., 2003). This relationship between the time of light exposure and the phase shift of the body clock that it produces is called a phase response curve (PRC). The size of the phase shifts produced also depends upon the intensity of the light; in the many individuals who nowadays have very little exposure to natural daylight, domestic lighting seems to be sufficient to shift the circadian clock and entrain it to a 24-h rhythm (Waterhouse et al., 1998).

Ingestion of melatonin, a hormone marking the biological night, can adjust the phase of the body clock. The shift produced depends on the timing of ingestion and tends to be the inverse of that produced by light (Lewy et al., 1998). Thus, ingestion in the afternoon and early evening advances the body clock and in the second half of sleep and during the early morning delays it. Since light inhibits endogenous melatonin secretion (normally highest during the darkness of the night and negligible during the bright light of daytime), the clock-shifting effects of light and melatonin reinforce each other; that is, bright light in the first hours after the temperature minimum advances the body clock, not only directly (via the PRC to light) but also indirectly (by suppressing melatonin secretion and so preventing the phase-delaying effect that melatonin would have exerted at this time).

Due to its position deep inside the brain, the body clock is difficult to study directly; 'clock markers' need to be used instead. Clock markers are rhythmic variables, the timing of which is bound closely to the activity of the body clock, so that the phase of the body clock can be inferred from the timing of the marker rhythm. The two markers used most frequently are core temperature and melatonin secretion. Core temperature is comparatively cheap to monitor, and continuous recording of rectal temperature is not difficult (though not always liked by the subjects!). The problem with this marker is that the exogenous component must be minimized. In practice, this means measuring core temperature whilst the subject is undergoing a constant routine – though methods to correct the temperature rhythm for the exogenous effects of the sleep-wake cycle have been developed (Waterhouse et al., 2000; Weinert et al., 2003). Melatonin is expensive to assay but its concentration can be measured in plasma (requiring continual blood sampling) or in the saliva, or its metabolite can be measured in the urine (requiring frequent emptying of the bladder) (Arendt, 1989). Since the rhythm of melatonin is little affected by sleep and activity, a constant routine is not required, but as melatonin secretion is suppressed by light, it is necessary for the subject to remain in dim light. Since melatonin is not normally secreted in the daytime, the time of onset of secretion (DLMO, dim light melatonin onset) is often used as the phase marker rather than the whole of the cycle (Lewy et al., 1998).

The body clock exerts two main influences upon the body's physiology. First, it promotes daytime activities (physical activity and cognition) and separates them from nocturnal sleep (when mental, physical and biochemical recovery and restitution occur). Second, it prepares individuals for going to sleep in the evening and waking up in the morning, these preparations requiring an ordered sequence of biochemical and physiological events to be accomplished (Waterhouse and DeCoursey, 2004a).

In short, we are rhythmic creatures attuned to our rhythmic environment: in the night, low core temperature and activity of the sympathetic nervous system (SNS) enable sleep and metabolism is biased towards fat metabolism and glucose conservation (for the brain); in the late night and early morning, the body clock prepares us for awakening; in the daytime, high levels of SNS activity and core temperature enable our physical and mental performance to be at their peak, and insulin secretion causes the metabolism of glucose and storage of excess calories in adipose tissue (Waterhouse et al., 1999); and in the evening, the body clock 'tones us down' in preparation for sleep. This rhythmicity is attained through integration between the body clock and the sleep-wake cycle, core temperature and melatonin secretion being important links (Krauchi and Wirz-Justice, 1994; Lack and Lushington, 1996; Murphy and Campbell, 1997; Shochat et al., 1997).

This integration between us and our environment has considerable inertia and protects against transient changes in our lifestyle (taking a daytime night or waking at night, for example) or in our environment (flashes of lightning at night or dark thunder clouds blacking out the daylight, for example), which do not alter the phase of the body clock. This robust property of the body clock has strong ecological value, but it causes problems when the individual's sleep-wake cycle is changed, as after a time-zone transition or during night work, for example (see 'Changes in cognitive performance after time-zone transitions and during night work' section).

Rhythms of cognitive performance and factors affecting them

To appreciate the problems that will be produced by time-zone transitions and night work, it is necessary to understand the normal relationship between cognitive performance, the body clock and the sleep-wake cycle. This topic is covered in detail in other reviews (Åkerstedt, 2007; Åkerstedt and Gillberg, 1981; Dinges, 1995; Valdez et al., 2008; Waterhouse et al., 2001) and chapters of this book, but the salient features are as follows.

A. The ease of falling asleep, the ability to maintain sleep and the likelihood of waking up are all associated with the rhythms of core temperature and melatonin secretion. Falling asleep and maintaining sleep are easiest when the core temperature is falling or low (melatonin is rising or high), and most difficult when core temperature is rising or high (melatonin is falling or low). Spontaneous waking is most likely when core temperature is rising (melatonin is falling). Based on these results, if individuals are to obtain about 7–8 h sleep each day, it follows that this is most likely if sleep is started around 23:00 h (core temperature falling rapidly and melatonin rising rapidly) and ends around 07:00 h (core temperature rising rapidly and melatonin falling rapidly) (see Fig. 1). In practice, this accords with the sleep-wake habits of most individuals (Dijk and Czeisler, 1995).
   This parallelism between sleep propensity and core temperature has been interpreted as evidence of causality (see, e.g. Kleitman, 1963) but such parallelism also exists with regard to the profiles of melatonin and adrenaline secretion. The current view is that all of these rhythms are acting as markers of the output of the SCN and that the detailed causes of the rhythms of sleep propensity remain to be established.

B. When exogenous influences have been standardized or kept constant, cognitive performance is mainly determined by the combination of effects due to a circadian component (originating from the body clock and parallel to the rhythm of core temperature) and time awake. This combination becomes the basis of many models predicting alertness and performance (Neri, 2004; Van Dongen, 2004).

One way to separate the contributions of these two components is to use a 'forced desynchronization' protocol. In this protocol, subjects live 'days' (defined as the period taken to complete an imposed sleep-wake cycle) of abnormal length, equal to 21, 27 or 28 solar hours, for example. With a 28-h 'day', the subjects' times of retiring, rising and eating meals, as well as all their daily activities and the imposed light–dark cycle, become 4 h later by solar time each 'day'. The body clock cannot adjust to such imposed zeitgeber periods and so shows a 'free-running' period just in excess of 24 h (see above). After about 6 imposed 'days', the sleep-wake cycle and body clock coincide once again (because $6 \times 28\ h = 7 \times 24\ h$); this length of time is called a beat cycle.

Data (cognitive performance results, for example) are collected regularly throughout at least one beat cycle. Each datum point can then be described both in terms of its phase in relationship to the body clock (circadian time) and in terms of its relationship to the sleep-wake cycle (time awake). In practice, results are put into 'bins' – say, 0–30° after the temperature maximum, 30–60° after the maximum etc. for the circadian bins and 0–2 h after waking, 2–4 h after waking etc. for the time-awake bins. All the results obtained from a beat cycle are treated in this way and the bins can then be averaged by two methods: (1) The results from each of the time-awake bins (0–2 h, 2–4 h etc.) can be averaged; this will have the effect of cancelling out the effects of the circadian component and so the effects of time awake alone can be shown by considering these averages. (2) The results from each of the circadian bins (0–30°, 30–60° etc.) can be averaged; this will have the effects of cancelling out the effects of the time-awake component and so the circadian component alone becomes manifest by considering these averages. Figure 2 illustrates this method, showing the example of mean subjective estimates of sleepiness by a group of subjects (Harrison et al., 2007).

Even though this protocol is currently the best experimental way to separate the influence of circadian and time-awake effects upon mood and cognitive performance rhythms, it is time consuming and repetitive sampling is required. It must be borne in mind that, for cognitive tasks, repetitive sampling requires a consideration of effects that might be due to practice and/or boredom (see, e.g. Chapter 51, Fulda and Schulz, 2010).

C. When the diurnal rhythms of performance tasks are considered, those of 'simple' tasks (with a comparatively small cognitive component) tend to parallel the rhythm of core temperature and peak in the late afternoon whereas those of more 'complex' tasks (with a larger cognitive component) tend to peak earlier in the day with an earlier and more marked fall afterwards (Folkard, 1990). If a cosine curve is fitted to the data, the maximum for the simple task will be close to that of core temperature but that of the complex task will peak earlier due to the earlier and more rapid fall after the peak.

A possible explanation of these different profiles is that, as in the two-process model of alertness (Åkerstedt and Folkard, 1991, 1997), performance profiles are a combination of a rhythmic component parallel to core temperature and a component that decrements with increasing time awake. It

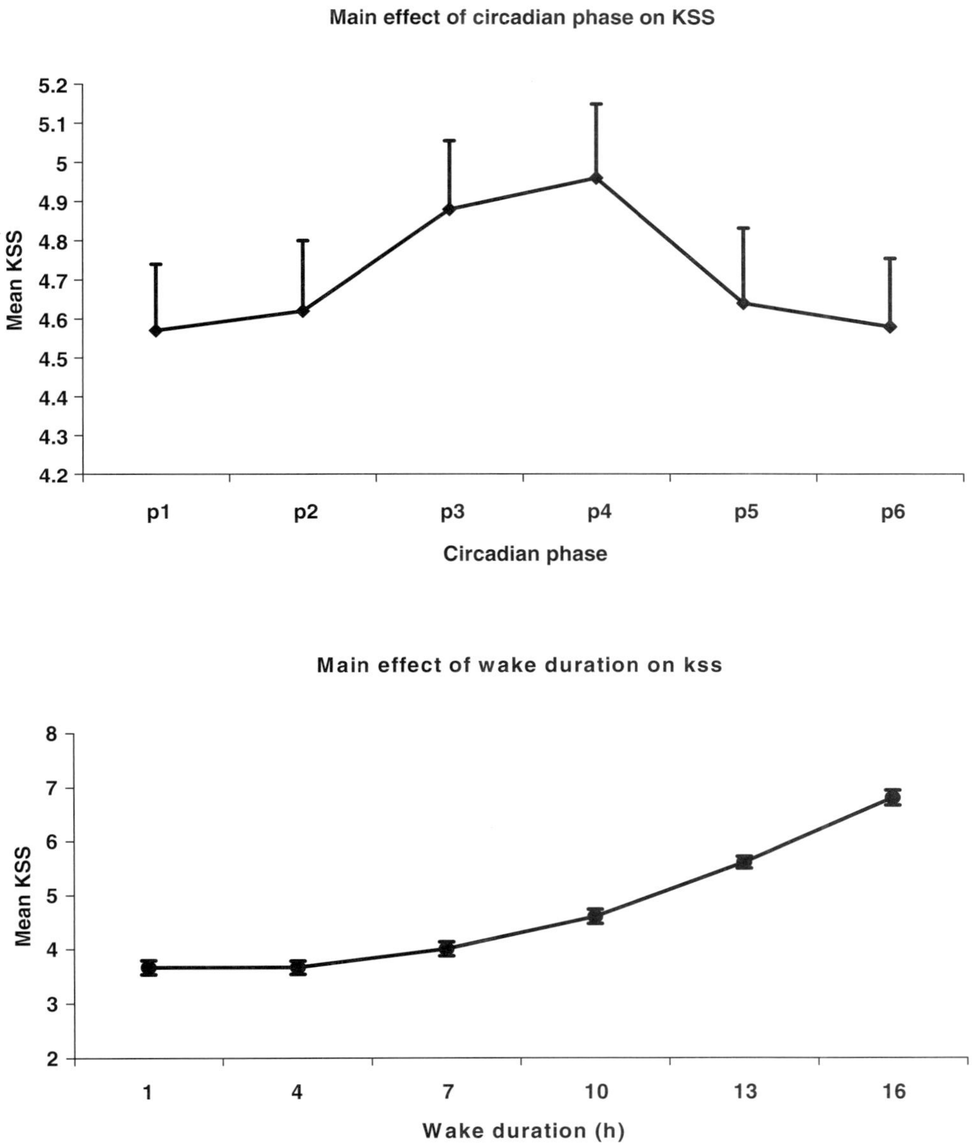

Fig. 2. Mean (+SE) scores for the Karolinska Sleepiness Scale (KSS) taken from subjects undergoing a forced desynchronization protocol (imposed 'days' of 28 h). Assessments of KSS were made 1, 4, 7, 10, 13 and 16 h after waking (total waking time was 18.67 h per 'day'). Top: Results shown relative to the circadian phase (p1–p6) of core temperature where p1 indicates a 60° 'bin' (where 360° equals the free-running period, tau) centred on the time of temperature maximum (30° before the maximum to 30° after the maximum), p2 indicates a bin 30–90° after this maximum, p3 indicates a bin 90–150° after this maximum, p4 indicates a bin 150–210° after this maximum (centred on the time of the temperature minimum), p5 indicates a bin 90–150° before the temperature maximum and p6 indicates a bin 30–90° before the temperature maximum. Bottom: Results shown relative to the number of hours awake. Taken from Harrison et al. (2007).

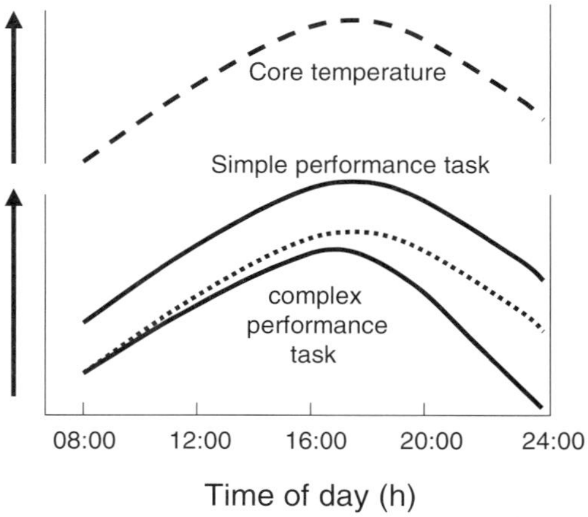

Fig. 3. Diagrammatic illustration of the diurnal rhythms of core temperature (top, dashed line) and 'simple' and 'complex' performance tasks (bottom, full lines). The upward arrows indicate higher temperature and better performance. For the simple performance task, the negative effect of time awake is small, and so the rhythm parallels that of core temperature. For the complex performance task, the effect of time awake is more marked; this makes the peak slightly earlier and the fall in performance after the peak more steep. The dotted line shows the time course the complex performance test would take in the absence of effects of time awake. For more details, see text. Based on Valdez et al. (2008).

is also supposed that the relative importance of these two factors depends upon the nature of the performance task, simple tasks being less influenced by the decrement due to time awake than are complex tasks (Fig. 3). Such a model predicts that the more important the decrement due to time awake, the sooner would the performance profile drop and the earlier would be the time of maximum of a cosine curve fitted to the profile. The degree to which time-awake effects depended upon the amount of cognition in a performance task could be investigated by separating the circadian and time-awake components using the forced desynchronization protocol (see Fig. 2). However, as far as the author is aware, those studies which have used the forced desynchronization protocol (see, e.g. Boivin et al., 1997; Harrison et al., 2007) have not systematically compared the rates of decrement of the time-awake component in tasks with different cognitive components.

An alternative test of the above explanation would be to investigate the fall in a variety of performance tests during a constant routine protocol. Several tasks requiring different amounts of cognition were investigated by Monk et al. (1997) using this protocol. However, the results were 'de-trended' before analysis, because the aim of the study was to compare circadian profiles of these tasks and any decrement due to time awake would have been a confounding factor. De-trending the results removed practice effects as well as those due to time awake, and so the amount of de-trending cannot be interpreted unambiguously.

D. Cognitive performance is also adversely affected by sleep loss, whether total or partial, acute or chronic (Åkerstedt, 2007; Dinges, 1995; Van Dongen and Dinges, 2005; Waterhouse et al., 2001). Since sleep loss of as little as 2 h can produce measurable decrements, these become a real possibility in subjects attempting sleep during the daytime when sleep is curtailed due to external disturbances and attempting sleep at a time that does not span the temperature minimum (see above).

E. In detail, individuals differ in the phasing of their lifestyle and circadian rhythms, and this determines their chronotype. An individual's chronotype score is measured by the Horne and Ostberg questionnaire (1976) which deals with individuals' preferred habits with respect to times of sleep, times when they feel most or least able to perform mentally or physically demanding tasks and times when they prefer to relax. The score shows a normal distribution but the 5–10% 'tails' of this are known as 'larks' (morning types) or 'owls' (evening types).

There is evidence that interpretation of individuals' scores requires knowledge of their cultural surroundings, but it has been a consistent finding that evening types show a greater sleep propensity in the morning and a later rise in sleep propensity in the evening (Lavie and Segal, 1989), and a later phasing of circadian rhythms of core temperature, cardiovascular variables and cognition (Kerkhof, 1985; Vidacek et al., 1988). The difference in phasing of core temperature is retained during a constant routine (Kerkhof and Van Dongen, 1996), indicating that it is at least partially due to the output of the body clock, regardless of differences in timing of the sleep-wake cycle.

Recent work indicates that polymorphisms exist in one of the human clock genes, PER3 (Archer et al., 2003; Mongrain and Dumont, 2007), and changes in part of this gene are associated with being an 'extreme lark' or 'extreme owl'. Extreme larks also suffer more adverse consequences of sleep deprivation and disruption, and the term 'trototype' has been coined to describe differences in susceptibility to sleep loss (see below).

Changes in cognitive performance after time-zone transitions and during night work

From these basic principles, changes in cognitive performance after time-zone transitions and during shift work can be predicted. In both circumstances, a brief explanation of the predictions will be given and then the current evidence relating to these predictions will be summarized.

Cognitive performance after time-zone transitions

After a time-zone transition, the body clock is slow to adjust and so, for some days after the journey, it is not adjusted to the new time zone (Dean et al., 2009; Haimov and Arendt, 1999; Waterhouse and DeCoursey, 2004b; Waterhouse et al., 1997, 2007). Adjustment of the body clock is brought about by the changed timing of the zeitgebers in the new time zone; adjustment is progressive and equivalent to 1–2 time zones per day. Before adjustment of the body clock has taken place, the normal synchrony between the endogenous and exogenous components of circadian rhythms will be absent (see Fig. 1 and associated text) – because only the exogenous component (due to the environment and individual's lifestyle) can be adjusted immediately in accord with timing in the new environment. This lack of synchrony will affect many aspects of the body's physiology and biochemistry and the individual will suffer from a group of symptoms known collectively as 'jet lag'. These symptoms regress as the body clock adjusts.

Some symptoms of jet lag recover more quickly than others. This difference can be explained in terms of the relative strengths of the adjusted exogenous and unadjusted endogenous components of the circadian rhythm for each variable. For those variables in which the exogenous component is stronger than the endogenous component (heart rate and appetite, for example), adjustment will appear to be more rapid; by contrast, for those variables with a stronger endogenous component (motivation, concentration and cognitive performance, for example), the rate of adjustment will be slower, in line with that of the body clock.

There are two reasons why deteriorations in cognitive performance are to be expected during the new daytime in the days immediately after the time-zone transition. First, after a flight across, say, eight time zones to the east, core temperature will not peak at 17:00 h by the new local time but rather at 01:00 h, and after a flight across eight time zones to the west, at 09:00 h. The component of the rhythm of cognitive performance that parallels core temperature will be phased in the same way. Second, the abnormality of timing of the body clock with regard to the new time zone will mean that sleep is more difficult to initiate and sustain during night at the new destination; subjects will feel most tired from 07:00 to 15:00 h after a flight across eight time zones to the east and from 15:00 to 23:00 h after flight across eight time zones to the west, in neither case feeling particularly tired when it is night in the new time zone. Consequently, sleep loss will be incurred, and this will independently produce performance decrement.

Data from batteries of tests of cognitive performance collected from field studies after time-zone transitions are comparatively rare. Not only is it difficult to perform such tests satisfactorily under field conditions but also most travellers will be attending important meetings or sightseeing rather than performing psychometric tests! Even so, there is a recent study on long-haul passengers (Vanttinen et al., 2008) and several studies on aircrew. For example, Graeber et al. (1986) measured sleep polysomnographically during layover days (rest days before the crew returned to their home time zone), and Samel et al. (1995) measured the electroencephalogram of crew members during long-haul flights. Also, measurements of eye blinking and wrist activity have been used and subjects have been studied in simulators (Beh and McLaughlin, 1991; Foushee et al., 1986; French et al., 1994; Rosekind et al., 1995). Nevertheless, due to the difficulties of measurement, most studies have entailed measurement of sleep diaries and subjective assessments of fatigue and alertness, measures that are quick to perform and intrude minimally upon work. Some important reviews include those by Graeber (1982, 1989), Winget et al. (1984), Åkerstedt (1995), Dinges (1995) and Srinivasan et al. (2008).

Long-haul flights to the south or north, in which there is no substantial change in the time zone (<3 time zones), do not produce changes in sleep pattern or fatigue unless they involve a night flight (see below); by contrast, it has been found that after long-haul flights to the east or west sleep-wake patterns (whether measured objectively or subjectively) are changed, that fatigue and sleepiness increase and that simple performance tasks are performed less quickly and/or with more errors (Ariznavarreta et al., 2002; Bourgeois-Bougrine et al., 2003; Carvalho-Bos et al., 2003; Gander et al., 1989; Graeber et al., 1986; Green, 1985; Lemmer et al., 2002; Lowden and Åkerstedt, 1998a, 1999; Nicholson et al., 1984, 1986; Richmond et al., 2004; Sasaki et al., 1993; Spencer et al., 1991; Stone et al., 1993; Takahashi et al., 2002). Also, in the study of Samel et al. (1995), which used the encephalogram to monitor brain activity during long-haul flights, there was an increased incidence of 'micro-events' (or 'micro-sleeps') during the cruise phase.

There is some evidence that chronic exposure to disruptions from time-zone transitions leads to long-term cognitive problems and psychiatric morbidity (Cho, 2001; Katz et al., 2002). There is evidence that increasing age is sometimes, but not always, associated with increased performance impairment (Gander et al., 1993; Monk, 2005; Monk et al., 2000) and that some person-specific traits (chronotype: Paine et al., 2006; rigidity of habits: Flower et al., 2003) alter the amount of jet lag and general disruption that are experienced.

Westward and eastward flights do not produce identical responses in the traveller in terms of changes in the sleep-wake cycle, amount of fatigue or frequency of micro-sleeps (Carvalho-Bos et al., 2003; Graeber et al., 1986; Samel et al., 1995; Takahashi et al., 2002); westward time-zone transitions are more often followed by an appropriate shift of the sleep-wake cycle (a delay equal to the number of time zones crossed), less fatigue and more rapid recuperation than are eastward flights (which require an advance of the sleep-wake cycle). The explanation generally offered (Waterhouse et al., 1997, 2007) invokes more than one reason: sleep after a westward flight is delayed (and so easier to achieve as the traveller is tired); the (free-running) body clock tends to run 'slow' and so can adjust more rapidly to the required delay; and the zeitgeber effect of the natural light–dark cycle at the destination tends to act to delay the body clock.

After westward flights, it is common for a single sleep of about normal length to be taken during the new night time; after eastward flights, by contrast, even though a single nocturnal sleep taken in phase with the new time zone is sometimes found, it is not uncommon for sleep to be split into two sessions (one in phase with home time and the other with destination time – an ‘anchor-sleep’ schedule), or even for it to remain in accord with the *home* time zone (Carvalho-Bos et al., 2003; Graeber et al., 1986). Retaining home time for hours of sleep is often found if the return flight takes place soon after the outward flight (see Lowden and Åkerstedt, 1998b, for example). The concept of split sleeps will be dealt with in detail in ‘Irregular sleeps and “anchor” sleeps’ section.

One difficulty with interpreting these results is that long-haul flights generally include overnight travel. That is, the aircrew will be performing night work as well as undergoing a time-zone transition, and the effects of these two abnormalities can be difficult to separate.

Cognitive performance during night work

During night work, problems similar to those after a time-zone transition are found, and for similar reasons; again, the requirement to work at night and sleep during the daytime does not accord with the timing of the body clock. A set of symptoms similar to those of jet lag is present, ‘shiftworker’s malaise’, and their cause is similar. Even so, the symptoms are not transient, and in individuals particularly susceptible to them, their persistence can lead to the individual having to leave night work. The difficulties are less transient because night work might constitute a substantial proportion of work hours over the course of years.

With night work, the problems that exist are worse because adjustment of the body clock is slower than that after a time-zone transition. This difference is because different zeitgebers no longer give unambiguous information with regard to the appropriate timing of circadian rhythms. Thus, even if an individual takes steps to adjust to the demands of night work (adjusting sleep times, altering the pattern of meals, being active during free time, for example), some zeitgebers, including the light–dark cycle and social inputs from the majority of the population, do not adjust in the same way. The night worker is likely to feel a ‘loner’, therefore, and problems with partners, the family and close friends are common. The problem is exacerbated during rest days since there is then a strong tendency for the individual to conform with the rest of society; if this happens then ALL zeitgebers act to adjust the body clock to ‘normal’ time, any partial and hard-won adjustment of the body clock during night work rapidly being lost during rest days. These general principles are reviewed in Waterhouse and DeCoursey (2004b).

Deterioration in performance at cognitive tasks is to be expected for several reasons: (1) Individuals will be working at a time closer to the temperature trough than its peak, and so poorer performance is likely. (2) For the same reason, individuals will feel sleepy whilst at work. (3) Daytime sleep will be more difficult to initiate and sustain (even if the bedroom is darkened, the phone is turned off, the rest of the household is quiet and so on) due to the inappropriately timed temperature rhythm. Partial sleep loss will occur, therefore, increasing fatigue and further decrementing cognitive performance. (4) There is also a more subtle problem associated with night work. During day work, individuals tend to work in the first part of their waking day and to relax with friends and family during the second part. By contrast, in order to spend some time with the family, night workers tend to sleep in the morning after returning from work and then meet their family in the evening before going to work. That is, they work in the second part of their wake span and so cognitive tasks will be negatively affected by the increased time awake (Fig. 3).

Measures of on-site performance during the night shift are rare, though two recent studies (Adam et al., 2007; Fullick et al., 2009) have investigated the quality of life in night workers. There are several reasons for this dearth of performance data: (1) the difficulty of assessing quantitatively many of the tasks that are performed during a duty period (e.g. the efficacy with which decisions are taken or negotiations carried out); (2) problems in standardizing the conditions under which a task is carried out; (3) and time and safety constraints preclude making accurate and controlled experimental measurements. Nevertheless, some pioneering studies have been performed, measuring errors made in the workplace (summarized by Hildebrandt et al., 1975; Minors and Waterhouse, 1981a). As predicted, performance at night was generally poorer than that during the daytime but difficulties of interpretation (lighting conditions, amount of sleep deprivation of the subjects) often precluded unambiguous interpretation of the results.

Strictly speaking, measurements of errors need not be exact markers of levels of cognitive performance, but it is generally assumed that poorer performance will lead to more errors and accidents and, anyway, a reduction of the frequency of these is a major aim, of course. However, poorer performance need not inevitably lead to an error or accident, and some accidents do not involve 'human error'. For a discussion of this issue, see Folkard (1990).

Recent studies of shift work have often concentrated on tests that are quick and easy to perform in the workplace, such as subjective assessments of mood, sleepiness and alertness. Alternatively, laboratory-based simulations of night work have been performed upon volunteers, when elaborate tests of cognitive performance can be carried out under standardized conditions and with control of prior sleep loss. Simulations might suffer from artefacts due to the tests being rather short and/or being examined for a period of time that is too short; it has been argued that performance decrement in some tasks, particularly those that are repetitive, might not be apparent unless performed for days and for several hours each day – as found in the real situation. The results will be a truer reflection of the real world only when such 'novelty' effects have worn off. Moreover, the subjects know that the test is not 'real' and this might affect the results obtained; they might try harder (because they know that their performance is being scrutinized) or less hard (because 'failure' is unimportant – the person in the driving simulator will not really crash and be injured, or incorrect responses to a task will not lead to catastrophe).

There have been several recent reviews of the problems associated with shift work (see, e.g. Åkerstedt, 1995; Balkin et al., 2008; Dinges, 1995; Graeber, 1989; Owens, 2007; Signal and Gander, 2007; Walker, 2008). All reviews and studies stress the negative effects of night work upon mood, sleepiness, alertness and cognitive performance, as well as the large contribution to the problem from sleep loss. Performance decrements that have been measured include poorer prefrontal executive function (Killgore et al., 2009), decreased alertness measured polysomnographically (Signal et al., 2009), worse performance at a psychomotor vigilance task (Kubo et al., 2007; Santhi et al., 2007; Signal et al., 2009; Smith et al., 2007; Smith-Coggins et al., 2006; Swann et al., 2006; Vgontzas et al., 2007), poorer memory (Diekelmann et al., 2008; Smith-Coggins et al., 2006; Tucker and Fishbein, 2008), increased visual simple reaction time (Miccoli et al., 2008), increased frequency of false alarms and misses when checking 'dangerous' baggage in a simulation of an airport X-ray screening system (Basner et al., 2008), decreased powers of logical reasoning (Kubo et al., 2007) and poorer visual search (Santhi et al., 2007). One exception to this general decrement in performance was maintenance of visuospatial perception following sleep loss (Killgore et al., 2007).

There is a tendency for the possibility of performance decrement due to sleep loss and/or working at the wrong circadian time to be mentioned whenever an accident occurs (Waterhouse and DeCoursey, 2004b), but it is often difficult to disentangle the possible role played by these factors from that due to the many others that might have been present at the time of the accident.

Comparatively new areas of research have concentrated on, first, inter-individual differences in susceptibility to the deleterious effects of sleep loss. Recent reviews include those by Van Dongen (2006), Czeisler (2009), Van Dongen and Belenky (2009). It appears that genetic polymorphisms are a contributory factor (King et al., 2009) and the term 'trototype' has been coined to describe the difference in susceptibility (Van Dongen et al., 2005). A second new area of research is to investigate the cellular and biochemical mechanisms by which sleep loss exerts its widespread effects (Bodenmann et al., 2009; Czeisler, 2009; Halassa et al., 2009; Meerlo et al., 2009). The current view is that astrocytes, dopaminergic mechanisms and hippocampal neurogenesis all have important roles to play, but further details are required. A third area of interest has been attempts to model the effects of chronic sleep loss upon cognitive performance more effectively than was achieved in earlier models (reviewed by Neri, 2004; Van Dongen, 2004); a recent contribution is that by McCauley et al. (2009). All these issues are covered in detail in other chapters of this book.

Accepting the need for night work and the inevitable problems associated with it, attempts to ameliorate these difficulties remain a priority. As well as continuing attempts to find the 'best' shift system (in terms of length of shift, direction of rotation, number of shifts before rotating), other possibilities include pharmacological methods of promoting daytime sleep and nocturnal alertness (covered elsewhere in this book), instituting systems to check the health of the workforce, particularly with regard to sleep hygiene (Czeisler, 2009; Gander and Signal, 2008), and comparing the efficacy of advancing or delaying the body clock by altering times of sleep and light exposure (Santhi et al., 2008). However, one of the most important methods is to use naps to 'top up' lost sleep. These naps can take place in the daytime (outside work hours) or during night work itself. What needs to be known is the effectiveness of such naps and how efficacy is affected by their length and timing. This important area is covered in detail in Chapter 9 in this book (Lovato and Lack, 2010).

Irregular sleeps and 'anchor' sleeps

Even though the sleep-wake cycle is changed both after a time-zone transition and during night work, the change does not take place every day (except with a very rapid rotation of shifts) and can generally be predicted. A different circumstance might arise in a military environment, when the sleep-wake cycle of those on active service can change on a daily basis and in an unpredictable way (Nicholson et al., 1984). Moreover, operational demands might render it impossible to take a single 8-h sleep per day, two 4-h sleeps per day being an alternative that fits better with military manoeuvres.

The basic 'anchor-sleep' protocols

A series of experiments was performed in an isolation unit to investigate the effect of irregular sleep times upon the circadian rhythms of core temperature and excretion of urinary constituents (Minors and Waterhouse, 1981b). The basic protocol (Protocol A) is shown in Fig. 4A. In this protocol, all experiments began with a control phase (days 1–5), during which subjects took 8-h sleeps from midnight to 08:00 h. The experimental phase consisted of a set of 8 days (days 7–14) during which an 8-h sleep was taken at a different time each day. The sleep times were randomly arranged, there being no overall trend for them to delay or advance during the experimental phase. A variant of this protocol (Protocol B) was to split the 8-h sleep into two 4-h sleeps separated by 12 h (Fig. 4B), one of each pair of sleeps being centred at the same time as in the basic protocol of Fig. 4A.

The times and composition of meals were kept as normal as possible throughout both the control and experimental phases of the experiment. Rectal temperature was recorded at hourly intervals throughout the protocol and urine samples were taken on rising from sleep and at 2-h intervals during the waking periods. These samples were analysed for rates of excretion of water, sodium, potassium, calcium, phosphate and urate. Cosine curves with a period of 24 h were fitted to the results for all variables, using 72-h moving 'windows' that were incremented by 24 h, the peak time for each curve (acrophase) being analysed.

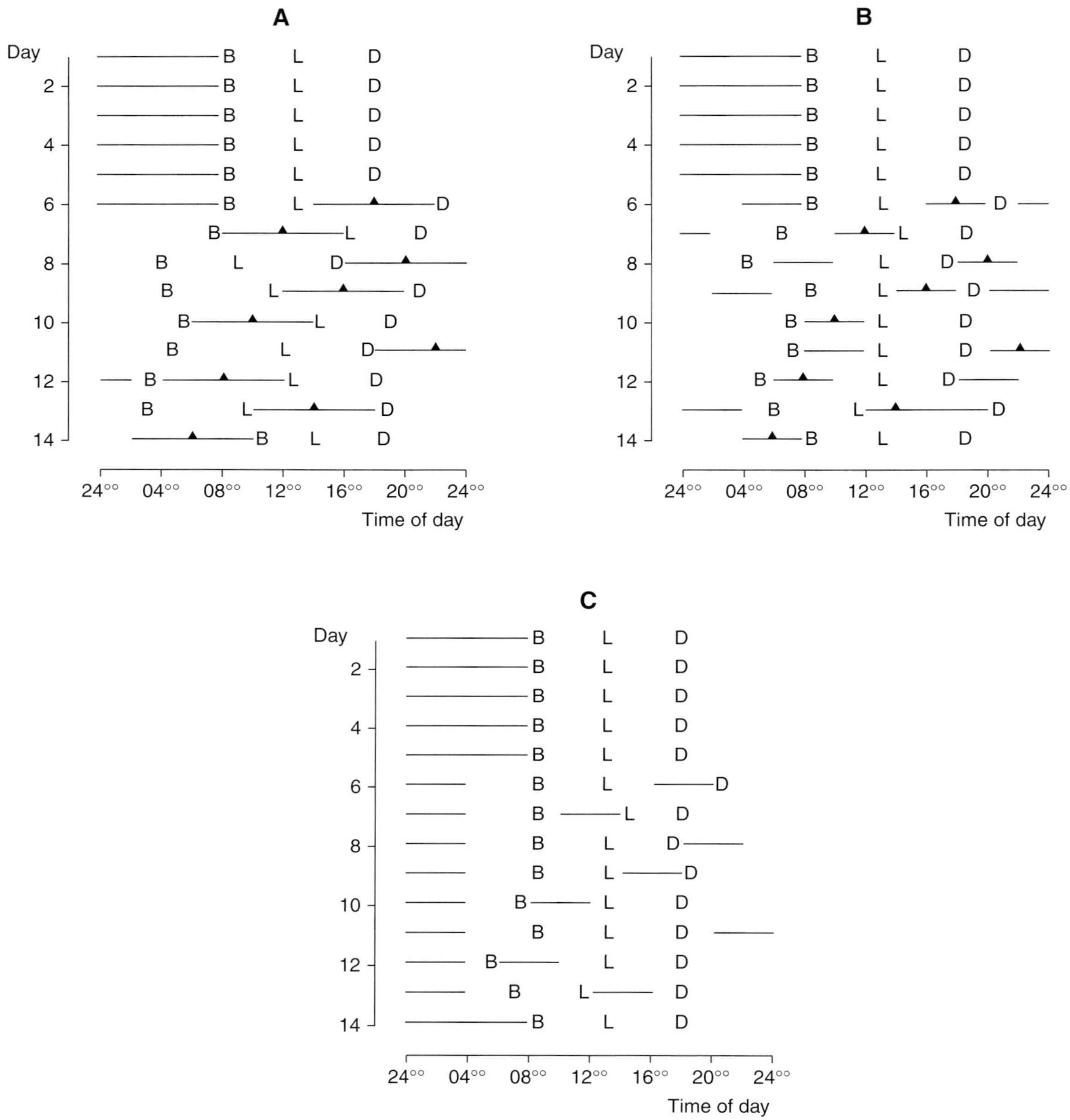

Fig. 4. Some of the protocols used for the 'anchor-sleep' studies. Successive days in the isolation unit shown from above downwards, sleeps being indicated by horizontal lines. Meals indicated as B (breakfast), L (lunch) and D (dinner). Protocol A: Basic protocol with irregular 8-h sleeps. Protocol B: Modification of Protocol A, each sleep being divided into two 4-h sleeps separated by 12 h and one of them being centred at the same time as in Protocol A. Protocol C: One of the 4-h sleeps is the same as in Protocol B but the other is always taken between midnight and 04:00 h. Triangles in Protocols A and B indicate the midpoints of the irregularly placed sleeps. For more details, see text. From Minors and Waterhouse (1981b).

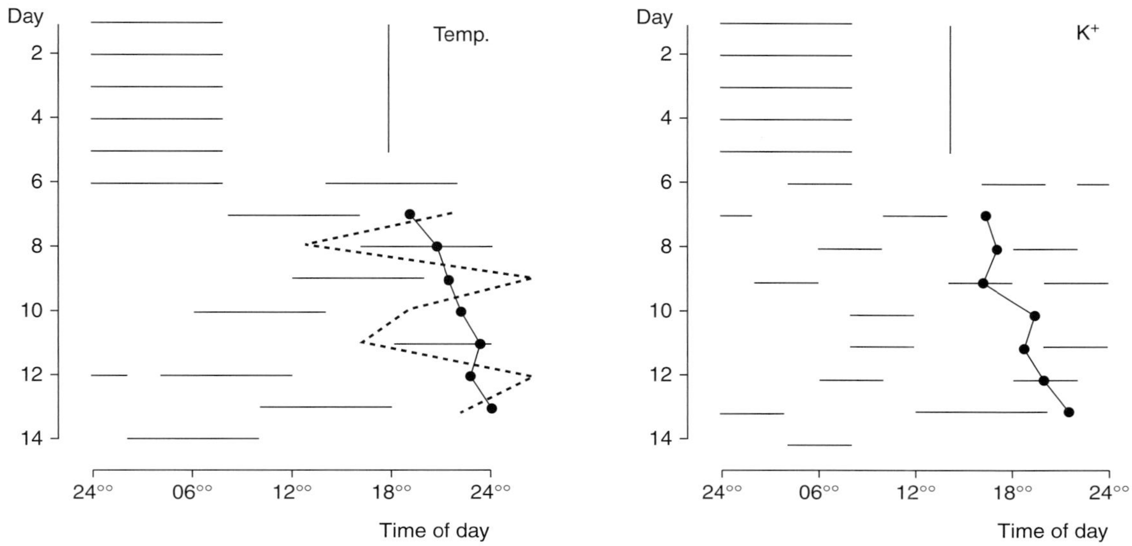

Fig. 5. Left: Acrophases of 24-h cosine curves, fitted to 72 h of data and advanced by 24-h increments, shown for rectal temperature rhythm (full line) and urinary calcium rhythm (dashed line) in a subject undergoing Protocol A. Right: Acrophases of urinary potassium rhythm in a subject undergoing Protocol B. Vertical lines show acrophase of cosine curve fitted to all control data. For more details, see text. Based on Minors and Waterhouse (1981b).

With both protocols, the overall trend of the circadian rhythms was to show a period of 25–26 h (Fig. 5). This result indicated that the regular timing of meals was not a sufficiently strong zeitgeber to maintain entrainment in the face of an irregular sleep-wake schedule (associated with which were irregular timings of light exposure). That is, the rhythms appeared to 'free run'. In addition to this progressive delay in timing, there was a tendency for the acrophases to 'zig-zag' so that they were in the waking rather than sleeping periods, a zig-zag that was more marked for rhythms with a larger exogenous component (urinary water, urate and calcium excretion, for example), as illustrated by the dashed line in the left-hand panel of Fig. 5.

A second variant of the basic protocol (Protocol C) was to retain the irregular timing of one of the 4-h sleeps but always to schedule the other sleep from midnight to 04:00 h (Fig. 4C). In this case, results showed that there was no overall delay in the rhythms, the rhythms appearing to remain entrained to the 24-h day (Fig. 6). As with Protocols A and B, a daily 'zig-zag', smaller for rhythms with a larger endogenous component (rectal temperature and urinary potassium excretion) and more marked for those rhythms with a stronger exogenous component (urinary water, urate and calcium excretion), was superimposed upon this stable rhythm.

Further experiments were performed using three variants of Protocol C in which the times of both the irregular and the regular sleeps were delayed by 4, 8 or 12 h. That is, the regular sleeps were taken at 04:00–08:00 h (Protocol D), 08:00–12:00 h (Protocol E) or 12:00–16:00 h (Protocol F). Protocols E and F are illustrated in Fig. 7. Figure 7 indicates that the circadian rhythms initially delayed from the control phase but then stabilized about 6 or 8 h later, respectively, than during the control phase. When the regular sleep was taken at 04:00–08:00 h (Protocol D), the rhythms stabilized

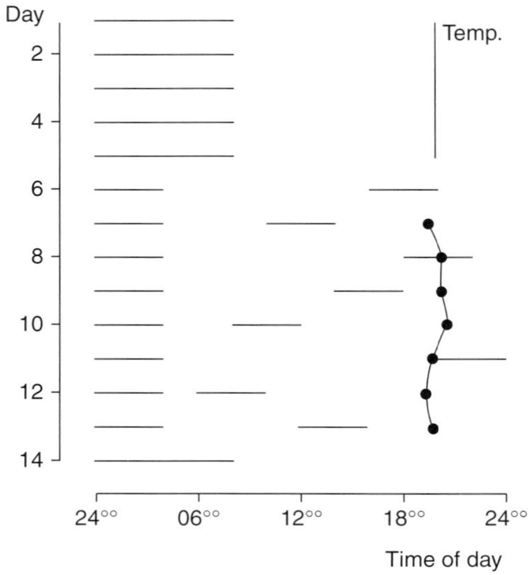

Fig. 6. Acrophases of 24-h cosine curves, fitted to 72 h of data and advanced by 24-h increments, for rectal temperature rhythm in a subject undergoing Protocol C. Vertical line shows acrophase of cosine curve fitted to all control data. For more details, see text. From Minors and Waterhouse (1981b).

about 2 h later than in the control phase (results not illustrated). That is, the phases of the rhythms were stabilized at a later time that corresponded to the delay in sleep times (though it could not be ascertained if the delay corresponded most closely to the delay of sleep onset, mid-sleep or sleep offset).

Two explanations of the stable phase of the circadian rhythms observed in these experiments suggest themselves a direct result of shifting the exogenous component of the rhythm or an effect due to entrainment of the body clock (by exposure to the delayed light–dark cycle, for example). It was the latter possibility that gave rise to the concept of 'anchor sleep', implying that exposure to a regular sleep-wake cycle of only 4 h (and its concomitants, including light exposure) acted as a sufficiently strong zeitgeber to stabilize the timing of the body clock. The slow delay of the circadian rhythms followed by their stabilization at a new delayed phase (see Fig. 7) supports this concept of an anchor sleep, the body clock free running until it became entrained (adjusted) to the delayed sleep-wake cycle. By contrast, the alternative view – that the delayed phase was a direct result of delaying the exogenous component of the circadian rhythm – would be expected to cause an immediate phase delay. Even so, further experiments were required to distinguish between these two possible explanations.

Further 'anchor-sleep' protocols and those incorporating constant routines

Therefore, a protocol (Protocol G) in which the sleep times were advanced by 4 h (the 'anchor sleep' being taken between 20:00 h and midnight) was used (Minors and Waterhouse, 1983). With this protocol, a stabilized rhythm advanced by 4–8 h (depending upon whether sleep onset, mid-sleep or sleep termination was the important change) would indicate either entrainment of the body clock or a direct effect of the exogenous component of the rhythms, whereas a delayed component would indicate that the body clock had not been entrained but rather was free running.

Results from this protocol showed that the phase shift varied according to the variable under consideration. The urinary excretory rhythms with a larger exogenous component (water, urate and calcium) tended to show two components – one advanced (by up to 4 h) and another delayed by up to 8 h; those with smaller exogenous components (potassium and core temperature) showed mainly a delay of up to 8 h. This finding does not support the view that the advanced sleep times acted as an anchor sleep; it suggests, instead, that the phase-advanced component, when present, reflected the exogenous component of the rhythms and that the body clock itself had not been advanced but rather delayed (due to a free-running period greater than 24 h, see Fig. 5).

What was happening to the endogenous components of the rhythms was tested more directly by

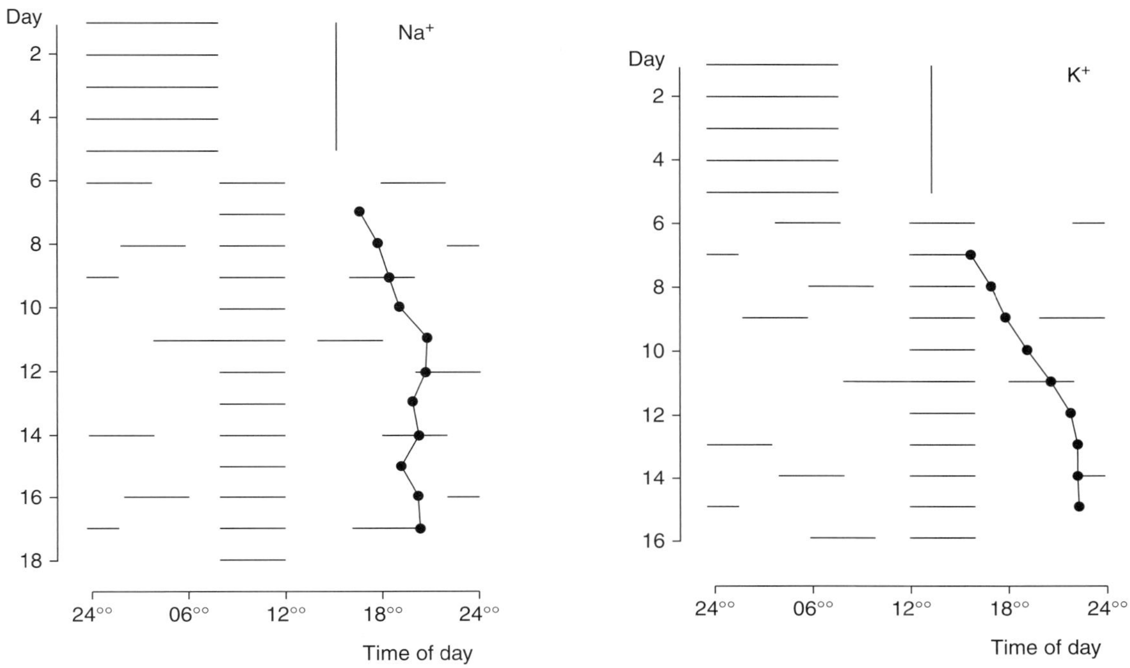

Fig. 7. Left: Urinary sodium rhythm in a subject undergoing Protocol E. Right: Urinary potassium rhythm in a subject undergoing Protocol F. Acrophases of 24-h cosine curves fitted to 72 h of data and advanced by 24-h increments. Vertical lines show acrophases of cosine curves fitted to all control data. For description of the variants, see text. From Minors and Waterhouse (1981b).

incorporating constant routine protocols into two of the protocols (Minors and Waterhouse, 1983). Two constant routines were incorporated, one at the end of the control phase (control constant routine) and the other, 8 days later, at the end of the experimental phase (experimental constant routine). During these, core temperature and urine samples were measured hourly.

Two protocols were used: Protocol C (Figs. 4C and 6, with the anchor sleep between midnight and 04:00 h) and Protocol G (where all sleeps were advanced by 4 h in comparison with Protocol C, the 'anchor sleep' being taken between 20:00 h and midnight). Rhythms from the two constant routines were compared by a two-component cross-correlation analysis which was devised especially for the purpose (for details, see Minors and Waterhouse, 1983). Briefly, in this analysis, the hourly data from the control constant routine were shifted by 0–23 h in hourly increments to produce 24 data sets, called D1, each of 24 hourly points. The control constant routine data were also shifted a second time by 0–23 h in hourly increments to produce another 24 data sets, called D2, again each of 24 hourly points. Each of the data sets D1 and D2 could then be combined in the ratios 0:10, 1:9, 2:8, . . . , 8:2, 9:1 and 10:0, giving a total of 3036 combinations. Each combination was compared with the data from the experimental constant routine by cross-correlation, the highest positive correlation being sought.

This analysis enabled the data from the experimental constant routine to be described in terms of the relative size of two shifted components derived from the control constant routine. A delayed component would indicate the presence of an unadjusted, free-running body clock; entrainment of the body clock by the 'anchor sleep' would produce a phase advance of 0–4 h in Protocol C (depending upon whether it was sleep onset, mid-sleep or sleep offset that determined the exact timing of the body clock) and a phase advance of 4–8 h with Protocol G. Any advanced component of the rhythms could NOT be attributed to effects of an exogenous component, as had been the case in the previous experiments, since this component had been removed by the constant routine protocol.

Figure 8 shows the outcome when this analysis was applied to Protocol C, the results from all variables being combined. There was a marked peak at zero shift and a smaller one showing a delay of about 8 h, but little evidence of a peak in the region of phase advances. The peak at zero hours was less marked with variables possessing a smaller exogenous component; this peak probably reflects in part a direct effect of the starts of the constant routines, when the subjects woke up and began hourly fluid and food intakes. (The two constant routines started at the same clock time. An improved protocol would have used longer constant routines – 30 h, for example – and ignored the results from the first 6 h, when these effects of waking up and 'settling into the routine' might be present.) With Protocol G also, there were two peaks, also centred round a zero shift and a delay of about 8 h; again, the peak at zero shift was more marked for variables with a larger exogenous component and there was no clear peak showing phase advances in the region of 4–8 h.

Such findings do not support the hypothesis that the body clock had been phase advanced by the 'anchor sleep' in these two protocols; instead, the body clock appears to have delayed by about 4 h, suggesting a 'free-running' period during the 8 days of the protocol of about 24.5 h. Whilst this finding suggests that 'anchor sleep' might be a

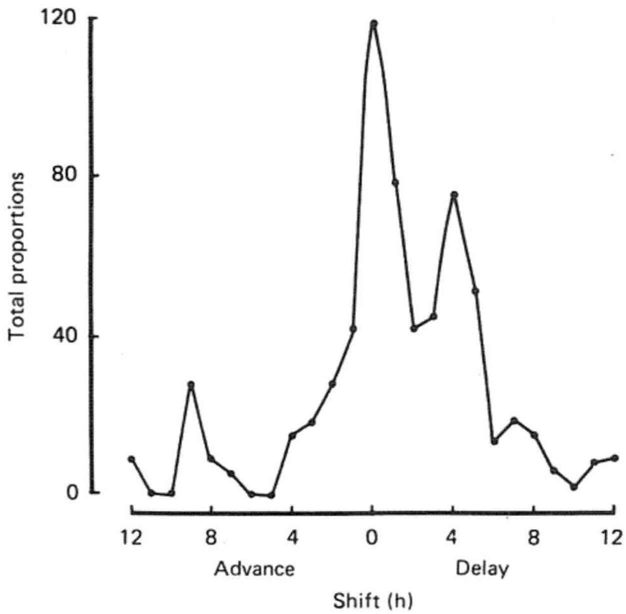

Fig. 8. Subjects undertaking Protocol C (Figs. 4C and 6) but with two constant routines incorporated into the end of the control and experimental phases. Total proportions and phase shifts of all variables from the control constant routine that yielded the highest positive correlation coefficient when compared with the experimental constant routine are shown. For more details, see text. From Minors and Waterhouse (1983).

misnomer, this is not necessarily the case. Even though it might not be strong enough to advance the body clock, it remains a possibility that a 4-h sleep taken 20:00 h–midnight could 'catch' and 'hold' a circadian rhythm, as illustrated for Protocols E and F in Fig. 7. That is, it might be that a regular sleep advanced by 4 h could entrain the body clock after it had delayed about 20 h, and so justify the use of 'anchor sleep'. This possibility remains to be investigated.

Implications of 'anchor sleep' and split sleeps

The application of the above findings to cognitive performance is not known, since such variables were not measured in the experiments just described. However, insofar as a component of cognitive performance parallels core temperature, it seems a reasonable speculation that the findings do have some applicability. Even if taking a 4-h sleep at the same time each day does not stabilize the body clock, there are two effects that certainly result from this regimen. First, the *measured* rhythm (which includes the exogenous component) is stabilized and this might apply equally to rhythms of cognitive performance. The second advantage of taking sleep in two 4-h blocks is that the time spent awake between sleeps decreases and this will decrease time-awake and fatigue effects upon cognitive performance (Stampi, 1992; Van Dongen, 2004). Possible applications of both these effects will now be considered briefly.

The stability of phase of measured circadian rhythms might be of application to night workers. Regularly taking a 4-h sleep during the late morning on rest days (the remainder of their sleep being taken when convenient) might enable night workers to maintain any adjustment to night work during these days of rest. Anchor sleep might also be of value to others whose sleep times are continually changing due to time-zone transitions. This problem can be marked for aircrew on duty tours involving long-distance flights, where night work and the time-zone transitions are present. Inspection of sleep logs and actimetry records indicates that sleep is often fractionated and some sleep is taken during the hours of night *as measured on home time*, regardless of what this time corresponds to on local time (Carvalho-Bos et al., 2003; Graeber et al., 1986; Lowden and Åkerstedt, 1998b). Whether such sleeps help stabilize the circadian rhythms of cognitive performance to home time, and if this is desirable, are issues that have not been researched. However, such sleep habits might be an example of a 'self-selection' by individuals who can deal most effectively with the problems posed by their lifestyle.

The other advantage of 'anchor sleep' is that it means that more than one shorter sleep can be taken each day. Not only does this practice mean that time awake (since the last sleep) tends to be decreased but also it might fit better with complex work schedules (Stampi, 1992). The concept of 'split sleep' has been investigated in some detail in the context of assessing deterioration in performance of a variety of cognitive performance tasks associated with sleep loss (Mollicone et al., 2007, 2008). These authors systematically varied the length of a nocturnal 'anchor sleep' as well as the length of a diurnal nap (Mollicone et al., 2008). They showed that the deterioration of cognitive performance was a function of the total amount of sleep lost per day regardless of whether the sleep was taken in one or two sessions. This work complemented earlier studies in which it was shown that sleep efficiency was not adversely affected by taking more than one sleep per day and the deterioration in cognitive performance due to sleep loss could be opposed as effectively by a split-sleep schedule as one involving a single sleep of equal length (Mollicone et al., 2007). Mollicone et al. (2008) concluded: 'Thus, split sleep schedules are feasible and can be used to enhance the flexibility of sleep/work schedules for space operations involving restricted nocturnal sleep due to mission-critical task scheduling. These results are generally applicable to any continuous industrial operation that involves sleep restriction, night operations, and shift work'.

References

Adam, A., Courthiat, M., Vespignani, H., Emser, W., & Hannarth, B. (2007). Comparison of the effects of permanent vs. rotating work schedules on sleep, vigilance and quality of life in French and German shift workers. *Archives des Maladies Professionelles et d l'Environnement, 68*, 482–493.

Åkerstedt, T. (1995). Work hours sleepiness and accidents. *Journal of Sleep Research, 4*(Suppl. 2); 1–3.

Åkerstedt, T. (2007). Altered sleep/wake patterns and mental performance. *Physiology & Behavior, 90*, 209–218.

Åkerstedt, T., & Folkard, S. (1991). A three process model of the regulation of alertness and sleepiness. In: Ogilvie, R., Broughton, R. (Eds.), *Sleep, arousal and performance: Problems and promises*. Birkhäuser, Boston, pp. 11–26.

Åkerstedt, T., & Folkard, S. (1997). The three-process model of alertness and its extension to performance, sleep latency, and sleep length. *Chronobiology International, 14*, 115–123.

Åkerstedt, T., & Gillberg, T. (1981). The circadian variation of experimentally displaced sleep. *Sleep, 4*, 159–169.

Archer, S., Robilliard, D., & Skene, D., et al., (2003). A length polymorphism in the circadian clock gene Per3 is linked to delayed sleep phase syndrome and extreme diurnal preference. *Sleep, 26*, 413–415.

Arendt, J. (1989). Melatonin and the pineal gland. In: Arendt, J., Minors, D., Waterhouse, J. (Eds.), *Biological rhythms in clinical practice*. Wright, London, pp. 184–206.

Ariznavarreta, C., Cardinali, D., & Villanua, M. (2002). Circadian rhythms in airline pilots submitted to long-haul transmeridian flights. *Aviation, Space, and Environmental Medicine, 73*, 445–455.

Balkin, T., Rupp, T., Picchioni, D., & Wesensten, N. (2008). Sleep loss and sleepiness – Current issues. *Chest, 134*, 653–660.

Basner, M., Rubinstein, J., Fomberstein, K., Coble, M., Ecker, A., & Avinash, D., et al., (2008). Effects of night work, sleep loss and time on task on simulated threat detection performance. *Sleep, 31*, 1251–1259.

Beh, H., & McLaughlin, P. (1991). Mental performance of air crew following layovers on transzonal flights. *Ergonomics, 34*, 123–135.

Bodenmann, S., Xu, S., Luhmann, U., Arand, M., Berger, W., & Jung, H., et al., (2009). Pharmacogenetics of Modafinil after sleep loss: Catechol-O-methyltransferase genotype modulates waking functions but not recovery sleep. *Clinical Pharmacology & Therapeutics, 85*, 296–304.

Boivin, D., Czeisler, C., Dijk, D., Duffy, J., Folkard, S., & Minors, D., et al., (1997). Complex interaction of the sleep-wake cycle and circadian phase modulates mood in healthy subjects. *Archives of General Psychiatry, 54*, 145–152.

Bourgeois-Bougrine, S., Carbon, P., Gounelle, C., Mollard, R., & Coblentz, A. (2003). Perceived fatigue for short- and long-haul flights: A survey of 739 airline pilots. *Aviation, Space, and Environmental Medicine, 74*, 1072–1077.

Carvalho-Bos, S., Waterhouse, J., Edwards, B., Simons, R., & Reilly, T. (2003). The use of actimetry to assess changes to the rest–activity cycle. *Chronobiology International, 20*, 1039–1059.

Cho, K. (2001). Chronic 'jet lag' produces temporal lobe atrophy and spatial cognitive deficits. *Nature Neuroscience, 4*, 567–568.

Clayton, J., Kyriacou, C., & Reppert, S. (2001). Keeping time with the human genome. *Nature, 409*, 829–831.

Czeisler, C. (2009). Medical and genetic differences in the adverse impact of sleep loss on performance: Ethical considerations for the medical profession. *Transactions of the American Clinical and Climatological Association, 120*, 249–285.

Dean, D., Forger, D., & Klerman, E. (2009). Taking the lag out of jet lag through model-based schedule design. *PLoS Computational Biology, 5*(6); e1000418.

Diekelmann, S., Landolt, H., Lahl, O., Born, J., & Wagner, U. (2008). Sleep loss produces false memories. *PLoS ONE, 3* (10); .

Dijk, D. -J., & Czeisler, C. (1995). Contribution of the circadian pacemaker and the sleep homeostat to sleep propensity, sleep structure, electroencephalographic slow waves, and spindle activity in humans. *Journal of Neuroscience, 15*, 3526–3538.

Dinges, D. (1995). An overview of sleepiness and accidents. *Journal of Sleep Research, 4*(Suppl. 2); 4–14.

Flower, D., Irvine, D., & Folkard, S. (2003). Perception and predictability of travel fatigue after long-haul flights: A retrospective study. *Aviation, Space, and Environmental Medicine, 74*, 173–179.

Folkard, S. (1990). Circadian performance rhythms: Some practical and theoretical implications. *Philosophical Transactions of the Royal Society of London, B, 327*, 543–553.

Foushee, H., Lauber, J., Baetge, M., & Acomb, D. (1986). Operational significance of exposure to short-haul air transport operations. NASA Technical Memorandum, 88322.

French, J., Bisson, R., Neville, K., Mitcha, J., & Storm, W. (1994). Crew fatigue during simulated, long duration B-1B bomber missions. *Aviation, Space, and Environmental Medicine, 65*(5 Suppl.); A1–A6.

Fulda, S., & Schulz, H. (2010). How treatment affects cognitive deficits in patients with sleep disorders: Methodological issues and results. Kerkhof, G., Van Dongen, H. (Eds.), *Human sleep and cognition, progress in brain research. Vol. 185*, Elsevier, Amsterdam.

Fullick, S., Grindey, C., Edwards, B., Morris, C., Reilly, T., & Richardson, D., et al., (2009). Relationships between leisure-time energy expenditure and individual coping strategies for shift-work. *Ergonomics, 52*, 448–455.

Gander, P., & Signal, L. (2008). Who is too old for shift work? Developing better criteria. *Chronobiology International, 25*, 199–213.

Gander, P., Myhre, G., Graeber, R., Anderson, H., & Lauber, J. (1989). Adjustment of sleep and circadian rhythm temperature rhythm after flights across nine time zones. *Aviation, Space, and Environmental Medicine*, *60*, 733–744.

Gander, P., Nguyen, D., Rosekind, M., & Connell, L. (1993). Age, circadian rhythms and sleep loss in flight crews. *Aviation, Space, and Environmental Medicine*, *64*, 189–195.

Graeber, R. (1982). Alterations in performance following rapid transmeridian flight. In: Brown, F., Graeber, R. (Eds.), *Rhythmic aspects of behaviour*. Lawrence Erlbaum Associates, Hillsdale, pp. 173–212.

Graeber, R. (1989). Jet lag and sleep disruption. In: Krugger, M., Roth, T., Dement, C. (Eds.), *Principles and practice of sleep medicine*. WB Saunders Co, Philadelphia, pp. 324–331.

Graeber, R., Dement, W., Nicholson, A., Sasaki, M., & Wegmann, H. (1986). International cooperative study of aircrew layover sleep; operational summary. *Aviation, Space, and Environmental Medicine*, *57*, B10–B13.

Green, R. G. (1985). Stress and accidents. *Aviation, Space, and Environmental Medicine*, *56*, 638–641.

Haimov, I., & Arendt, J. (1999). The prevention and treatment of jet lag. *Sleep Medicine Reviews*, *3*, 229–240.

Halassa, M., Florian, C., Fellin, T., Munoz, J., Lee, S., & Abel, T., et al., (2009). Astrocytic modulation of sleep homeostasis and cognitive consequences of sleep loss. *Neuron*, *61*, 213–219.

Harrison, Y., Jones, K., & Waterhouse, J. (2007). The influence of time awake and circadian rhythm upon performance on a frontal lobe task. *Neuropsychobiologia*, *45*, 1996–1972.

Hildebrandt, G., Rohmert, W., & Rutenfranz, J. (1975). The influence of fatigue and rest period on the circadian variation of error frequency in shift workers (engine drivers). In: Colquhoun, P., Folkard, S., Knauth, P., Rutenfranz, J. (Eds.), *Experimental studies on shiftwork*. Westdeutschen Verlag, Opladen, pp. 177–187.

Horne, J., & Ostberg, O. (1976). A self-assessment questionnaire to determine morning-eveningness. *International Journal of Chronobiology*, *4*, 97–110.

Katz, G., Knobler, H., Laibel, Z., Strauss, Z., & Durst, R. (2002). Time zone change and major psychiatric morbidity: The results of a 6-year study in Jerusalem. *Comprehensive Psychiatry*, *43*, 37–40.

Kerkhof, G. (1985). Inter-individual differences in the human circadian system: A review. *Biological Psychology*, *20*, 83–112.

Kerkhof, G., & Van Dongen, H. (1996). Morning-type and evening-type individuals differ in the phase position of their endogenous circadian oscillator. *Neuroscience Letters*, *218*, 153–156.

Khalsa, S., Jewett, M., & Cajochen, C. (2003). A phase response curve to single bright light pulses in human subjects. *Journal of Physiology*, *549*, 945–952.

Killgore, W., Kendall, A., Richards, J., & McBride, S. (2007). Lack of degradation in visuospatial perception of line orientation after one night of sleep loss. *Perceptual and Motor Skills*, *105*, 276–286.

Killgore, W., Grugle, N., Reichardt, R., Killgore, D., & Balkin, T. (2009). Executive functions and the ability to sustain vigilance during sleep loss. *Aviation, Space, and Environmental Medicine*, *80*, 81–87.

King, A., Belenky, G., & Van Dongen, H. (2009). Performance impairment consequent to sleep loss: Determinants of resistance and susceptibility. *Current Opinion in Pulmonary Medicine*, *15*, 559–564.

Kleitman, N. (1963). *Sleep and wakefulness.* University of Chicago Press, Chicago.

Krauchi, K., & Wirz-Justice, A. (1994). Circadian rhythm of heat production, heart rate, and skin and core temperature under unmasking conditions in man. *American Journal of Physiology (Regulatory, Integrative and Comparative Physiology)*, *267*, R819–R828.

Kubo, T., Takeyama, H., Matsumoto, S., Ebara, T., Murata, K., & Tachi, N., et al., (2007). Impact of nap length, nap timing and sleep quality on sustaining early morning performance. *Industrial Health*, *45*, 552–563.

Lack, L., & Lushington, K. (1996). The rhythms of sleep propensity and core body-temperature. *Journal of Sleep Research*, *5*, 1–11.

Lavie, P., & Segal, S. (1989). Twenty-four-hour structure of sleepiness in morning and evening persons investigated by ultrashort sleep-wake cycle. *Sleep*, *12*, 522–528.

Lemmer, B., Kern, R., Nold, G., & Lohrer, H. (2002). Jet lag in athletes after eastward and westward time-zone transition. *Chronobiology International*, *19*, 743–764.

Lewy, A., Bauer, V., & Ahmed, S. (1998). The human phase response curve (PRC) to melatonin is about 12 hours out of phase with the PRC to light. *Chronobiology International*, *15*, 71–83.

Lovato, N., & Lack, L. (2010). The effects of napping on cognitive functioning. Kerkhof, G., Van Dongen, H. (Eds.), *Human sleep and cognition, progress in brain research. Vol. 185*, Elsevier, Amsterdam.

Lowden, A., & Åkerstedt, T. (1998a). Sleep and wake patterns in aircrew on a 2-day layover on westward long distance flights. *Aviation, Space, and Environmental Medicine*, *69*, 596–602.

Lowden, A., & Åkerstedt, T. (1998b). Retaining home-base sleep hours to prevent jet lag in connection with a westward flight across nine time zones. *Chronobiology International*, *15*, 365–376.

Lowden, A., & Åkerstedt, T. (1999). Eastward long distance flights, sleep and wake patterns in air crews in connection with a two-day layover. *Journal Sleep Research*, *8*, 15–24.

McCauley, P., Kalachev, L., Smith, A., Belenky, G., Dinges, D., & Van Dongen, H. (2009). A new mathematical model for the homeostatic effects of sleep loss on neurobehavioral performance. *Journal of Theoretical Biology*, *256*, 227–239.

Meerlo, P., Mistiberger, R., Jacobs, B., Heller, H., & McGinty, D. (2009). New neurons in the adult brain: The role of sleep and consequences of sleep loss. *Sleep Medicine Reviews*, *13*, 187–194.

Miccoli, L., Versace, F., Koterle, S., & Cavallero, C. (2008). Comparing sleep-loss sleepiness and sleep inertia: Lapses make the difference. *Chronobiology International, 25*, 725–744.

Mills, J., Minors, D., & Waterhouse, J. (1978). Adaptation to abrupt time shifts of the oscillator(s) controlling human circadian rhythms. *Journal of Physiology, 285*, 455–470.

Minors, D., & Waterhouse, J. (1981a). *Circadian rhythms and the human.* John Wright, Bristol.

Minors, D., & Waterhouse, J. (1981b). Anchor sleep as a synchronizer of rhythms on abnormal routines. *International Journal of Chronobiology, 7*, 165–188.

Minors, D., & Waterhouse, J. (1983). Does anchor sleep entrain circadian-rhythms? Evidence from Constant Routine studies. *Journal of Physiology (London), 345*, 451–467.

Mollicone, D., Van Dongen, H., & Dinges, D. (2007). Optimizing sleep/wake schedules in space: Sleep during chronic with and without diurnal naps. *Acta Astronautica, 60*, 354–361.

Mollicone, D., Van Dongen, H., Rogers, N., & Dinges, D. (2008). Response surface mapping of neurobehavioral performance: Testing the feasibility of split sleep schedules for space operations. *Acta Astronautica, 63*, 833–840.

Mongrain, V., & Dumont, M. (2007). Increased homeostatic response to behavioral sleep fragmentation in morning types compared to evening types. *Sleep, 30*, 773–780.

Monk, T. (2005). Aging human circadian rhythms: Conventional wisdom may not always be right. *Journal of Biological Rhythms, 20*, 366–374.

Monk, T., Buysse, D., Carrier, J., & Kupfer, D. (2000). Inducing jet-lag in older people: Directional asymmetry. *Journal of Sleep Research, 9*, 101–116.

Monk, T., Buysse, D., Reynolds, C., Berga, A., Jarrett, D., & Begley, A., et al., (1997). Circadian rhythms in human performance and mood under constant conditions. *Journal of Sleep Research, 6*, 9–18.

Murphy, P., & Campbell, S. (1997). Nighttime drop in body temperature: A physiological trigger for sleep onset? *Sleep, 20*, 505–511.

Neri, D. (2004). Proceedings of the Fatigue and Performance Modeling Workshop, June 13–14, 2002, Seattle, Washington. *Aviation, Space, and Environmental Medicine, 75*(Section II, Suppl.); A1–A199.

Nicholson, A., Pascoe, P., Spencer, M., Stone, B., & Green, R. (1986). Nocturnal sleep and daytime alertness of aircrew after transmeridian flights. *Aviation, Space, and Environmental Medicine, 57*, B42–B52.

Nicholson, A., Stone, B., Borland, R., & Spencer, M. (1984). Adaptation to irregularity of rest and activity. *Aviation, Space, and Environmental Medicine, 55*, 102–112.

Owens, J. (2007). Sleep loss and fatigue in healthcare professionals. *Journal of Perinatal and Neonatal Nursing, 21*, 92–100.

Paine, S., Gander, P., & Travier, N. (2006). The epidemiology of morningness/eveningness: Influence of age, gender, ethnicity, and socioeconomic factors in adults (30–49 years). *Journal of Biological Rhythms, 21*, 68–76.

Reilly, T., Atkinson, G., & Waterhouse, J. (1997). *Biological rhythms and exercise.* Oxford University Press, Oxford.

Reppert, S., & Weaver, D. (2001). Molecular analysis of mammalian circadian rhythms. *Annual Review of Physiology, 63*, 647–678.

Richmond, L., Dawson, B., Hillman, D., & Eastwood, P. (2004). The effect of interstate travel on sleep patterns of elite Australian Rules footballers. *Journal of Sports Science and Medicine, 7*, 186–196.

Rosekind, M., Smith, R., Miller, D., Co, E., Gregory, K., & Webbon, L., et al., (1995). Alertness management; strategic naps in operational settings. *Journal of Sleep Research, 4* (Suppl. 2); 62–66.

Samel, A., Wegmann, H., & Vejvoda, M. (1995). Jet-lag and sleepiness in aircrew. *Journal of Sleep Research, 4*(Suppl. 2); 30–36.

Santhi, N., Aeschbach, D., Horowitz, T., & Czeisler, C. (2008). The impact of sleep timing and bright light exposure on attentional impairment during night work. *Journal of Biological Rhythms, 23*, 341–352.

Santhi, N., Horowitz, T., Duffy, J., & Czeisler, C. (2007). Acute sleep deprivation and circadian misalignment associated with transition onto the first night of work impairs visual selective attention. *PLoS ONE, 2*(11); BP e1233.

Sasaki, M., Kurosaki, Y., Spinweber, C., Graeber, R., & Takahashi, T. (1993). Flight crew sleep during multiple layover polar flights. *Aviation, Space, and Environmental Medicine, 64*, 641–667.

Shanahan, T., & Czeisler, C. (2000). Physiological effects of light on the human circadian pacemaker. *Seminars in Perinatology, 24*, 299–320.

Shochat, T., Luboshitzky, R., & Lavie, P. (1997). Nocturnal melatonin onset is phase locked to the primary sleep gate. *American Journal of Physiology (Regulatory, Integrative and Comparative Physiology), 273*, R364–R370.

Signal, T., & Gander, P. (2007). Rapid counterclockwise shift rotation in air traffic control: Effects on sleep and night work. *Aviation, Space, and Environmental Medicine, 78*, 878–885.

Signal, T., Gander, P., Anderson, H., & Brash, S. (2009). Scheduled napping as a countermeasure to sleepiness in air traffic controllers. *Journal of Sleep Research, 18*, 11–19.

Smith, S., Kilby, S., Jorgensen, G., & Douglas, J. (2007). Napping and nightshift work: Effects of a short nap on psychomotor vigilance and subjective sleepiness in health workers. *Sleep and Biological Rhythms, 5*, 117–125.

Smith-Coggins, R., Howard, S., Mac, D., Wang, C., Kwan, S., & Rosekind, M., et al., (2006). Improving alertness and performance in emergency department physicians and nurses: The use of planned naps. *Annals of Emergency Medicine, 48*, 596–604.

Spencer, M., Stone, B., Rogers, A., & Nicholson, A. (1991). Circadian rhythmicity and sleep of aircrew during polar schedules. *Aviation, Space, and Environmental Medicine*, *62*, 3–13.

Srinivasan, V., Spence, D., Pandi-Perumal, S., Trakht, I., & Cardinali, D. (2008). Jet lag: Therapeutic use of melatonin and possible application of melatonin analogs. *Travel Medicine and Infectious Disease*, *6*, 17–28.

Stampi, C. (1992). The effects of polyphasic and ultrashort sleep schedules. In: Stampi, C. (Ed.), *Why we nap: Evolution, chronobiology, and functions of polyphasic and ultrashort sleep*. Birkhauser, Boston, pp. 137–179.

Stone, B., Spencer, M., Rogers, A., Nicholson, A., Barnes, R., & Green, R. (1993). Influence of polar route schedules on the duty and rest patterns of aircrew. *Ergonomics*, *36*, 1465–1477.

Swann, C., Yelland, G., Redman, J., & Rajaratnam, S. (2006). Chronic partial sleep loss increases the facilitatory role of a masked prime in a word recognition task. *Journal of Sleep Research*, *15*, 23–29.

Takahashi, M., Nakata, A., & Arito, H. (2002). Disturbed sleep-wake patterns during and after short-term international travel among academics attending conferences. *International Archives of Occupational and Environmental Health*, *75*, 435–440.

Tucker, M., & Fishbein, W. (2008). Enhancement of declarative memory performance following a daytime nap is contingent on strength of initial task acquisition. *Sleep*, *31*, 197–203.

Valdez, P., Reilly, T., & Waterhouse, J. (2008). Rhythms of mental performance. *Mind, Brain, and Education*, *2*, 7–16.

Van Dongen, H. (2004). Comparison of mathematical model predictions to experimental data of fatigue and performance. *Aviation, Space, and Environmental Medicine*, *75*(Suppl.); A15–A36.

Van Dongen, H. (2006). Shift work and inter-individual differences in sleep and sleepiness. *Chronobiology International*, *23*, 1139–1147.

Van Dongen, H., & Belenky, G. (2009). Individual differences in vulnerability to sleep loss in the work environment. *Industrial Health*, *47*, 518–526.

Van Dongen, H., & Dinges, D. (2005). Sleep, circadian rhythms, and psychomotor vigilance. *Clinics in Sports Medicine*, *24*, 237–252.

Van Dongen, H., Vitellaro, K., & Dinges, D. (2005). Individual differences in adult human sleep and wakefulness: Leitmotif for a research agenda. *Sleep*, *28*, 479–496.

Vanttinen, T., Jiang, Y., Baca, A. & Zhang, H. (2008). Athletes' jet-lag as a consequence of traveling across six time zones. *Proceedings of the First Joint International Pre-Olympic Conference on Sports Science and Sport Engineering*, Vol. 1, pp. 402–405.

Vgontzas, A., Pejovic, S., Zoumakis, E., Lin, H., Bixler, E., & Basta, M., et al., (2007). Daytime napping after a night of sleep loss decreases sleepiness, improves performance, and causes beneficial changes in cortisol and interleukin-6 secretion. *American Journal of Physiology (Endocrinology and Metabolism)*, *292*, E253–E261.

Vidacek, S., Kaliterna, L., Radosevic-Vidacek, B., & Folkard, S. (1988). Personality differences in the phase of circadian rhythms: A comparison of morningness and extraversion. *Ergonomics*, *31*, 873–888.

Walker, M. (2008). Cognitive consequences of sleep and sleep loss. *Sleep Medicine*, *9*, S29–S34.

Waterhouse, J., & DeCoursey, P. (2004a). Human circadian organization. In: Dunlap, J., Loros, J., DeCoursey, P. (Eds.), *Chronobiology. Biological timekeeping*. Sinauer, Sunderland, pp. 291–323.

Waterhouse, J., & DeCoursey, P. (2004b). The relevance of circadian rhythms for human welfare. In: Dunlap, J., Loros, J., DeCoursey, P. (Eds.), *Chronobiology. Biological timekeeping*. Sinauer, Sunderland, pp. 325–356.

Waterhouse, J., Åkerstedt, T., Lennernas, M., & Arendt, J. (1999). Chronobiology and nutrition: Internal and external factors. *Canadian Journal of Diabetes Care*, *23*(Suppl. 2); 82–88.

Waterhouse, J., Atkinson, G., & Reilly, T. (1997). Jet lag. *Lancet*, *350*, 1611–1616.

Waterhouse, J., Minors, D., Åkerstedt, T., Reilly, T., & Atkinson, G. (2001). Rhythms of human performance. In: Takahashi, J., Turek, F., Moore, R. (Eds.), *Handbook of behavioral neurobiology: Circadian clocks*. Kluwer Academic/Plenum Publishers, New York, pp. 571–601.

Waterhouse, J., Minors, D., Folkard, S., Owens, D., Atkinson, G., & MacDonald, I., et al., (1998). Light of domestic intensity produces phase shifts of the circadian oscillator in humans. *Neuroscience Letters*, *245*, 97–100.

Waterhouse, J., Reilly, T., Atkinson, G., & Edwards, B. (2007). Jet lag: Trends and coping strategies. *Lancet*, *369*, 1117–1129.

Waterhouse, J., Weinert, D., Minors, D., Folkard, S., Owens, D., & Atkinson, G., et al., (2000). A comparison of some different methods for purifying core temperature data from humans. *Chronobiology International*, *17*, 539–566.

Weinert, D., Nevill, A., Weinandy, R., & Waterhouse, J. (2003). The development of new purification methods to assess the circadian rhythms of body temperature in Mongolian gerbils. *Chronobiology International*, *20*, 249–270.

Winget, C., deRoshia, C., Markley, L., & Holley, D. (1984). A review of human physiological and performance changes associated with desynchronosis of biological rhythms. *Aviation, Space, and Environmental Medicine*, *55*, 1085–1096.

G. A. Kerkhof and H. P. A. Van Dongen (Eds.)
Progress in Brain Research, Vol. 185
ISSN: 0079-6123

CHAPTER 9

The effects of napping on cognitive functioning

Nicole Lovato and Leon Lack*

School of Psychology, Flinders University, Adelaide, SA, Australia

Abstract: Naps (brief sleeps) are a global and highly prevalent phenomenon, thus warranting consideration for their effects on cognitive functioning. Naps can reduce sleepiness and improve cognitive performance. The benefits of brief (5–15 min) naps are almost immediate after the nap and last a limited period (1–3 h). Longer naps (>30 min) can produce impairment from sleep inertia for a short period after waking but then produce improved cognitive performance for a longer period (up to many hours). Other factors that affect the benefits from the nap are the circadian timing of the nap with early afternoon being the most favourable time. Longer periods of prior wakefulness favour longer naps over brief naps. Those who regularly nap seem to show greater benefits than those who rarely nap. These conclusions, however, need to be accepted cautiously until more comprehensive research programmes are conducted in which all these parameters are varied. Research is also needed to test the benefits of brief naps taken more naturalistically at the time when sleepiness becomes intrusive. The significant benefits of a brief nap, containing virtually no slow wave EEG activity, are not predicted by the present theory of homeostatic sleep drive (Process S). A new biological process (Process O) suggests that sleep onset followed by only 7–10 min of sleep can result in a substantial increase of alertness because it allows the rapid dissipation of inhibition in the 'wake-active' cells associated with the 'sleep-switch' mechanism rather than the dissipation of Process S.

Keywords: Naps; cognitive performance benefits; nap length; sleep inertia; sleep homeostasis; Process O

Overview

A nap is commonly referred to as a 'short sleep', more specifically a sleep which is distinct from and substantially shorter than an individual's normal sleep episode (Dinges, 1989). Dinges et al. (1987) define a nap in more quantitative terms as 'any sleep period with a duration of less than 50% of the average major sleep period of an individual' (p. 313). The briefest naps may consist of only a few

* Corresponding author.
Tel.: (+) 618 8201 2391; Fax: (+) 618 8201 3877.
E-mail: Leon.lack@flinders.edu.au

DOI:10.1016/B978-0-444-53702-7.00009-9

minutes of sleep and the longest up to several hours of sleep. Most commonly nap lengths range from 30 to 90 min (Dinges, 1989). Napping is considered a global phenomenon that occurs during infancy and persists into adulthood for a large proportion of the world's population (Stampi, 1992). Dinges (1989) conducted a comprehensive review of studies which investigated the prevalence of napping among the adult population. The prevalence of regular napping (at least once per week) was reported to vary greatly across countries from 33 to 84%, with the greatest prevalence among countries located close to the equator (Dinges, 1989). More recently, Pilcher et al. (2001) reported similar rates of napping, indicating that approximately 74% of young and middle-aged adults living in the United States reported napping at least once per week.

A multitude of research has investigated the effects of napping and has consistently demonstrated that naps can counteract the effects of sleepiness by enhancing subjective and objective alertness, improving cognition, vigilance and psychomotor ability. This chapter will review the current literature investigating the effects of naps, outline several factors that can affect the recuperative value of a nap, and will discuss potential applications for napping within industry and health care. The chapter will also explain how the recuperative benefits of brief naps cannot be explained by the present conceptualization of homeostatic sleep drive and thus requires a new sleep process (Process O) in addition to the three-process model (Åkerstedt and Folkard, 1997).

For many individuals, napping offers a practical solution to reduce sleepiness. Naps taken for this reason are referred to as replacement or compensatory naps. This type of napping strategy is common among shift workers, individuals suffering from sleep disorders associated with excessive daytime sleepiness and those who have a restricted main sleep episode (Dinges, 1992; Dinges et al., 1981). However, researchers have acknowledged that this is not the only reason individuals may nap. In some circumstances, individuals may choose to nap in anticipation of sleep loss, or to avoid feelings of sleepiness later on. This type of napping is referred to as prophylactic, and is common among shift workers particularly before beginning extended shifts (Stampi, 1992). Although the majority of experimental research has focused on these types of napping, it has also been reported that some people nap in the absence of sleep loss, due to feelings of boredom or for enjoyment. Åkerstedt et al. (1989) have termed this type of napping as appetitive or recreational.

Benefits of naps

The high prevalence rates of napping around the globe alone are suggestive that napping is beneficial (Brooks and Lack, 2006; Dinges, 1989). The benefits of naps have been supported by a number of experimental research paradigms (Betrus, 1986; Bonnet, 1991; Brooks and Lack, 2006; Hayashi and Hori, 1997; Hayashi et al., 2003; Lovato et al., 2009; Milner et al., 2006; Takahashi and Arito, 2000; Tietzel and Lack, 2001, 2003; Tucker and Fishbein, 2008). Naps have not only been shown to reduce subjective and objective sleepiness but can also improve cognitive functioning and psychomotor performance and enhance short-term memory and mood (Brooks and Lack, 2006; Hayashi and Hori, 1997; Takahashi and Arito, 2000; Tamaki et al., 2000; Tietzel and Lack, 2003; Tucker and Fishbein, 2008).

Research has also investigated whether the effects of napping are comparable to other countermeasures commonly used to reduce sleepiness and performance impairments, such as caffeine and stimulant medications. Bonnet et al. (1995) showed that a prophylactic nap produced improvements to performance, mood and alertness which were longer lasting and less variable when compared to improvements following caffeine. Mednick et al. (2008) reported that naps significantly improved declarative verbal memory relative to both caffeine and a placebo. In a similar study, Reyner and Horne (1997) assessed the efficacy of a 15-min nap, caffeine intake or a combination of both on performance using a driver-simulator task. Caffeine taken in conjunction with the nap resulted in a threefold reduction in accidents when compared to caffeine alone.

Limited research has investigated the benefits of naps relative to currently available stimulant medications such as modafinil. Batejat and Lagarde (1999) assessed the effects of naps, modafinil or a combination of both, on cognitive functioning during sleep deprivation. The naps were found to significantly improve psychomotor performance; however, these benefits were strengthened when naps were taken in conjunction with modafinil.

The restorative effects of naps have been well established across a variety of alertness and performance domains, with improvements evident across a wide range of objective and subjective sleepiness measures and cognitive performance measures. Naps are found to have alerting benefits that are comparable, and often superior, to other countermeasures against sleepiness and performance decrements (Batejat and Lagarde, 1999; Bonnet et al., 1995; Mednick et al., 2008; Reyner and Horne, 1997). However, there are a number of factors to consider when aiming to optimize the beneficial effects of a nap, including the duration of the nap and circadian timing of the nap.

Duration of the nap and sleep inertia

Research has demonstrated that the length of a nap can determine its effect on alertness and cognition (Bonnet, 1991; Kubo et al., 2007; Tietzel and Lack, 2001). Naps of all durations (from 5 min to 2 h) have been shown to have some benefits to cognition (Brooks and Lack, 2005). However, it is the way in which these benefits emerge over the period following the nap that produces the most evident differences between different length naps. The benefits of a brief nap (e.g. 10 min of sleep) emerge almost immediately following the nap and can last up to 3 h (Brooks and Lack, 2006). However, immediately following long naps (e.g. 2 h) performance can actually decline for a period with eventual improvements that can last up to 24 h (Achermann et al., 1995; Jewett et al., 1999; Lumley et al., 1986). Figure 1 illustrates the tentative conclusions we can draw about the general time course of negative and positive effects on cognition for brief (e.g. 10 min), short (e.g. 30 min)

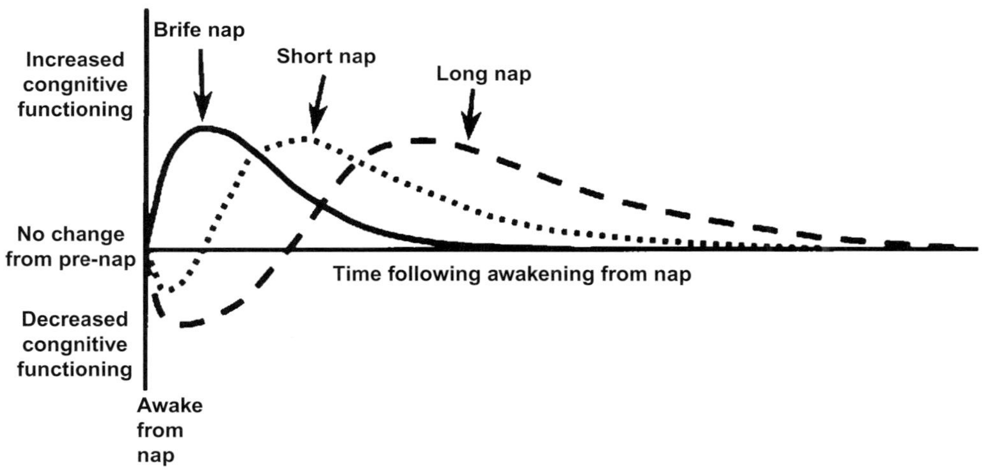

Fig. 1. Relative changes in detrimental and beneficial effects of brief, short and long naps following awakening from the nap.

and long (e.g. 2 h) naps. Still needed is a systematic parametric programme of research in which length of nap, time of nap and amount of prior sleep restriction are all varied while using a comprehensive set of outcome measures of alertness and cognitive performance administered over at least a 3-h period following the nap.

The temporary deterioration of performance immediately following long naps has been attributed to sleep inertia. Naitoh and Angus (1989) describe sleep inertia as 'inferior task performance and/or disorientation occurring immediately after awakening' (p. 226). Sleep inertia reflects a transition from a sleep state to a wake state and is characterized by electroencephalography patterns, which resemble Stage 1 sleep patterns (Naitoh and Angus, 1989) rather than wake (Naitoh et al., 1993).

The magnitude of sleep inertia is dependent on several factors the most important of which is the quantity of slow-wave sleep (SWS) contained within the napping episode (Åkerstedt and Folkard, 1991). Although the quantity of SWS is positively correlated with the recuperative value of a nap, particularly when considering improvements to short-term memory performance (Schmidt et al., 2006; Tucker et al., 2006), it is also positively correlated with the intensity and duration of sleep inertia (Åkerstedt and Folkard, 1991). Since SWS normally develops gradually over time asleep, longer naps, at least up to the point of maximum slow-wave activity (SWA) in a sleep cycle, are expected to result in longer and more intense periods of sleep inertia.

The magnitude of sleep inertia is also influenced by prior sleep debt, circadian time and sleep stage at awakening (Tassi and Muzet, 2000). Sleep inertia is the most persistent from sleep episodes taken during the circadian nadir, under conditions of high sleep debt and waking from SWS (Tassi and Muzet, 2000). The substantial sleep inertia arising from these longer naps can be ameliorated to some extent by consuming caffeine on awakening (Bonnet and Arand, 1994; Schweitzer et al., 2006; Van Dongen et al., 2001).

Brief naps (less than 20 min) have been shown to ameliorate sleepiness and improve performance after both a restricted nocturnal sleep and a nocturnal sleep of normal duration (Hayashi et al., 2005; Tamaki et al., 2000; Tietzel and Lack, 2002, 2003). A number of researchers have demonstrated that naps as brief as 10 min in duration can improve subjective and objective alertness, increase feelings of vigour and decrease fatigue, in addition to improving accuracy and speed on a number of cognitive tasks (Brooks and Lack, 2006; Horne and Reyner, 1996; Takahashi and Arito, 2000; Tietzel and Lack, 2002). One study has found that a nap as brief as 7 min is beneficial for restoring alertness (Takahashi et al., 1998). Unlike long naps, the beneficial effects of brief naps are evident almost immediately after waking (Tietzel and Lack, 2002). Brief naps are associated with shorter periods of sleep inertia, and in some instances, no sleep inertia (Tietzel and Lack, 2002).

Although research suggests that both brief and long naps are beneficial for improving alertness, few studies have used the same protocol and outcome measures to directly compare the benefits of brief and long naps. This remains an important research programme to be pursued. Nevertheless, it is suggested that for sleep restricted individuals and individuals who have experienced normal nocturnal sleep duration, brief naps and long naps produce comparable benefits to alertness (Brooks and Lack, 2006; Takahashi et al., 1998; Taub et al., 1976; Tietzel and Lack, 2001). It is only in the case of total sleep deprivation that naps of a longer duration (1–2 h) have been demonstrated to elicit greater alerting benefits than brief naps (Helmus et al., 1997; Lumley et al., 1986).

Circadian placement of the nap

The recuperative value of a nap is also dependent on when the nap is taken with respect to the 24-h circadian rhythm (e.g. as reflected in core body temperature). The three-process model of alertness (Åkerstedt and Folkard, 1991) proposes that the maximum period of circadian sleepiness occurs in the early hours of the morning (0300–0600 h). A secondary period of sleepiness occurs in the mid-afternoon (1300–1600 h), referred to as the post-lunch dip period (Åkerstedt and Folkard, 1991). Experimental studies using both continuous wakefulness and sleep/wake ultradian routines across the 24-h day, have also reported peaks in sleepiness and napping at these times (Broughton, 1989; Lack and Lushington, 1996; Lack et al., 2009; Lavie, 1989). Since most individuals take their main sleep nocturnally across the maximum period of circadian sleepiness, the preferred time to nap is usually reported to be during the post-lunch dip period between 1300 and 1600 h (Broughton, 1989).

Research has indicated that naps taken during the post-lunch dip period have a greater recuperative value than when naps are taken in the early morning, late morning or evening (Naitoh and Angus, 1989; Taub et al., 1978). Researchers have further established the optimum time to nap during the 3-h post-lunch dip period. Hayashi et al. (1999a, 1999b) compared a 20-min nap taken at noon or 1400 h relative to a no-nap control condition. The 20-min nap scheduled at 1400 h produced both greater and longer lasting benefits to mood, fatigue, objective performance, self-rated performance and objective alertness, when compared to the 20-min nap scheduled at noon.

Naps taken during the circadian nadir (approximately 0400 h) produce less recuperative value when compared to naps taken during the day or in the early hours of the morning. Sallinen et al. (1998) found that 30- and 50-min naps taken by shift workers at 0100 h improved objective alertness; however, when the same naps were taken closer to the circadian nadir at 0400 h, no alerting benefits were observed. Purnell et al. (2002) reported benefits in performance after a 20-min nap when taken at either 0100 or 0300 h, while Saito and Sasaki (1996) found that 1-h naps ending at either 0400 or 0500 h had no alerting benefits for subjective fatigue. It is still difficult at present to come to confident conclusions about the effect of circadian phase on napping effects from the sparse evidence available from a few studies using different measures and methodologies. This strengthens the earlier point about the need for a comprehensive research programme testing a variety of circadian times with a variety of nap lengths.

Other factors: prior wake time and experience with napping

Research has also suggested that other factors such as prior wake time and experience with napping can contribute to the duration and magnitude of alerting benefits (Dinges, 1995; Dinges et al., 1987; Rosa et al., 1983). Several researchers have demonstrated that naps taken after long periods of wakefulness (e.g. 18 h) are less effective and have shorter-lasting benefits than naps taken after shorter periods of wakefulness (Dinges, 1995; Dinges et al., 1987). Additionally, research has concluded that the longer an individual has been awake, the longer a nap needs to be to improve alertness (Dinges, 1995; Dinges et al., 1987).

A limited amount of research has been conducted on the impact experience with napping can have on the recuperative effects of a nap. Taub and colleagues (Taub, 1979; Taub and Berger, 1973; Taub et al., 1976, 1977, 1978) conducted several studies investigating the alerting benefits of naps for individuals who habitually nap (one or more times per week for at least 2 years). Taub and Berger (1973) reported that an afternoon nap improved the mood and performance of habitual nappers. Evans et al. (1977) extended Taub and Berger's (1973) work to compare the benefits of a nap for habitual nappers and non-nappers. In this study, participants who regularly napped reported feeling more satisfied and less sleepy and tired following an afternoon nap when compared to participants who did not nap on a regular basis. Recently, Milner et al. (2006) reported that a short nap improved motor learning performance for individuals who regularly napped, but was detrimental for those who were not habitual nappers. Contrary to these findings, other studies have demonstrated no significant differences in performance for habitual and non-habitual nappers following an afternoon nap (Daiss et al., 1986; Keyes, 1989). Further research is required to clarify the differential effects of naps for habitual and non-habitual nappers (Milner and Cote, 2008). Perhaps habitual nappers choose to nap on a regular basis because they experience a greater benefit from the nap. Habitual nappers may be chronically sleep restricted and require naps to achieve acceptable alertness levels during the day. Differences between regular nappers and non-nappers could thus be compared after several nights of unlimited sleep opportunity in order to eliminate any residual effects of sleep restriction.

Can experiments capture the naturalistic use of napping?

There is considerable experimental support for the ability of brief naps to increase alertness as evidenced in measures of subjective feelings, objective sleep latency and objective measures of cognitive performance. All of these studies administered nap opportunities at scheduled times in fixed experimental protocols. They were not self-selected times that, in a more naturalistic situation, would usually determine the timing of a nap. In practice, an individual is likely to take a nap when sleepiness becomes so intense that it interferes with ongoing activity and when opportunity or conditions (physical and social) allow. Most of us in our mildly sleep-restricted lives have experienced occasional drowsiness and the struggle to remain awake whether it is during an uninteresting lecture or meeting, some quiet reading or study in the early afternoon, or in front of the television in the evening (Johns, 1991). A common anecdotal report is that a brief nap at that time can remarkably remove the drowsiness feeling and restore cognitive functioning. The experimental evidence supports these reports. We predict that an experiment that allowed a self-selected nap time at the point of heightened drowsiness would show even more impressive improvements in subjective alertness as well as objective cognitive performance.

Theoretical implications of brief nap benefits

The research confirming the benefits of brief naps not only has applied importance but it can also contribute to theoretical biological models of sleep propensity. The apparent rapid reversal of sleepiness following a brief nap suggests the need for a biological mechanism additional to the presently accepted three-process model that includes sleep homeostasis (Process S), circadian phase (Process C) and sleep inertia (Process W) (Åkerstedt and Folkard, 1997). The three-process model would suggest that if the circadian factor was kept relatively constant and any sleep inertia were allowed to dissipate, any benefits of a brief sleep would be entirely dependent on the decrease of homeostatic sleep drive (Process S) following sleep onset. The original simplified conceptualization of the dissipation of Process S was represented by an exponential decaying function in which the rate of decay was maximal following sleep onset (Daan et al., 1984). However, the model was then revised to indicate that the decrease of homeostatic sleep drive during sleep is entirely dependent of the amount of SWA that varies across sleep with an ultradian rhythm of an approximately 90-min period length (Achermann and Borbély, 1990). Thus, Process S would dissipate most rapidly when SWA is at a maximum, but this would not occur immediately at sleep onset. It would increase gradually over 20–70 min with the gradual increase in SWA. The ultradian rhythm of SWA during sleep and the predicted decrease of Process S is illustrated in Fig. 2.

This dissipation function of Process S during sleep would suggest that the longer the sleep or the nap, especially the more SWA included in the sleep, the greater the benefit for alertness or decrease of sleepiness. However, the data suggest considerable benefits to alertness from very brief

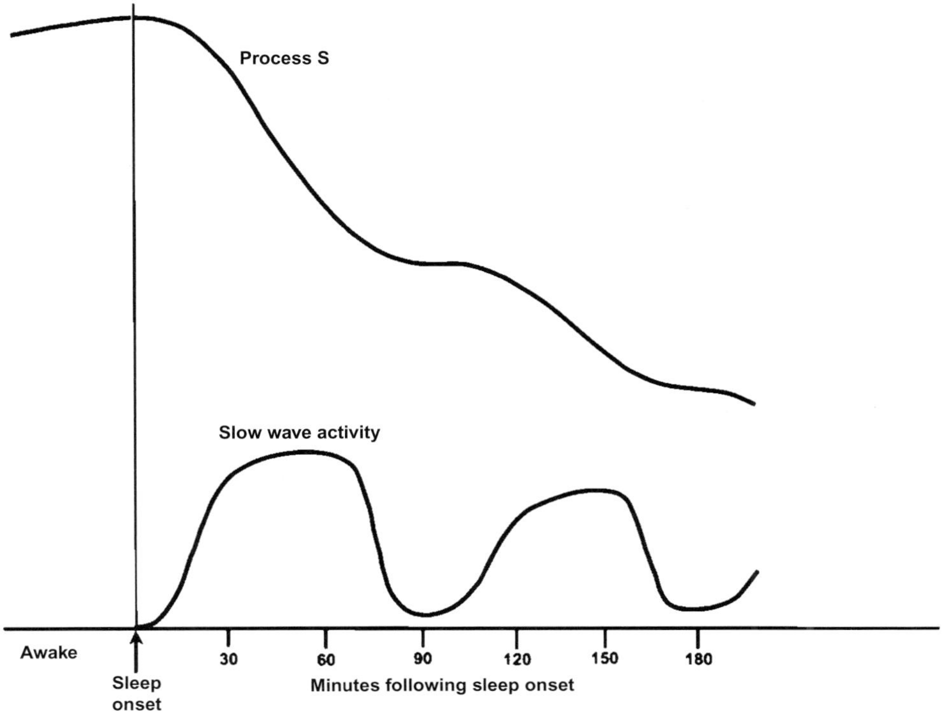

Fig. 2. Revised dissipation of homeostatic sleep drive (Process S) as a function solely of slow-wave activity during the sleep period illustrating very little decrease of Process S for brief (<15 min of sleep) naps.

(7–10 min of sleep) naps. Yet, in terms of satisfying accumulated homeostatic sleep drive, such a brief and light sleep with virtually no SWA should result in virtually no decrease in Process S and thus provide almost no benefit. For example, Fig. 2 shows very little decrease of Process S in the first 15 min of sleep. However, in comparison with longer naps (20–60 min of sleep) containing much more SWA, the benefits following brief naps are surprisingly comparable. These benefits are maintained even after allowing for the dissipation of the negative effects of sleep inertia immediately following a longer sleep. This suggests some other mechanism, apart from homeostatic sleep drive, determines the improvement of alertness and performance following brief naps.

This additional process may incorporate what Saper et al. (2001) have termed as a 'sleep-switch' mechanism. This is a bi-stable, 'flip-flop' circuit that spends little time in transition and promotes stability of either sleep or wake. Evidence suggests the sleep-switch mechanism involves nuclei of sleep-active neurons and opposing nuclei of wake-active neurons with mutual inhibitory connections. When the balance is tipped in favour of sleep, as a result of accumulated homeostatic sleep drive, high circadian sleep propensity or sleep-conducive circumstances, the sleep-active nuclei increase their activity and thus increase their inhibition of the wake-active neurons. With the decreased activation of the wake-active neurons there would be less inhibitory feedback to the sleep-active neurons and the switch to sleep would occur quickly and then tend to be maintained by strong inhibition of the wake-active neurons. The process is analogous to the switches that occurs when breathing (from inspiration to expiration and the opposite change), these also being controlled by groups of mutually inhibitory neurons.

An additional sleep process (Process 'O')

We suggest that alertness can be increased a constant amount simply through the process of sleep onset (or Process O) (Lack and Tietzel, 2000). What exactly constitutes sleep onset in this sense and how brief the period of sleep needs to be and still satisfy this process has already been explored to some extent. It appears to require more than the onset of Stage 1 sleep since ultra-brief naps of 30–90 s of sleep produce no measurable benefit (Tietzel and Lack, 2002). Hayashi et al. (2005) have suggested that it is not the onset of Stage 2 but the presence of at least 3 min of Stage 2 sleep following 4–5 min of Stage 1 sleep that provides the benefits of a brief nap. More recently, Brooks and Lack (2006), by comparing different nap lengths (5, 10, 20 and 30 min sleep), obtained data that suggested an elapsed amount of sleep (about 10 min) or the onset of some SWA are potential candidates for the benefits of Process O.

This proposed mechanism may be intrinsic to the sleep switch itself rather than an 'external' factor (elsewhere in the brain) playing upon it such as Process S or C. As Saper et al. (2001) describe, when the switch 'flops' to the sleep state, the sleep nuclei become active and the wake-active nuclei are inhibited and, as a result, become inactive. The mechanism we suggest would incorporate a fatigue or adaptation process that builds up slowly over the period of activation with a time constant in the order of hours. This would gradually decrease the excitability of the active neural centre. However, with a flip or flop of the sleep switch, the previously active centre is turned off during which the accumulated fatigue or satiation (lowered excitability) dissipates relatively rapidly with a time constant more in the order of minutes. Thus, during a brief (e.g. 10 min) sleep, excitability returns almost entirely to the now inactive wake centre. If an awakening then occurs, the wake-active nuclei have regained most of their maximal excitability and provide a significant increase of alertness or decrease of the prior sleepiness. This would account for the relatively rapid improvement in alertness following a brief nap and its benefits lasting in the order of 2–3 h as fatigue slowly builds again in the wake-active nuclei.

This return of excitability to the wake-active centre during a brief nap does not flip the switch back to awake on its own, since it is still being inhibited by the still active sleep centre. Therefore, if one desires to limit the length of a nap to a brief 10–15 min it would be advisable, particularly for inexperienced nappers, to use a timed alarm. Interestingly, there are anecdotal reports from experienced brief nappers that they are usually able to awake spontaneously to ensure a brief nap only. This is an interesting question that deserves some research to explore its applied utility.

The existence of differential time constants between reduction of excitability during activation and return of excitability at the cessation of activity is not a novel mechanism in physiology and behaviour. There are other analogues of this process such as sensory adaptation, habituation and reactive inhibition (Hull, 1951). These processes have similarities with a relatively slow build up of inhibition during activation and a relatively rapid dissipation of this inhibition or return of excitability following cessation of activity (Duncan, 1956). As a further example, the time-constants are very different between activation and de-activation of sodium and potassium voltage-gated channels during the generation of an action potential in excitable tissues.

The anecdotal scenario described above, in which strong drowsiness is alleviated following a brief nap, could be explained in terms of Process O which is intrinsic to the 'sleep-switch' mechanism of Saper et al. (2001). The strong drowsiness feeling would be an indication that the input to the sleep switch from situational and behavioural variables was moving the switch closer to the threshold of sleep or tipping the position of the switch very close to a 'flop' into sleep. Then allowing sleep to occur for the few minutes to maximally satisfy Process O would return excitability to the 'wake-active' nuclei and result in noticeably increased alertness upon awakening.

We are not suggesting that this dissipation of 'fatigue' or recovery of excitability of the wake-active nuclei is enough on its own to overcome Process S, which has decreased very little during this brief sleep. The maximum effect of this intrinsic mechanism, Process O, in comparison with Process S needs to be investigated by considerably more research. However, our guess is that it is significantly weaker than the effect of accumulated Process S during 16 h of wakefulness in a normal day. We suggest that this Process O is similar in operation to Process S but with a much shorter time scale and smaller maximum intensity. Thus, although it accumulates fatigue much more slowly than it dissipates it, the time scale to maximum fatigue would be in the order of 2–3 h and dissipation complete in 8–15 min. In contrast, Process S can accumulate sleep pressure over days of total sleep deprivation and require over 10–12 h of sleep to dissipate entirely.

Parenthetically, the most parsimonious assumption of the operation of this process on the sleep switch is that it operates symmetrically for brief awakenings during the major sleep period as it would for brief sleeps during the major wake period. That is a brief (5–10 min) awakening from the major sleep period should rapidly dissipate fatigue from the sleep-active nuclei thus facilitating the re-establishment of sleep when it recurs. Such a re-establishment of sleep, in conjunction with Process W, sleep inertia (still potent only after 5–10 min of wakefulness) and maximal sleepiness from Process C towards the end of the normal sleep period, should all help to maintain the continuity of the major sleep period (Dijk and Czeisler, 1994).

Relative impacts of brief and long naps on subsequent nocturnal sleep and clinical implications

The substantial SWS contained in longer naps has been demonstrated to disturb the duration and architecture of the subsequent nocturnal sleep period (Åkerstedt et al., 1989; Dinges, 1989). For this reason, behavioural treatments of insomnia, such as stimulus control therapy and bedtime restriction therapy, that rely upon the increase of sleep drive in the early stages of treatment, recommend avoiding daytime naps that would lower the therapeutic benefits of this temporarily raised sleep pressure. On the other hand, brief afternoon naps have not been shown to affect the length or quality of the subsequent night sleep (Purnell et al., 2002). Therefore, brief naps during the day to temporarily reduce daytime sleepiness that may accumulate during the initial stages of insomnia treatment may be permissible. If successful at relieving the sleepiness, the use of brief naps may improve the compliance with these sometimes onerous therapies. In addition, the adoption of this brief nap strategy may provide the insomniac with a tool to counteract the tiredness following a poor night of sleep. Therefore, this new napping skill could reduce the negative daytime consequences of poor sleep and thus help to ameliorate the insomnia.

Applications for napping

The benefits of napping have been well established and can be utilized in many situations to minimize sleepiness and regain alertness. Naps of brief duration are particularly ideal for use within the workplace as they can be taken during the employees' break time (Anthony and Anthony, 2005; Signal and Gander, 2002). The minimal sleep inertia produced by brief naps also allows for maximum productivity to resume almost immediately after waking from the nap. Research has suggested that brief naps can temporarily relieve the excessive levels of daytime sleepiness experienced by narcolepsy suffers (Mullington and Broughton, 1993; Roehrs et al., 1986; Rogers and Aldrich, 1993; Schulz et al., 1992). Also, sleep apnoea patients with high levels of daytime sleepiness regularly take naps to alleviate bouts of sleepiness.

The use of napping is also recommended for trans-meridian travel to allow the biological clock to adapt en route (Kerkhof, 2009). Kerkhof (2009) has also recently reported the use of multiple 10-min naps by a solo sailor during long legs of a journey when opportunities for longer sleeps were not possible. Therefore, brief naps (power naps) have anecdotal and research support for their effectiveness in relieving sleepiness as well as becoming a prompt for revising our theoretical models of sleep.

References

Achermann, P., & Borbély, A. A. (1990). Simulation of human sleep: Ultradian dynamics of electroencephalographic slow-wave activity. *Journal of Biological Rhythms*, *5*(2); 141–157.

Achermann, P., Werth, E., Dikj, D. J., & Borbély, A. (1995). Time course of sleep inertia after nighttime and daytime sleep episodes. *Archives Italiennes de Biologie*, *134*, 109–119.

Åkerstedt, T., & Folkard, S. (1991). A three process model of the regulation of alertness and sleepiness. In: Ogilvie, R., Broughton, R. (Eds.), *Sleep, arousal and performance: Problems and promises*. Birkhäuser, Boston, pp. 11–26.

Åkerstedt, T., & Folkard, S. (1997). The three-process model of alertness and its extension to performance, sleep latency, and sleep length. *Chronobiology International*, *14*, 115–123.

Åkerstedt, T., Torsvall, L., & Gillberg, M. (1989). Shift work and napping. In: Dinges, D., Broughton, R. (Eds.), *Sleep and alertness: Chronobiological, behavioural and medical aspects of napping*. Raven Press, New York, pp. 205–220.

Anthony, W., & Anthony, C. (2005). The napping company: Bringing science to the workplace. *Industrial Health*, *43*, 209–212.

Batejat, D. M., & Lagarde, D. P. (1999). Naps and modafinil as countermeasures for the effects of sleep deprivation on cognitive performance. *Aviation, Space, and Environmental Medicine*, *70*, 493–498.

Betrus, P. (1986). Afternoon naps: Immediate and delayed effects on performance and mood. *Dissertation Abstracts International*, *46*, 3630–3631.

Bonnet, M. (1991). The effect of varying prophylactic naps on performance, alertness and mood throughout a 52-hour continuous operation. *Sleep*, *14*, 307–315.

Bonnet, M., & Arand, D. L. (1994). The use of prophylactic naps and caffeine during a continuous operation. *Ergonomics*, *37*(6); 1009–1020.

Bonnet, M., Gomez, S., Wirth, O., & Arand, D. (1995). The use of caffeine versus prophylactic naps in sustained performance. *Sleep*, *18*, 97–104.

Brooks, A., & Lack, L. C. (2005). Naps. In: Kushida, C. A. (Ed.), *Sleep deprivation: Clinical issues, pharmacology, and sleep loss effects*. Marcel Dekker, Inc, New York, pp. 457–474.

Brooks, A., & Lack, L. (2006). A brief afternoon nap following nocturnal sleep restriction: Which nap duration is most recuperative? *Sleep*, *29*, 831–840.

Broughton, R. J. (1989). Chronobiological aspects and models of sleep and napping. In: Dinges, D. F., Broughton, R. J. (Eds.), *Sleep and alertness: Chronobiological, behavioural and medical aspects of napping*. Raven Press, New York, pp. 71–98.

Daan, S., Beersma, D. G. M., & Borbély, A. A. (1984). Timing of human sleep: Recovery process gated by a circadian pacemaker. *American Journal of Physiology*, *246*, R161–R178.

Daiss, S., Bertelson, A., & Benjamin, L. (1986). Napping versus resting: Effects on performance and mood. *Psychophysiology*, *23*, 82–88.

Dijk, D., & Czeisler, C. (1994). Paradoxical timing of the circadian rhythms of sleep propensity serves to consolidate sleep and wakefulness in humans. *Neuroscience Letters*, *166*, 63–68.

Dinges, D. F. (1989). Napping patterns and effects in human adults. In: Dinges, D. F., Broughton, R. J. (Eds.), *Sleep and alertness: Chronobiological, behavioural and medical aspects of napping*. Raven Press, New York, pp. 171–204.

Dinges, D. F. (1992). Adult napping and its effects of ability to function. In: Stampi, C. (Ed.), *Why we nap: Evolution, chronobiology and functions of polyphasic and ultrashort sleep*. Birkhauser, Boston, pp. 118–132.

Dinges, D. (1995). An overview of sleepiness and accidents. *Journal of Sleep Research*, *4*(Suppl. 2); 4–14.

Dinges, D., Orne, M., Orne, E., & Evans, F. (1981). Behavioural patterns in habitual nappers. [Abstract only]. *Journal of Sleep Research,* 136

Dinges, D., Orne, E., Whitehouse, W., & Orne, M. (1987). Temporal placement of a nap for alertness: Contributions of circadian phase and prior wakefulness. *Sleep*, *10*, 313–329.

Duncan, C. P. (1956). On the similarity between reactive inhibition and neural satiation. *American Journal of Psychology*, *69*, 227–235.

Evans, F., Cook, M., Cohen, H., Orne, E., & Orne, M. (1977). Appetitive and replacement naps: EEG and behaviour. *Science*, *197*, 687–689.

Hayashi, M., & Hori, T. (1997). The effects of a 20-minute nap in the early afternoon. [Abstract only]. *Psychiatry and Clinical Neurosciences*, *51*, 558.

Hayashi, M., Fukushima, H., & Hori, T. (2003). The effects of short daytime naps for five consecutive days. *Sleep Research Online*, *5*, 13–17.

Hayashi, M., Ito, S., & Hori, T. (1999a). The effects of a 20-min nap at noon on sleepiness, performance and EEG activity. *International Journal of Psychophysiology*, *32*, 173–180.

Hayashi, M., Motoyoshi, N., & Hori, T. (2005). Recuperative power of a short daytime nap with or without stage 2 sleep. *Sleep*, *28*, 829–836.

Hayashi, M., Watanabe, M., & Hori, T. (1999b). The effects of a 20 min nap in the mid-afternoon on mood performance and EEG activity. *Clinical Neurophysiology*, *110*, 272–279.

Helmus, T., Rosenthal, L., Bishop, C., Roehrs, T., Syron, M., & Roth, T. (1997). The alerting effects of short and long naps in narcoleptic, sleep-deprived and alert individuals. *Sleep*, *20*, 251–257.

Horne, J., & Reyner, L. (1996). Counteracting driver sleepiness: Effects of napping, caffeine and placebo. *Psychophysiology*, *33*, 306–309.

Hull, C. L. (1951). *Essentials of behavior.* Greenwood, Westport, CT.

Jewett, M., Wyatt, J., Cecco, A., Khalsa, S., Dijk, D., & Czeisler, C. (1999). Time course of sleep inertia dissipation in human performance and alertness. *Journal of Sleep Research*, *8*, 1–8.

Johns, M. (1991). A new method for measuring daytime sleepiness: The Epworth Sleepiness Scale. *Sleep*, *14*, 540–545.

Kerkhof, G. (2009). Transmeridian sailing. *Mind Open: Insights in Psychology*4–5

Keyes, K. (1989). Effects of sleep quality and daytime naps on the mood and functioning of older persons. *Dissertation Abstracts International*, *58*, 2350–2351.

Kubo, T., Takeyama, H., Matsumoto, S., Ebara, T., Murata, K., & Tachi, N., et al., (2007). Impact of nap length, nap timing and sleep quality on sustaining early morning performance. *Industrial Health*, *45*, 552–563.

Lack, L., & Lushington, K. (1996). The rhythms of sleep propensity and core body-temperature. *Journal of Sleep Research*, *5*, 1–11.

Lack, L., & Tietzel, A. (2000). Do the benefits of brief naps suggest a fourth biological process determining sleepiness? *Sleep*, *23*(Suppl. 2); A56.

Lack, L., Bailey, M., Lovato, N., & Wright, H. (2009). Chronotype differences in circadian rhythms of temperature, melatonin, and sleepiness as measured in a modified constant routine protocol. *Nature and Science of Sleep*, *1*, 1–8.

Lavie, P. (1989). To nap, perchance to sleep – Ultradian aspects of napping. In: Dinges, D., Broughton, R. (Eds.), *Sleep and alertness: Chronobiological, behavioural and medical aspects of napping*. Raven Press, New York, pp. 99–120.

Lovato, N., Lack, L., Ferguson, S., & Tremaine, R. (2009). The effects of a 30-min nap during night shift following a prophylactic sleep in the afternoon. *Sleep and Biological Rhythms*, *7*, 34–42.

Lumley, M., Roehrs, T., Zorick, F., Lamphere, J., & Roth, T. (1986). The alerting effects of naps in sleep-deprived subjects. *Psychophysiology*, *23*, 403–408.

Mednick, S., Cai, D., Kanady, J., & Drummond, S. (2008). Comparing the benefits of caffeine, naps and placebo on verbal, motor and perceptual memory. *Behavioural Brain Research*, *193*, 79–86.

Milner, C., & Cote, K. (2008). Benefits of napping in healthy adults: Impact of nap length, time of day, age, and experience with napping. *Journal of Sleep Research*, *18*(2); 272–281.

Milner, C., Fogel, S., & Cote, K. (2006). Habitual napping moderates motor performance improvements following a short daytime nap. *Biological Psychology*, *73*, 141–156.

Mullington, J., & Broughton, R. (1993). Scheduled naps in the management of daytime sleepiness in narcolepsy-cataplexy. *Sleep*, *16*, 444–456.

Naitoh, P., & Angus, R. (1989). Napping and human functioning during prolonged work. In: Dinges, D., Broughton, R. (Eds.), *Sleep and alertness: Chronobiological, behavioral and medical aspects of napping*. Raven Press, New York, pp. 221–246.

Naitoh, P., Kelly, T., & Babkoff, H. (1993). Sleep inertia: Best time not to wake up? *Chronobiology International*, *10*, 109–118.

Pilcher, J., Michalowski, K., & Carrigan, R. (2001). The prevalence of daytime napping and its relationship to nighttime sleep. *Behavioral Medicine*, *27*, 71–76.

Purnell, M., Feyer, M., & Herbison, G. (2002). The impact of a nap opportunity during the night shift on performance and alertness of 12-h shift workers. *Journal of Sleep Research*, *11*, 219–227.

Reyner, L., & Horne, J. (1997). Suppression of sleepiness in drivers: Combination of caffeine with a short nap. *Psychophysiology*, *34*, 721–725.

Roehrs, T., Zorick, F., Wittig, R., Paxton, C., Sicklesteel, J., & Roth, T. (1986). Alerting effects of naps in patients with narcolepsy. *Sleep*, *9*, 194–199.

Rogers, A., & Aldrich, M. (1993). The effect of regularly scheduled naps on sleep attacks and excessive daytime sleepiness associated with narcolepsy. *Nursing Research*, *42*, 111–117.

Rosa, R., Bonnet, M., & Warm, J. (1983). Recovery of performance during sleep following sleep deprivation. *Psychophysiology*, *20*, 152–159.

Saito, Y., & Sasaki, T. (1996). The effect of length of a nocturnal nap on fatigue feelings during subsequent early morning hours. *Journal of Science Labour*, *72*, 15–23.

Sallinen, M., Harma, M., Åkerstedt, T., Rosa, R., & Lillqvist, O. (1998). Promoting alertness with a short nap during a night shift. *Journal of Sleep Research*, *7*, 240–247.

Saper, C. B., Chou, T. C., & Scammell, T. E. (2001). The sleep switch: Hypothalamic control of sleep and wakefulness. *Trends in Neurosciences*, *24*, 726–731.

Schmidt, C., Peigneux, P., Muto, V., Schenkel, M., Knoblauch, V., & Munch, M. (2006). Encoding difficulty promotes post-learning changes in sleep spindle activity during napping. *Journal of Neuroscience*, *26*, 8976–8982.

Schulz, H., Wilde-Frenz, J., Volk, S., & Geisler, P. (1992). Narcolepsy and the pathological aspects of multiple napping. In: Stampi, C. (Ed.), *Why we nap: Evolution, chronobiology and functions of polyphasic and ultrashort sleep*. Birkhauser, Boston, pp. 258–270.

Schweitzer, P. K., Randazzo, A. C., Stone, K., Erman, M., & Walsh, J. K. (2006). Laboratory and field studies of naps and caffeine as practical countermeasures for sleep-wake problems associated with night work. *Sleep*, *29*(1); 39–50.

Signal, L., & Gander, P. (2002). Psychomotor performance improvements with a short workplace nap on the night shift: Benefits of stage 1 sleep. [Abstract only]. *Sleep*, *25*, 116.

Stampi, C. (1992). Evolution, chronobiology and functions of polyphasic and ultrashort sleep: Main issues. In: Stampi, C. (Ed.), *Why we nap: Evolution, chronobiology and functions of polyphasic and ultrashort sleep*. Birkhauser, Boston, pp. 1–20.

Takahashi, M., & Arito, H. (2000). Maintenance of alertness and performance by a brief nap after lunch under prior sleep deficit. *Sleep*, *23*, 813–819.

Takahashi, M., Fukuda, H., & Arito, H. (1998). Brief naps during post-lunch rest: Effects on alertness, performance and autonomic balance. *European Journal of Applied Physiology*, *78*, 93–98.

Tamaki, M., Shirota, A., Hayashi, M., & Hori, T. (2000). Restorative effects of a short afternoon nap (<30 min) in the elderly on subjective mood, performance and EEG activity. *Sleep Research Online*, *3*, 131–139.

Tassi, P., & Muzet, A. (2000). Sleep inertia. *Sleep Medicine Reviews*, *4*(4); 341–353.

Taub, J. (1979). Effects of habitual variations in napping on psychomotor performance, memory and subjective states. *International Journal of Neuroscience*, *9*, 97–112.

Taub, J., & Berger, R. (1973). Performance and mood following variations in the length and timing of sleep. *Psychophysiology*, *10*, 559–570.

Taub, J., Hawkins, D., & Van de Castle, R. (1978). Temporal relationships of napping behaviour to performance, mood states and sleep physiology. *Sleep Research*, *7*, 164.

Taub, J., Tanguay, P., & Clarkson, D. (1976). Effects of daytime naps on performance and mood in a college student population. *The Journal of Abnormal Psychology*, *85*, 210–217.

Taub, J., Tanguay, P., & Rosa, R. (1977). Effects of afternoon naps on physiological variables, performance and self-reported activation. *Biological Psychology*, *5*, 191–210.

Tietzel, A., & Lack, L. (2001). The short-term benefits of brief and long naps following nocturnal sleep restriction. *Sleep*, *24*, 293–300.

Tietzel, A., & Lack, L. (2002). The recuperative value of brief and ultra-brief naps on alertness and cognitive performance. *Journal of Sleep Research*, *11*, 213–218.

Tietzel, A., & Lack, L. (2003). The objective alerting effects of brief naps following eight hours of nocturnal sleep. [Abstract only]. *Sleep*, *26*, 431.

Tucker, M., & Fishbein, W. (2008). Enhancement of declarative memory performance following a daytime nap is contingent on strength of initial task acquisition. *Sleep*, *31*, 197–203.

Tucker, M., Hirota, Y., Wamsley, E., Lau, H., Chaklader, A., & Fishbein, W. (2006). A daytime nap containing solely non-REM sleep enhances declarative but not procedural memory. *Neurobiology of Learning and Memory*, *86*, 241–247.

Van Dongen, H., Price, N. J., Mullington, J. M., Szuba, M. P., Kapoor, S. C., & Dinges, D. (2001). Caffeine eliminates psychomotor vigilance deficits from sleep inertia. *Sleep*, *24*(7); 813–819.

G. A. Kerkhof and H. P. A. Van Dongen (Eds.)
Progress in Brain Research, Vol. 185
ISSN: 0079-6123

CHAPTER 10

Sleep, intelligence and cognition in a developmental context: differentiation between traits and state-dependent aspects

Anja Geiger[†,§], Peter Achermann[‡,§] and Oskar G. Jenni[†,§,*]

[†]*Child Development Center, University Children's Hospital Zürich, Zürich, Switzerland*
[‡]*Institute of Pharmacology and Toxicology, University of Zürich, Zürich, Switzerland*
[§]*Zürich Center for Integrative Human Physiology (ZIHP), University of Zürich, Zürich, Switzerland*

Abstract: This article addresses associations between sleep, cognition and intelligence in a developmental context and clarifies the terminology. Research must differentiate between aspects related to general underlying traits and those aspects that are characterized by state-dependent fluctuations.

Keywords: Sleep; cognitive performance; intelligence; trait; state; intra-individual stability; ability; electroencephalogram

Introduction

Sleep is a behavioural state which covers a large part of everyone's life. Sleep is also a focus of interest for many scientific disciplines such as medicine and psychology and bears substantial relevance for the entire society. For example, sleep deprivation or chronic sleep restriction is known to impair the performance of individuals, their health and well being (Banks and Dinges, 2007; Carskadon et al., 2004).

A number of hypotheses have been proposed to explain the functions of sleep. Among these theories, one is currently dominating the field: sleep plays a fundamental role in memory consolidation, learning and brain plasticity (Dang-Vu et al., 2006; Tononi and Cirelli, 2006; Walker, 2009) and thus, affects the individual's cognitive functioning during wakefulness (Diekelmann and Born, 2010). Indeed, sleep deprivation or restriction is associated with impaired cognitive performance, which is

[*]Corresponding author.
Tel.: (+) 41 44 266 77 51; Fax: (+) 41 44 266 71 64.
E-mail: Oskar.Jenni@kispi.uzh.ch

DOI:10.1016/B978-0-444-53702-7.00010-5

hypothesized to be of particular relevance for those cognitive domains that mainly rely on the frontal cortex such as executive functions and working memory (Durmer and Dinges, 2005; Jones and Harrison, 2001). On the other hand, learning processes also exert influence on sleep. For instance, activation of circumscribed brain areas with a visuomotor-learning task resulted in a local increase of slow-wave activity [SWA or delta power, corresponding to spectral power of the sleep electroencephalogram (EEG) in the range of 0.75–4.5 Hz] of non-rapid-eye-movement (NREM) sleep during the initial phase of the subsequent night. This local increase of SWA was located above those brain areas that were previously challenged (Huber et al., 2004).

This chapter presents an overview about sleep, cognition and intelligence, clarifies the terminology, describes developmental aspects and finally offers a concept that differentiates between underlying traits and state-dependent aspects.

Developmental aspects of sleep

Sleep changes substantially during development, in particular early in life. These changes occur on the physiological as well as on the behavioural level, and involve quantitative and qualitative aspects. For example, sleep duration is known to decrease in the course of childhood [from more than 50% of the 24-h day in the newborn (Iglowstein et al., 2003) to approximately 8 h per 24 h in adults]. This decline in sleep duration is paralleled by the following alterations of the sleep structure: a gradual change from a poly- to a monophasic sleep pattern (Anders et al., 1995), a decrease in rapid-eye-movement (REM)-sleep compared to NREM-sleep (Coons and Guilleminault, 1982) and alterations in the circadian and homeostatic sleep regulation (Carskadon et al., 2004; Jenni et al., 2005a). For instance, the circadian phase undergoes a delay in the course of puberty and the build-up of homeostatic sleep pressure during wakefulness is slower in mature adolescents than in prepubertal children (Carskadon et al., 2004; Jenni et al., 2005a).

EEG power and power within specific frequency bands of the sleep EEG (Tarokh and Carskadon, 2010), as well as the topographical distribution of sleep EEG power also varies with age (Jenni et al., 2005b; Kurth et al., 2010). For instance, recent findings suggest that SWA shifts from posterior to anterior regions (Kurth et al., 2010) which may parallel developmental changes in brain morphology, with brain regions that are associated with basic sensory or motor functions maturing first, followed by those involved in more complex behaviour and cognitive functions (for review, see Casey et al., 2005). In particular, the maturation of the frontal lobe is known to follow a specific time course characterized by a preadolescent increase followed by a post-adolescent decrease in cortical grey matter (Shaw et al., 2006; Sowell et al., 2004). Both, the time course of synaptic density (Giedd, 2004; Huttenlocher, 1979) and SWA (Campbell and Feinberg, 2009; Feinberg, 1982) follow an inverted U-shaped time course. This striking similarity has led to the assumption that SWA reflects cortical maturation and plasticity during development (Buchmann et al., in press; Campbell and Feinberg, 2009; Feinberg and Campbell, 2010; Kurth et al., 2010).

Because these age-related changes are highly specific for sleep physiology as well for brain morphology and thus for cognitive development, it may be suggested that common underlying processes are involved.

Cognition, learning and intelligence

Evolving from different schools of thoughts and research traditions, cognition and intelligence have been unrelated terms for a long time, but simultaneously been used as synonyms. Cognition can be described as basic information processing, the application of knowledge and distinct cognitive processes, whereas intelligence relates to individual differences in mental ability, often conceptualized as a general factor, the so-called g-factor (Spearman, 1927). Thus, cognitive psychologists were primarily interested in 'lower order' processes of the mind, whereas the study of individual differences in intelligence examined 'higher order' and metacognitive abilities (Pretz and Sternberg, 2005). As such, 'learning' may be considered as an example of a single cognitive process on a lower order level. According to Baddeley (1999), 'the term *learning* can be legitimately used for [...] remembering a personal incident, acquiring new information, mastering a new skill, or developing a new habit'.

Including a developmental perspective, Anderson (2005) highlighted another important aspect which at the same time offers an elegant way to differentiate between the two concepts cognition and intelligence: Cognitive processes are subjected to an age-dependent performance increase (on a quantitative and qualitative level), whereas intelligence refers to individual differences that remain constant across development.

Despite these inherent conceptual differences between bottom-up (based on 'lower order' cognitive processes) and top-down (related to 'higher order' intellectual ability) approaches, however, there is a vagueness of definitions and terminology which deserves clarification. It is essential to differentiate between two concepts: Intelligence is conceptualized as a *trait*, whereas cognitive processes are conceived as *state*-dependent. In general, a trait represents a behavioural or biological disposition which is empirically or statistically established (Allport, 1931), not specific to certain situations or tasks and fairly stable over time. Intelligence is characterized by a high long-term intra-individual stability, with stability coefficients for general intelligence ranging from 0.89 to 0.96 (Hertzog and Schaie, 1986). Furthermore, based on comparisons in mono- versus dizygotic twins, a considerably large genetic foundation of intelligence was reported (Deary et al., 2009), with heritability estimates of 40–50% during childhood and 80% in adulthood (Baltes et al., 1999). Overall, intelligence fits the general definition of a trait on the psychological and biological level. In contrast, cognitive processes, such as the performance in a perceptual motor-learning task or a verbal learning paradigm, are characterized by situational fluctuations and may therefore be considered as *state*-dependent.

Although (higher-order) intelligence and (lower-order) cognitive processes are mutually dependent and influenced by each other, there is an important distinction; whereas cognitive processes are influenced by the underlying trait intelligence as well as by additional external and internal factors (e.g. the current setting, intrinsic motivation, level of concentration, alertness etc.), intelligence should co-vary with lower-order cognitive processes, but not basically with situational factors.

The term 'intelligence' has been used by several disciplines (e.g. psychology, behaviourism, computer science) and in different contexts (e.g. emotional, practical and social intelligence) (see Weber and Westmeyer, 2001). However, most research in the field of intelligence has been related to what can be described as 'academic intelligence'. 'Intelligence, by definition, is what intelligence tests measure' (Jensen, 1972). This prominent definition, circular in nature and unhelpful in specifying the concept, is nevertheless worth keeping in mind because it is making the point that performance in a given test always depends on the underlying concept and assessment tool. Other definitions link intelligence to overt intelligent behaviour, for instance intelligence as 'the ensemble of abilities which is common to all successful individuals of a given culture' (Hofstaetter, 1957). Although there may be as many definitions of intelligence as there are researchers working in the field, there exists a certain consensus on which most of them would agree. Intelligence is an umbrella term for adaptive behaviour, for the ability to reason or to solve problems (Gottfredson, 1997).

Assessment of cognitive processes and intelligence

Lower-order cognitive processes may be considered as a heterogeneous group of various cognitive functions (e.g. perceptual motor learning, visual short-term memory, selective attention etc.). Thus, there is no unitary-assessment approach. The evaluation of cognitive processes ranges from simple reaction times (RTs) measure to the query of strategies adopted during problem-solving tasks, and depends on the particular problem. For example, mirror tracing is a visual motor task to measure visual integration, hand–eye coordination and learning of new motor skills. During skill acquisition, subjects have to copy a figure, but with their hand being placed behind a barrier. Feedback from their copying performance is only visible in a mirror. Because a detailed description of cognitive assessments would go beyond the scope of this article, we will exclusively focus on the assessment of intelligence.

Intelligence can only indirectly be inferred. Basically, three main approaches may be distinguished (1) inference from an external criterion, (2) psychometric testing [e.g. the classical intelligence test, resulting in intelligence quotient (IQ) scores] and (3) inference from neurobiological correlates.

Intelligence can be inferred from apparent behaviour or linked to an external criterion. Usually, professional success is assumed to reflect the underlying intelligence. Intelligence correlates positively with professional success, income or career advancement, and seems to be the single best predictor for the later position in society (Brody, 1992). According to a meta-analysis by Fraser et al. (1987), correlation coefficients between intelligence scores and school marks vary from 0.34 to 0.51, depending on the type of school and years of education. Thus, intelligence only moderately correlates with school performance (Cohen, 1992), reflecting the fact that intelligence does not exactly mirror school performance, and limiting the significance of intelligence testing for prognostic use in the prediction of individual school careers. In fact, many aspects such as concrete learning opportunity, individual support and personality factors (e.g. achievement motivation), have an impact on external criteria such as school marks which explains the moderate nature of correlations between intelligence scores and school marks.

Psychometric testing is the standard approach to infer about intelligence. Specific tasks, which are assumed to reflect individual differences in intellectual ability, are applied. Introduced by Albert Binet and published as the Simon–Binet test in 1905 (Binet and Simon, 1905), the first tool for the assessment of intelligence was aimed to detect and support children with special needs. The items included in this test battery reflected age-appropriate intellectual ability. Individual items ranked for chronological age (CA) allowed for inference about children's mental age (MA). Accordingly, the individual mental ability score for a given child was related to its CA, thus providing a mean to evaluate its general state of intellectual development – advance or delay. With the transformation of the original difference score (MA minus CA) into a quotient score (MA/CA $\times$ 100) by William Stern (1912), the well-known IQ score was born. Two basic principles from this seminal work are still present in today's IQ tests: (1) adaptive testing, that is the principle to start with items assumed to match approximately the intellectual level of a given subject, with a subsequent gradual progression of item difficulty and (2) relation of individual test scores to age-standardized population norms which is based on the assumption that intellectual ability just as many other human characteristics should be normally distributed in the general population.

Finally, intelligence can be inferred from neurobiological correlates. Early anthropometric approaches from the 19th century used total brain weight and volume as correlates of intelligence, assuming that bigger brains are better brains. Even though, there are in fact positive correlations between total brain volume and IQ scores, correlation coefficients are only small to moderate ($r \sim 0.3$) (McDaniel, 2005), and there is no causal relation. Besides, many of these approaches were biased by sexual and racial aspects, frequently suiting scientifically justified racism (Gould, 1994). Summarizing studies that are based on voxel-based morphometry, Jung and Haier (2007) elaborated and upgraded the original idea of linking grey matter volume to intelligence. The *parieto-frontal integration theory* (P-FIT) implies that networks of grey matter volumes in specific brain areas (local aspects) and interactions dependent on the connecting fibre tracts are the biological substrates of individual differences in intelligence.

A different approach, the so-called *mental-speed approach* is based on the assumption that speed of processing in elementary cognitive tasks is related to psychometric intelligence. In general, RTs are slower with increasing load of information. However, subjects with higher IQ scores need less extra time to process additional information. In fact, the increase in RT with increasing load of information correlates about −0.18 to −0.23 with IQ scores (Jensen, 1987). Techniques such as positron emission tomography (PET), EEG and functional magnetic resonance imaging (fMRI) have considerably contributed to a refinement of the mental-speed approach. A seminal study was performed by Richard Haier et al. (1988). Subjects engaged in a non-verbal IQ test were simultaneously scanned for their glucose metabolism rate (GMR). Surprisingly, those that reached the highest IQ scores displayed the lowest GMR. In other words, the higher the IQ score, the lower the cognitive effort or demand, which has become known as the principle of *neural efficiency*. Haier interpreted his finding as follows '... intelligence is not a function of how hard the brain works, but rather of how efficiently it works'. (Haier et al., 1992). Since then, many studies have replicated and further characterized neural efficiency which is modulated by the level of task complexity and a task–sex interaction (for review, see Neubauer and Fink, 2009).

In sum, over the past decades common lines emerged regarding the neurobiology of intelligence. First, general statements are formulated for specific abilities rather than global aptitude. Second, neurobiological correlates are related to the local, instead of the global anatomical level. Third, the focus is on dynamic rather than static aspects of processing. As a notion of caution, it has to be mentioned that neurobiological correlates are easily mistaken as a direct measurement of intelligence. There is, however, no causal relationship between physiological parameters and psychometrically assessed intelligence. Furthermore, there is no solid theoretical model linking physiological parameters of the central nervous system to intelligence as a behavioural trait and the reported magnitude of correlations between IQ scores and physiological parameters of the waking brain (e.g. waveforms of event-related potentials, cerebral metabolic rates) are only moderate ($r \sim 0.4$) (Deary and Caryl, 1997).

Sleep: a trait and state-dependent perspective

Considering the relationship between sleep, cognition and intelligence, it is essential to differentiate clearly between the two fundamental concepts *trait* and *state*. As mentioned earlier, intelligence is considered a *trait* whereas cognitive performances are *state*-dependent. The distinction between traits and states is, however, also important for sleep.

Many studies allude to the influence of experimental manipulations on the sleep pattern and sleep EEG at the state level. For example, total or partial sleep deprivation and sleep fragmentation are known to result in changes of sleep latency, slow-wave sleep (SWS) and the spectral composition of the sleep EEG (Borbély et al., 1981; Van Dongen et al., 2003). Beyond the effects of experimental manipulation on subsequent sleep, sleep restriction and deprivation may also impair cognitive processes such as working memory or executive functions (Durmer and Dinges, 2005; Ratcliff and Van Dongen, 2009).

However, the human sleep pattern also qualifies for a trait with characteristic individual sleep durations and chronotypes (Van Dongen et al., 2005). It is assumed that specific aspects of sleep architecture and regulation are also genetically determined (for recent reviews, see Andretic et al., 2008; Cirelli, 2009). Polysomnographic studies demonstrated that a significant proportion of the variance in stage 2, stage 4, SWS and the density of REMs in REM sleep are in part under genetic control

(Linkowski et al., 1989; Merica and Gaillard, 1985). Spectral analyses of the sleep EEG in twins revealed that the sleep EEG is among the most heritable traits in humans (Ambrosius et al., 2008; De Gennaro et al., 2008). For example, heritability for the amount of NREM sleep in humans is estimated at about 50% (Linkowski, 1999). The trait-like stability of sleep stages (Tucker et al., 2007) is surpassed by the individual pattern of sleep EEG power spectra (Buckelmüller et al., 2006; De Gennaro et al., 2005). Furthermore, the intra-individual stability of spectral power maps largely exceeded the effects that are caused by experimental manipulations such as sleep deprivation (Finelli et al., 2001). For instance, spindle frequency activity (SFA or sigma power, i.e. spectral power in the 12–15 Hz range) is highly variable across, but highly stable within individuals (Werth et al., 1997), thus representing a trait or phenotype of a given subject. Based on data of sleep EEG recordings in mono- versus dizygotic twins, a heritability estimate of 96% for NREM sleep power spectra for frequencies between 8 and 16 Hz was found (De Gennaro et al., 2008). The spectral composition of NREM sleep EEG was even proposed as constituting endophenotypes (Ambrosius et al., 2008). In summary, the human sleep EEG has repeatedly been characterized as a 'fingerprint'-like trait, probably reflecting the underlying brain anatomy (Finelli et al., 2001).

However, despite converging evidence for sleep as a 'fingerprint' in adults, there is only a single study pointing towards similar trait-like characteristics of the children's sleep EEG, with high *intra-individual* similarity, but high *inter-individual* variability of sleep EEG power spectra for children aged 8–12 years old (Geiger et al., in press).

Sleep and cognitive processes – the state approach

Generic aspects

Many studies have demonstrated that sleep can enhance performance of tasks learned during prior wakefulness. Evidence of sleep-dependent memory consolidation has accumulated in humans and animals (e.g. Born et al., 2006; Peigneux et al., 2001; Walker and Stickgold, 2004), applying a variety of paradigms for different types of learning. Given the extensive amount of literature on sleep and learning/memory, this chapter will only briefly touch on the state-dependent relationship between sleep, learning and cognitive processes.

In adults, several studies have highlighted the importance of specific sleep EEG variables and in particular sleep spindles or SFA for learning. Sleep spindles, the hallmark of stage 2 NREM sleep involve short waxing and waning synchronous bursts of activity. Based on animal models, single cell recordings and anatomical studies of the spindle-generating thalamocortical system, it was speculated that sleep spindles may play a dominant role in gating plastic changes during sleep and thus may be considered a candidate physiological mechanism for memory consolidation (Sejnowski and Destexhe, 2000; Steriade et al., 1993). For example, performance in a procedural learning task (Tamaki et al., 2008), and declarative memory retention after a night of sleep (Clemens et al., 2005; Gais et al., 2002) and after a short nap (Schmidt et al., 2006), positively correlated with SFA. Moreover, by demonstrating locally increased SFA over areas that have been challenged by a motor-learning task, it was shown that SFA does not only reflect learning improvement on a global level but also on a local level (Nishida and Walker, 2007).

However, there is also evidence for an important role of the EEG slow waves in learning processes. A visuomotor-learning task activating circumscribed right parietal cortical areas resulted in a local increase of SWA in NREM sleep during the subsequent night. Furthermore, this localized increase in SWA was shown to correlate with a performance increase after motor learning, suggesting that the increase in SWA reflects synaptic potentiation triggered by learning (Huber et al., 2004). To directly test predictions from this study, subjects were explicitly deprived from sleep slow waves by acoustic stimulation after performing on the visuomotor-learning task and compared with subjects in a control condition. Those in the control condition improved over night, whereas those that were deprived from sleep slow waves did not (Landsness et al., 2009). Likewise, performance in texture discrimination, a specific form of perceptual learning, was shown to be impaired by SWA suppression (Aeschbach et al., 2008). This was interpreted in light of the synaptic homeostasis hypothesis (Tononi and Cirelli, 2006), which states that plastic processes occurring during wakefulness result in a net increase in synaptic strength. In this hypothesis, EEG slow waves are suggested to be an opponent mechanism to downscale the synaptic strength to baseline levels, thus providing an efficient synaptic load in terms of space and energy and optimizing the signal-to-noise ratio of synaptic transmission. Although this appealing hypothesis is supported by several lines of evidence, it is still a matter of debate whether the synaptic homeostasis hypothesis represents a general functional correlate of learning in the classical sense or whether it only applies to rather specific forms of learning, such as implicit learning.

Developmental aspects

Despite the vast amount of literature about the relationship between sleep and learning or cognitive processes in adults and animals (for a recent review, see Walker, 2009), there are only little data in children. Basically two different approaches were taken to examine the sleep/cognition relationship in children. First, studies on the associations between sleep and cognitive processes in clinical populations and second, studies using experimental sleep manipulations to assess the associations between sleep and cognitive processes.

Several clinical populations are characterized by disturbed sleep patterns concordant with cognitive impairments. For example, sleep-related breathing disorders show negative effects on children's attention capacity and academic achievement (Blunden et al., 2001). Many studies in the clinical context lack, however, the clear distinction between state-effects of sleep on learning and trait-like associations between sleep and general intellectual ability. Furthermore, even though clinical studies consistently point towards a close relationship between sleep and a variety of cognitive processes such as learning, perceptual speed, working memory and executive functions, it remains unclear whether the relationship also holds for healthy children. In general, inference from clinical to normal populations has to be regarded with caution because the underlying structural and functional conditions may be fundamentally different between these groups and thus not comparable.

More direct insights into the associations between sleep and cognition during development are provided by studies which experimentally restrict sleep and determine cognitive processes. Randazzo et al. (1998) compared school age children restricted to sleep only 5 h with a control group which was allowed to sleep 11 h and found impaired cognitive processes (verbal creativity and cognitive flexibility) in the restricted group. Similarly, Sadeh et al. (2003) compared a control group over three consecutive nights with two groups of school age children whose sleep was either restricted or extended by 1 h per night. Children with a sleep extension performed significantly better in a continuous performance test and a simple RT task than those with sleep restriction or no intervention. Comparing pre- to post-sleep performance without prior sleep restriction, several other studies argued for an important role of sleep for learning in children and infants (e.g. Backhaus et al., 2008; Gomez et al., 2006). A recent review by Kopasz et al. (2010) summarizes studies about the impact of sleep on children's and adolescent's performance of working memory and memory consolidation. The authors highlight the importance of sleep for memory consolidation, and conclude that higher order brain functions may be more susceptible to sleep deprivation than performance in simple memory tasks.

Sleep and intellectual ability – the trait approach

Generic aspects

In adults, few studies have examined the relationship between sleep and intellectual ability. On the physiological level, the following variables of the sleep EEG have been included: distribution of sleep stages, percentage of NREM sleep, number of sleep cycles and EEG power within specific frequency bands. SFA or sleep spindles have been the main candidate in the search of a physiological variable for the relationship between sleep and intelligence on the trait level. Total number of sleep spindles (Fogel et al., 2007), the density of fast spindles at specific electrode sites (Bódizs et al., 2005), sigma power (Fogel et al., 2007; Schabus et al., 2006, 2008) and the percentage of total sleep time spent in stage 2 NREM (Bódizs et al., 2005) correlate with full-scale IQ scores. Interestingly, reported effects are all positive in nature – the higher the SFA, the higher the IQ scores. Correlation coefficients between physiological variables of the sleep EEG and full-scale IQ scores are of a moderate to substantial magnitude and vary between 0.44 (Schabus et al., 2006) and 0.76 (Fogel et al., 2007), which is remarkably higher than those reported for the waking brain. It may be that high correlation coefficients for the sleeping brain trace back to the fact that interference with external cognitive or sensory stimulation during sleep is minimized. Thus, physiological variables assessed during sleep may be more reliable as correlates for psychometric intelligence than physiological measures during waking.

Developmental aspects

In children, only a single study in a non-clinical population points towards the same direction: Busby and Pivik (1983) reported higher percentage of stage 2 NREM sleep in 10-year old boys with superior IQ scores compared to those with average IQ scores, indirectly supporting the association between sleep spindles and intellectual ability.

In the clinical context, the pattern of the sleep EEG has been used to predict developmental outcome and later IQ scores in pre-term infants (Beckwith and Parmelee, 1986) as well as in healthy infants (Scher et al., 1996). For example, Becker and Thoman (1981) reported a positive relationship between the occurrence of intense REMs (REM storms) during REM sleep at the age of 6 months and later intellectual functioning at age 1 year. SFA and sleep spindles have also been associated with intellectual ability in developmentally delayed children (Bixler and Rhodes, 1968; Shibagaki and Kiyono, 1983) and it has been suggested that children with mental retardation exhibit either large amounts of SFA or virtually none (Bixler and Rhodes, 1968). In light of the earlier mentioned positive association between IQ scores and SFA in healthy subjects, increased SFA in children with mental retardation appears contra-intuitive on a first glance. However, Fogel et al. (2010) postulated that the relationship between intelligence and SFA may not be linear, but rather U-shaped or curvilinear, which would reconcile contradictory results in the field.

In contrast to clinical studies of children with neurological or genetic disorders, where the sleep EEG was used as physiological correlate of intellectual ability, research in healthy children has largely been based on behavioural parameters of sleep in association with intellectual or psychosocial outcome variables. Sleep duration, sleep quality and daytime sleepiness have been suggested as potential modulators of children's daytime performance and intellectual ability. Several authors have concluded that a minimal amount of sleep is necessary for adequate behavioural and cognitive functioning in school age children (Dahl, 1996; Nixon et al., 2008; Touchette et al., 2007). The assumption that sleep and in particular sufficiently long sleep duration is critically important for the developing brain is quite common. This was already prominently expressed in 1904 by G. Stanley Hall: '... no one should be allowed to go to school at all without (at least) nine hours of sleep . . .' (Hall, 1904).

Intuitively, the dogma of 'the longer the sleep duration, the better the intellectual performance' makes sense, but on the other hand, there are several popular science reports and anecdotes about gifted children which appear to require very little sleep (Grubar, 1985). Interestingly, earlier publications from the 1930s indeed reported negative correlations between sleep duration and intellectual ability in children (reviewed in Geiger et al., 2010a). A recent study from our own group replicated these findings and reported a negative association between sleep duration and IQ scores in healthy children (Geiger et al., 2010a). Two explanations may be considered, first, children with a short sleep duration benefit from a long waketime, which offers constant opportunities for cognitive stimulation, social interactions and multisensory input. Because children's sleep duration shows large inter-individual variability as well as intra-individual stability (Jenni et al., 2007), we may assume that children characterized by a short sleep duration were more stimulated over the years compared to those with longer sleep duration. Finally, it may be speculated that those with shorter habitual sleep duration may benefit from this extra wake-time in terms of higher scores on IQ testing. An alternative explanation relates to the *neural efficiency theory* (see above, Haier et al., 1988). In the view that children spend a considerable time of the 24-h period asleep, our results may argue for an extension of this original theory – referring not only to daytime but also to nighttime behaviour. Children with higher cognitive efficiency, reflected by higher IQ scores, may also display higher nighttime efficiency (i.e. more efficient neuronal recovery) reflected by shorter sleep duration.

So far, the only systematic review on the influence of sleepiness, sleep duration and quality on children's daytime performance exclusively focused on school performance. Moreover, even though the reported effects in this meta-analysis were significant, they were rather small (ranging from $r = 0.069$ for the relationship between school performance and sleep duration to -0.133 for the relationship between school performance and sleepiness) (Dewald et al., 2010).

Thus, the relationship between sleep duration, cognitive processes and intellectual ability may be more complex than common sense and intuitive beliefs may imply (the longer, the better). Furthermore, the assumed causality that sleep duration affects intellectual ability does not necessarily resist a critical analysis and may actually be misleading. In fact, a recent study in adolescents demonstrated that not sleep duration per se determined daytime executive functioning, but rather subjective sleepiness (Anderson et al., 2009). Moreover, inter-individual differences in sleepiness and neurobehavioural deficits due to sleep deprivation are characterized by a strong trait component (Van Dongen et al., 2004). Thus, the cognitive and neurobehavioural impairments after sleep deprivation may not exclusively be of a universal nature but also be modulated by a strong individual component.

Conclusions and implications

There is no theoretical framework that bridges the findings of the neurobiology of intelligence and cognition with those from developmental sciences and sleep research. However, this review from a psychologist, a sleep researcher and a developmental paediatrician emphasizes important conceptual issues: research about the relationship between cognition, intelligence and sleep must differentiate between aspects related to general underlying traits and those that are characterized by state-dependent fluctuations.

From a clinical point of view, many assumptions about the association between sleep, intellectual ability and cognitive processes are shaped by intuitive beliefs rather than by scientific evidence which may be particularly problematic for children because they are usually not autonomous for choosing their sleep schedule. Given that sleep behaviour has a strong trait-like component, sleep duration may not be easily adapted to culturally defined sleep norms and parental expectations. The popular assumption that sleep is necessary for optimal cognitive functioning and development may finally result in a poor fit between parental expectations (favouring long sleep duration to foster cognitive functioning and development) and characteristics of the individual child, and may even create sleep problems, sleep onset difficulties and bedtime struggles. Thus, it is neither recommended to purposely increase nor recommended to restrict sleep. When children are healthy, it may well be presumed that their individual sleep need meets what is necessary for adequate cognitive functioning. Thus, we call for accepting children's sleep need and matching sleep schedules according to their needs (Jenni and O'Connor, 2005).

Acknowledgements

This work was supported by research grants of the Center for Integrative Human Physiology (ZIHP) of the University of Zurich (to PA and OGJ), the Schüller Foundation (to OGJ), and the Swiss National Science Foundation (32473B-129956 to OGJ and 320030-130766 to PA).

References

Aeschbach, D., Cutler, A. J., & Ronda, J. M. (2008). A role for non-rapid-eye-movement sleep homeostasis in perceptual learning. *Journal of Neuroscience*, *28*, 2766–2772.

Allport, G. W. (1931). What is a trait of personality. *Journal of Abnormal and Social Psychology*, *25*, 368–372.

Ambrosius, U., Lietzenmaier, S., Wehrle, R., Wichniak, A., Kalus, S., & Winkelmann, J., et al., (2008). Heritability of sleep encephalogram. *Biological Psychology*, *64*, 344–348.

Anders, T. F., Sadeh, A., & Appareddy, V. (1995). Normal sleep in neonates and children. In: Ferber, R., Kryger, M. (Eds.), *Principles and practice of sleep medicine in the child*. W.B. Saunders Company, Philadelphia, PA.

Anderson, B., Storfer-Isser, A., Taylor, H. G., Rosen, C. L., & Redline, S. (2009). Associations of executive function with sleepiness and sleep duration in adolescents. *Pediatrics*, *123*, e701–e707.

Anderson, M. (2005). Marrying intelligence and cognition – A developmental view. In: Sternberg, R. J., Pretz, J. E. (Eds.), *Cognition & intelligence*. Cambridge University Press, New York.

Andretic, R., Franken, P., & Tafti, M. (2008). Genetics of sleep. *Annual Review of Genetics*, *42*, 361–388.

Backhaus, J., Hoeckesfeld, R., Born, J., Hohagen, F., & Junghanns, K. (2008). Immediate as well as delayed post learning sleep but not wakefulness enhances declarative memory consolidation in children. *Neurobiology of Learning and Memory*, *89*, 76–80.

Baddeley, A. (1999). When practice makes perfect. In: Baddeley, A. (Ed.), *Human memory, Revised edn. Psychology Press, Hove.*

Baltes, P. B., Staudinger, U. M., & Lindenberger, U. (1999). Lifespan psychology: Theory and application to intellectual functioning. *Annual Review of Psychology*, *50*, 471–507.

Banks, S., & Dinges, D. F. (2007). Behavioral and physiological consequences of sleep restriction. *Journal of Clinical Sleep Medicine*, *3*, 519–528.

Becker, P. T., & Thoman, E. B. (1981). Rapid eye movement storms in infants: Rate of occurrence at 6 months predicts mental development at 1 year. *Science*, *212*, 1415–1416.

Beckwith, L., & Parmelee Jr., A. H. (1986). EEG patterns of preterm infants, home environment, and later IQ. *Child Development*, *57*, 777–789.

Binet, A., & Simon, T. (1905). Methodes nouvelles pour le diagnostic du niveau intellectuel anormeaux. *Annee Psychologique*, *11*, 191–244.

Bixler, E. O., & Rhodes, J. M. (1968). Spindle activity during sleep in cultural-familial mild retardate. *Psychophysiology*, *5*, 212.

Blunden, S., Lushington, K., & Kennedy, D. (2001). Cognitive and behavioural performance in children with sleep-related obstructive breathing disorders. *Sleep Medicine Reviews*, *5*, 447–461.

Bódizs, R., Kis, T., Lazar, A. S., Havran, L., Rigo, P., & Clemens, Z., et al., (2005). Prediction of general mental ability based on neural oscillation measures of sleep. *Journal of Sleep Research*, *14*, 285–292.

Borbély, A. A., Baumann, F., Brandeis, D., Strauch, I., & Lehmann, D. (1981). Sleep deprivation: Effect on sleep stages and EEG power density in man. *Electroencephalography and Clinical Neurophysiology*, *51*, 483–495.

Born, J., Rasch, B., & Gais, S. (2006). Sleep to remember. *Neuroscientist*, *12*, 410–424.

Brody, N. (1992). *Intelligence.* Academic Press, San Diego, CA.

Buchmann, A., Ringli, M., Kurth, S., Schaerer, M., Geiger, A., & Jenni, O. G., et al., (2010). EEG sleep slow-wave activity as a mirror of cortical maturation. *Cerebral Cortex* Jul 12. [Epub ahead of print].

Buckelmüller, J., Landolt, H. P., Stassen, H. H., & Achermann, P. (2006). Trait-like individual differences in the human sleep electroencephalogram. *Neuroscience*, *138*, 351–356.

Busby, K., & Pivik, R. T. (1983). Sleep patterns in children of superior intelligence. *Journal of Child Psychology and Psychiatry*, *24*, 587–600.

Campbell, I. G., & Feinberg, I. (2009). Longitudinal trajectories of non-rapid eye movement delta and theta EEG as indicators of adolescent brain maturation. *Proceedings of the National Academy of Sciences of the United States of America*, *106*, 5177–5180.

Carskadon, M. A., Acebo, C., & Jenni, O. G. (2004). Regulation of adolescent sleep: Implications for behavior. *Annals of the New York Academy of Sciences*, *1021*, 276–291.

Casey, B. J., Tottenham, N., Liston, C., & Durston, S. (2005). Imaging the developing brain: What have we learned about cognitive development? *Trends in Cognitive Sciences*, *9*, 104–110.

Cirelli, C. (2009). The genetic and molecular regulation of sleep: From fruit flies to humans. *Nature Reviews Neuroscience*, *10*, 549–560.

Clemens, Z., Fabo, D., & Halasz, P. (2005). Overnight verbal memory retention correlates with the number of sleep spindles. *Neuroscience*, *132*, 529–535.

Cohen, J. (1992). A power primer. *Psychological Bulletin*, *112*, 155–159.

Coons, S., & Guilleminault, C. (1982). Development of sleep-wake patterns and non-rapid eye movement sleep stages during the first six months of life in normal infants. *Pediatrics*, *69*, 793–798.

Dahl, R. E. (1996). The impact of inadequate sleep on children's daytime cognitive function. *Seminars in Pediatric Neurology*, *3*, 44–50.

Dang-Vu, T. T., Desseilles, M., Peigneux, P., & Maquet, P. (2006). A role for sleep in brain plasticity. *Pediatric Rehabilitation*, *9*, 98–118.

Deary, I. J., & Caryl, P. G. (1997). Neuroscience and human intelligence differences. *Trends in Neurosciences*, *20*, 365–371.

Deary, I. J., Johnson, W., & Houlihan, L. M. (2009). Genetic foundations of human intelligence. *Human Genetics*, *126*, 215–232.

De Gennaro, L., Ferrara, M., Vecchio, F., Curcio, G., & Bertini, M. (2005). An electroencephalographic fingerprint of human sleep. *Neuroimage*, *26*, 114–122.

De Gennaro, L., Marzano, C., Fratello, F., Moroni, F., Pellicciari, M. C., & Ferlazzo, F., et al., (2008). The electroencephalographic fingerprint of sleep is genetically determined: A twin study. *Annals of Neurology*, *64*, 455–460.

Dewald, J. F., Meijer, A. M., Oort, F. J., Kerkhof, G. A., & Bögels, S. M. (2010). The influence of sleep quality, sleep duration and sleepiness on school performance in children and adolescents. A meta-analytic review. *Sleep Medicine Reviews*, *14*, 179–189.

Diekelmann, S., & Born, J. (2010). The memory function of sleep. *Nature Reviews Neuroscience*, *11*, 114–126.

Durmer, J. S., & Dinges, D. F. (2005). Neurocognitive consequences of sleep deprivation. *Seminars in Neurology*, *25*, 117–129.

Feinberg, I. (1982). Schizophrenia: Caused by a fault in programmed synaptic elimination during adolescence? *Journal of Psychiatric Research*, *17*, 319–334.

Feinberg, I., & Campbell, I. G. (2010). Sleep EEG changes during adolescence: An index of a fundamental brain reorganization. *Brain and Cognition*, *72*, 56–65.

Finelli, L. A., Achermann, P., & Borbely, A. A. (2001). Individual 'fingerprints' in human sleep EEG topography. *Neuropsychopharmacology*, *25*, S57–S62.

Fogel, S. M., Nader, R., Cote, K. A., & Smith, C. T. (2007). Sleep spindles and learning potential. *Behavioral Neuroscience*, *121*, 1–10.

Fogel, S. M., Smith, C. T., & Beninger, R. J. (2010). Too much of a good thing? Elevated baseline sleep spindles predict poor avoidance performance in rats. *Brain Research*, *1319*, 112–117.

Fraser, B. J., Walberg, H. J., Welch, W. W., & Hattie, J. A. (1987). Synthesis of productivity research. *International Journal of Educational Research*, *11*, 147–252.

Gais, S., Molle, M., Helms, K., & Born, J. (2002). Learning-dependent increases in sleep spindle density. *Journal of Neuroscience*, *22*, 6830–6834.

Geiger, A., Achermann, P., & Jenni, O. G. (2010a). Association between sleep duration and intelligence scores in healthy children. *Developmental Psychology*, *46*, 949–954.

Geiger, A., Huber, R., Kurth, S., Ringli, M., Jenni, O. G. & Achermann, P. The sleep EEG as a marker for intellectual ability in healthy children. *Sleep*, in press.

Giedd, J. N. (2004). Structural magnetic resonance imaging of the adolescent brain. *Annals of the New York Academy of Sciences*, *1021*, 77–85.

Gomez, R. L., Bootzin, R. R., & Nadel, L. (2006). Naps promote abstraction in language-learning infants. *Psychological Science*, *17*, 670–674.

Gottfredson, L. S. (1997). Mainstream science on intelligence: An editorial with 52 signatories, history, and bibliography (Reprinted from *The Wall Street Journal*, 1994). *Intelligence*, *24*, 13–23.

Gould, S. J. (1994). *Der falsch vermessene Mensch.* Suhrkamp, Frankfurt a. M.

Grubar, J. C. (1985). Sleep and mental efficiency. In: Freeman, J. (Ed.), *The psychology of gifted children.* Wiley, Chichester.

Haier, R. J., Siegel, B. V., Nuechterlein, K. H., Hazlett, E., Wu, J. C., & Paek, J., et al., (1988). Cortical glucose metabolic rate correlates of abstract reasoning and attention studied with positron emission tomography. *Intelligence*, *12*, 199–217.

Haier, R. J., Siegel, B. V., Tang, C., Abel, L., & Buchsbaum, M. S. (1992). Intelligence and changes in regional cerebral glucose metabolic rate following learning. *Intelligence*, *16*, 415–426.

Hall, G. S. (1904). *Adolescence, its psychology and its relations to physiology, anthropology, sociology, sex, crime, religion, and education.* Appleton, New York, NY.

Hertzog, C., & Schaie, K. W. (1986). Stability and change in adult intelligence: 1. Analysis of longitudinal covariance structures. *Psychology and Aging*, *1*, 159–171.

Hofstaetter, P. R. (1957). *Psychologie.* Fischer Lexikon, Frankfurt a. M.

Huber, R., Ghilardi, M. F., Massimini, M., & Tononi, G. (2004). Local sleep and learning. *Nature*, *430*, 78–81.

Huttenlocher, P. R. (1979). Synaptic density in human frontal cortex – developmental changes and effects of aging. *Brain Research*, *163*, 195–205.

Iglowstein, I., Jenni, O. G., Molinari, L., & Largo, R. H. (2003). Sleep duration from infancy to adolescence: Reference values and generational trends. *Pediatrics*, *111*, 302–307.

Jenni, O. G., Achermann, P., & Carskadon, M. A. (2005a). Homeostatic sleep regulation in adolescents. *Sleep*, *28*, 1446–1454.

Jenni, O. G., Molinari, L., Caflisch, J. A., & Largo, R. H. (2007). Sleep duration from ages 1 to 10 years: Variability and stability in comparison with growth. *Pediatrics*, *120*, e769–e776.

Jenni, O. G., & O'Connor, B. B. (2005). Children's sleep: An interplay between culture and biology. *Pediatrics*, *115*, 204–216.

Jenni, O. G., Van Reen, E., & Carskadon, M. A. (2005b). Regional differences of the sleep electroencephalogram in adolescents. *Journal of Sleep Research*, *14*, 141–147.

Jensen, A. R. (1972). *Genetics and education.* Methuen, London.

Jensen, A. R. (1987). Individual differences in the Hick paradigm. In: Vernon, P. A. (Ed.), *Speed of information processing and intelligence*. Ablex, Norwood, NJ.

Jones, K., & Harrison, Y. (2001). Frontal lobe function, sleep loss and fragmented sleep. *Sleep Medicine Reviews*, *5*, 463–475.

Jung, R. E., & Haier, R. J. (2007). The Parieto-Frontal Integration Theory (P-FIT) of intelligence: Converging neuroimaging evidence. *Behavioral and Brain Sciences*, *30*, 135–154 discussion 154–187.

Kopasz, M., Loessl, B., Hornyak, M., Riemann, D., Nissen, C., & Piosczyk, H., et al., (2010). Sleep and memory in healthy children and adolescents – a review. *Sleep Medicine Reviews*, *14*, 167–177.

Kurth, S., Ringli, M., Geiger, A., Lebourgeois, M., Jenni, O. G., & Huber, R. (2010). Mapping of cortical activity in the first two decades of life: A high-density sleep encephalogram study. *Journal of Neuroscience*, *30*, 13211–13219.

Landsness, E. C., Crupi, D., Hulse, B. K., Peterson, M. J., Huber, R., & Ansari, H., et al., (2009). Sleep-dependent improvement in visuomotor learning: A causal role for slow waves. *Sleep*, *32*, 1273–1284.

Linkowski, P. (1999). EEG sleep patterns in twins. *Journal of Sleep Research*, *8*(Suppl. 1); 11–13.

Linkowski, P., Kerkhofs, M., Hauspie, R., Susanne, C., & Mendlewicz, J. (1989). EEG sleep patterns in man: A twin study. *Electroencephalography and Clinical Neurophysiology*, *73*, 279–284.

McDaniel, M. A. (2005). Big-brained people are smarter: A meta-analysis of the relationship between in vivo brain volume and intelligence. *Intelligence*, *33*, 337–346.

Merica, H., & Gaillard, J. M. (1985). Statistical description and evaluation of the interrelationships of standard sleep variables for normal subjects. *Sleep*, *8*, 261–273.

Neubauer, A., & Fink, A. (2009). Intelligence and neural efficiency. *Neuroscience & Biobehavioral Reviews*, *33*, 1004–1023.

Nishida, M., & Walker, M. P. (2007). Daytime naps, motor memory consolidation and regionally specific sleep spindles. *PLoS ONE*, *2*, e341.

Nixon, G. M., Thompson, J. M. D., Han, D. Y., Clark, P. M., Robinson, E., & Waldie, K. E., et al., (2008). Short sleep duration in middle childhood: Risk factors and consequences. *Sleep*, *31*, 71–78.

Peigneux, P., Laureys, S., Delbeuck, X., & Maquet, P. (2001). Sleeping brain, learning brain. The role of sleep for memory systems. *Neuroreport*, *12*, A111–A124.

Pretz, J. E., & Sternberg, R. J. (2005). Unifying the field – cognition and intelligence. In: Sternberg, R. J., Pretz, J. E. (Eds.), *Cognition & intelligence*. Cambridge University Press, New York.

Randazzo, A. C., Muehlbach, M. J., Schweitzer, P. K., & Walsh, J. K. (1998). Cognitive function following acute sleep restriction in children ages 10-14. *Sleep*, *21*, 861–868.

Ratcliff, R., & Van Dongen, H. P. (2009). Sleep deprivation affects multiple distinct cognitive processes. *Psychonomic Bulletin & Review*, *16*, 742–751.

Sadeh, A., Gruber, R., & Raviv, A. (2003). The effects of sleep restriction and extension on school-age children: What a difference an hour makes. *Child Development*, *74*, 444–455.

Schabus, M., Hodlmoser, K., Gruber, G., Sauter, C., Anderer, P., & Klosch, G., et al., (2006). Sleep spindle-related activity in the human EEG and its relation to general cognitive and learning abilities. *European Journal of Neuroscience*, *23*, 1738–1746.

Schabus, M., Hoedlmoser, K., Pecherstorfer, T., Anderer, P., Gruber, G., & Parapatics, S., et al., (2008). Interindividual sleep spindle differences and their relation to learning-related enhancements. *Brain Research*, *1191*, 127–135.

Scher, M. S., Steppe, D. A., & Banks, D. L. (1996). Prediction of lower developmental performances of healthy neonates by neonatal EEG-sleep measures. *Pediatric Neurology*, *14*, 137–144.

Schmidt, C., Peigneux, P., Muto, V., Schenkel, M., Knoblauch, V., & Munch, M., et al., (2006). Encoding difficulty promotes postlearning changes in sleep spindle activity during napping. *Journal of Neuroscience*, *26*, 8976–8982.

Sejnowski, T. J., & Destexhe, A. (2000). Why do we sleep? *Brain Research*, *886*, 208–223.

Shaw, P., Greenstein, D., Lerch, J., Clasen, L., Lenroot, R., & Gogtay, N., et al., (2006). Intellectual ability and cortical development in children and adolescents. *Nature*, *440*, 676–679.

Shibagaki, M., & Kiyono, S. (1983). Duration of spindle bursts during nocturnal sleep in mentally retarded children. *Electroencephalography and Clinical Neurophysiology*, *55*, 645–651.

Sowell, E. R., Thompson, P. M., Leonard, C. M., Welcome, S. E., Kan, E., & Toga, A. W. (2004). Longitudinal mapping of cortical thickness and brain growth in normal children. *Journal of Neuroscience*, *24*, 8223–8231.

Spearman, C. (1927). *The abilities of man*. Macmillan, London.

Steriade, M., Mccormick, D. A., & Sejnowski, T. J. (1993). Thalamocortical oscillations in the sleeping and aroused brain. *Science*, *262*, 679–685.

Stern, W. (1912). *Die psychologischen Methoden der Intelligenzprüfung*. Barth, Leipzig.

Tamaki, M., Matsuoka, T., Nittono, H., & Hori, T. (2008). Fast sleep spindle (13-15 Hz) activity correlates with sleep-dependent improvement in visuomotor performance. *Sleep*, *31*, 204–211.

Tarokh, L., & Carskadon, M. A. (2010). Developmental changes in the human sleep EEG during early adolescence: A preliminary study. *Sleep*, *33*, 801–809.

Tononi, G., & Cirelli, C. (2006). Sleep function and synaptic homeostasis. *Sleep Medicine Reviews*, *10*, 49–62.

Touchette, E., Petit, D., Seguin, J. R., Boivin, M., Tremblay, R. E., & Montplaisir, J. Y. (2007). Associations between sleep duration patterns and behavioral/cognitive functioning at school entry. *Sleep*, *30*, 1213–1219.

Tucker, A. M., Dinges, D. F., & Van Dongen, H. P. (2007). Trait interindividual differences in the sleep physiology of healthy young adults. *Journal of Sleep Research*, *16*, 170–180.

Van Dongen, H. P., Baynard, M. D., Maislin, G., & Dinges, D. F. (2004). Systematic interindividual differences in neurobehavioral impairment from sleep loss: Evidence of trait-like differential vulnerability. *Sleep*, *27*, 423–433.

Van Dongen, H. P., Maislin, G., Mullington, J. M., & Dinges, D. F. (2003). The cumulative cost of additional wakefulness: Dose-response effects on neurobehavioral functions and sleep physiology from chronic sleep restriction and total sleep deprivation. *Sleep*, *26*, 117–126.

Van Dongen, H. P., Vitellaro, K. M., & Dinges, D. F. (2005). Individual differences in adult human sleep and wakefulness: Leitmotif for a research agenda. *Sleep*, *28*, 479–496.

Walker, M. P. (2009). The role of sleep in cognition and emotion. *Annals of the New York Academy of Sciences*, *1156*, 168–197.

Walker, M. P., & Stickgold, R. (2004). Sleep-dependent learning and memory consolidation. *Neuron*, *44*, 121–133.

Weber, H., & Westmeyer, H. (2001). Die Inflation der Intelligenzen. In: Stern, E., Guthke, J. (Eds.), *Perspektiven der intelligenzforschung*. Pabst Science Publishers, Lengerich.

Werth, E., Achermann, P., Dijk, D. J., & Borbely, A. A. (1997). Spindle frequency activity in the sleep EEG: Individual differences and topographic distribution. *Electroencephalography and Clinical Neurophysiology*, *103*, 535–542.

G. A. Kerkhof and H. P. A. Van Dongen (Eds.)
Progress in Brain Research, Vol. 185
ISSN: 0079-6123

CHAPTER 11

Do sleep complaints contribute to age-related cognitive decline?

Ellemarije Altena[†], Jennifer R. Ramautar[†], Ysbrand D. Van Der Werf[†,‡] and Eus J.W. Van Someren[†,§,**,*]

[†]*Department Sleep and Cognition, Netherlands Institute for Neuroscience (NIN), an Institute of the Royal Netherlands Academy of Arts and Sciences, Amsterdam, The Netherlands*
[‡]*Department of Anatomy and Neurosciences, VU University Medical Center, Amsterdam, The Netherlands*
[§]*Sleep Center Leiden, Departments of Neurology and Radiology, Leiden Institute for Brain and Cognition, Leiden University Medical Center, Leiden, The Netherlands*
[**]*Department of Integrative Neurophysiology, Faculty of Earth and Life Sciences, VU University Amsterdam, Amsterdam, The Netherlands*

Abstract: The cognitive changes that occur with ageing are usually referred to as 'age-related cognitive decline'. The most pronounced changes may be found in the executive functions that require integrity of the prefrontal cortical circuitry. With age, sleep also changes profoundly, with more sleep fragmentation, earlier awakenings and less slow wave sleep as its main features. Interestingly, experimental sleep deprivation studies in healthy young adults showed a particularly consistent effect on executive functions, suggesting that sleep problems might contribute to the cognitive changes accompanying older age. We here investigate this possibility by reviewing reports on age-related and insomnia-related changes in cognition and brain function and structure, as found in studies investigating subjective complaints, objective functioning in everyday life, neuropsychological assessment, psychometry, structural and functional magnetic resonance imaging, electroencephalography, positron emission tomography and transcranial magnetic stimulation. The chapter focuses on the 'normal' age-related sleep changes that are experienced as insomnia – that is, fragmentation of sleep, more superficial sleep, more wake after sleep onset and earlier awakenings – rather than on specific sleep disturbances as sleep-disordered breathing, restless legs or periodic limb movements during sleep, for all of which the risk increases with age. It turned out that relatively few studies directly addressed the question whether elderly with different degrees of sleep complaints are differentially affected by 'age-related cognitive decline'. Still, several similarities between age-related and insomnia-related cognitive and brain changes are apparent, notably with respect to

[*] Corresponding author.
Tel.: (+) 31 20 5665500; Fax: (+) 31 20 5666121.
E-mail: e.van.someren@nin.knaw.nl

DOI:10.1016/B978-0-444-53702-7.00011-7

performance requiring integrity of the prefrontal cortical system. We suggest that at least part of what we regard as age-related changes may, in fact, be due to poor sleep, which is in some cases a treatable condition. Further research directly comparing aged good sleepers versus aged insomniacs will need to elucidate how sleep disturbances are involved in the cognitive, structural and functional changes observed with increasing age. The findings suggest that discrimination of subtypes of poor sleep at high age will aid in understanding the mechanisms by which it affects cognition and brain function.

Keywords: Ageing; sleep; insomnia; cognition; brain imaging; performance

Introduction

Several changes in cognitive functioning have been reported to occur with ageing, perhaps most noticeably in the executive functions that require integrity of the prefrontal cortical circuitry (Daigneault et al., 1992). Sleep also changes profoundly with age, with more sleep fragmentation, earlier awakenings and less slow wave sleep as its main features (Bliwise, 1993). Older adults complain more about sleep problems than any other age group (Foley et al., 1995; Morphy et al., 2007). Interestingly, experimental sleep deprivation studies in healthy young adults show a particular sensitivity of executive functions (Buysse, 2008; Chesson et al., 2000; Lichstein et al., 2003; Zhang and Wing, 2006). Subjective sleep problems in later life predict cognitive decline (Jelicic et al., 2002). It thus seems worthwhile to investigate the triad sleep disturbances–ageing–prefrontal dysfunction to determine whether sleep problems contribute to, or aggravate, the cognitive changes accompanying older age. We here focus on the 'normal' age-related sleep changes that are experienced as insomnia – fragmentation of sleep, more superficial sleep, more wake after sleep onset, and earlier awakenings – rather than on specific sleep disturbances such as sleep-disordered breathing, restless legs or periodic limb movements during sleep, for all of which the risk increases with age. The chapter does not aim to be comprehensive on the age-related and insomnia-related changes in sleep and in cognitive function per se; many other reviews provide excellent sources (e.g. the chapter 'Chronic insomnia, sleepiness, and cognitive performance' by Kerkhof in the next volume). Rather, the present review aims to provide examples and discuss to what extent the age-related increase in the risk of sleep complaints could contribute to what we usually refer to as 'age-related cognitive decline'. This is systematically evaluated for subjective functioning, objective functioning in everyday life, neuropsychological test performance, computerized psychomotor test performance and several brain imaging modalities including structural and functional magnetic resonance imaging (MRI), positron emission tomography (PET), transcranial magnetic stimulation (TMS) and both background electroencephalography (EEG) and event-related potentials (ERP). Before doing so, some background on insomnia and its increasing prevalence in elderly people should be provided.

Insomnia: diagnosis, risk factors and its association with age

Depending on the criteria, estimates on the prevalence of insomnia vary between about 4 and 11%. Insomnia is more prevalent in women, but the most important risk factor appears to be age; estimates of insomnia in elderly people reach up to about 40% (Foley et al., 1995; Morphy et al., 2007; Van Someren, 2000; Zhang and Wing, 2006). Primary insomnia (PI) is defined by subjective problems of falling asleep (sleep onset problems) or waking up too frequently or early (sleep continuation problems), while these problems cannot be explained by a medical or psychiatric condition or another sleep disorder (Lichstein et al., 2003). If these problems persist for more than months, for at least three nights a week, we speak of chronic PI (Buysse, 2008). Until recently, chronic PI was diagnosed on the basis of subjective reports verified by sleep questionnaire scores and a structured interview based on the Diagnostic and Statistical Manual of Mental Disorders (DSM)-IV criteria (Chesson et al., 2000). A more precise diagnosis of insomnia, defined as psychophysiological insomnia, is given by the International Classification of Sleep Disorders (ICSD)-2 (American Academy of Sleep, 2000). Current criteria require a more elaborate diagnosis of insomnia, including polysomnography to exclude other sleep disorders such as restless legs and breathing problems (Buysse et al., 2006).

The '3P-model' of Spielman (1986) suggests three factors for the onset and course of insomnia. Predisposing personality traits (e.g. tendency to worry) are the first factor; precipitating events (e.g. work-related stress) the second; and perpetuating attitudes and practices (e.g. misconceptions about sleep) the third. According to this model, insomnia may become independent of its cause over time (Basta et al., 2007). Genetic factors may be involved in any of these 'three Ps'. Beaulieu-Bonneau et al. (2007) showed that a family history of insomnia is a predisposing factor for an individual to develop insomnia him/herself in later life in later life. Twin studies support the suggestion of a genetic component for sleep quality (Boomsma et al., 2008).

Predisposing factors for insomnia are depression, anxiety, excessive worrying (Pallesen et al., 2002) and disturbances of emotion regulation (Kales et al., 1987; Morin et al., 2003). Internalization of emotions, instead of expressing or acting on emotions, is a typical personality trait of insomnia patients (Kales et al., 1983). This trait has been proposed to induce physiological hyperarousal, indicated by an increased heart rate, peripheral vasoconstriction, elevated rectal temperature and increased skeletal muscle movements before and during sleep (Bonnet and Arand, 2003; Kales et al., 1987; Rodenbeck et al., 2002; Spielman, 1986; Vgontzas et al., 2001). A state of hyperarousal may be involved both in sleep onset problems and in difficulties returning to sleep after nighttime awakening (Basta et al., 2007). Evening levels of arousal indeed predict sleep quality (Lombardo et al., 2008). The pervasiveness of the hyperarousal condition, present 24 h a day, may also explain why insomniacs are significantly more alert during daytime than normal sleepers (Bonnet and Arand, 1995; Edinger et al., 2001; Stepanski et al., 1988).

Although showing a typical circadian pattern, average 24 h levels of the stress hormones adrenocorticotropic hormone (ACTH) and cortisol may be increased for insomniacs compared to controls, with the largest difference occurring during the evening and first half of the night (Basta et al., 2007; Vgontzas et al., 2002). Not all studies confirm a difference in cortisol levels between insomniacs and controls, however (Varkevisser and Kerkhof, 2005). Hyperarousal has also been confirmed in the subjective experience of insomniacs, as assessed with a dedicated Hyperarousal Scale (Pavlova et al., 2001).

Of note, the physiological and psychological characteristics of insomnia are usually not found after experimental sleep deprivation or sleep restriction (Kato et al., 2000; Landis et al., 1998; Muenter et al., 2000).

Age-related increased vulnerability to stress and hormonal changes could contribute to increased prevalence of insomnia in older adults. Middle-aged men are more sensitive to the arousing effects of corticotropin-releasing hormone (CRH), a hormone with an arousing/awaking effect, than young men. This suggests that not the increased exposure to stressful events but rather a higher sensitivity to the resulting arousal-producing stress hormones may initiate or perpetuate insomnia, specifically in older adults (Basta et al., 2007; Vgontzas et al., 2002). Women with insomnia scored higher on a psychological distress scale [the Symptom Check List-90 Revised (SCL90-R)] than women without insomnia, after correcting for objective stressfulness of the event (Shaver et al., 2002). Insomniacs generally rate the impact of daily minor stressors and the intensity of major negative life events higher than good sleepers and experience less control over stressful events (Morin et al., 2003). Another contribution to the age-related increase in poor sleep may be hormonal changes; post-menopausal women without hormone replacement therapy (HRT) showed longer sleep latencies and less slow wave sleep compared to post-menopausal women with HRT (Bixler et al., 2007; Lugaresi et al., 1987).

In some persons, both insomnia and psychiatric symptoms may develop, even enhancing each other. The most noted example of such a relationship is that of depression leading to insomnia, and conversely, insomnia causing or further aggravating depression (Chang et al., 1997; Ford and Kamerow, 1989). Since a major eliciting factor for depression is the accumulation of randomly occurring negative life events (der Werf et al., 2006), the higher perceived intensity of such life events may directly place insomniacs at an elevated risk of developing a depressive episode (Kaptein et al., 2007). Simultaneous treatment of both a mental disorder and a sleep disorder was therefore recently recommended (Sateia, 2009). In line with this, the term ‘secondary insomnia’ was replaced by ‘comorbid insomnia’ in the 2005 US National Institute of Health resolution (National Institutes of Health State of the Science Conference Statement, 2005). Indeed, the beneficial effects of cognitive behavioural therapy are shown not only for primary but also for comorbid insomnia (Stepanski and Rybarczyk, 2006).

Thus, with increasing age, there is a higher prevalence of sleep problems in general and insomnia in particular. Other age-related changes that may contribute are a higher sensitivity to stress, a higher chance of a stress-invoking life event such as the care of or loss of a loved one, or the aftermath of hormonal changes such as menopause. These factors can increase the severity of insomnia or provoke its onset and perpetuation.

It is thus conceivable that at least part of what we refer to as ‘age-related cognitive decline’ reflects ‘insomnia-related’ cognitive complaints and changes. The following paragraphs will therefore systematically discuss subjective and objective cognitive changes, as well as changes in brain function and structure, as reported to be associated with normal ageing on the one hand and insomnia on the other hand.

Subjective complaints about functioning in everyday life

A first possibility to address cognitive functioning is to obtain introspective reports. In structured or more open interviews and questionnaires, one may query people on their subjective experiences of cognitive functioning in everyday life.

Normal ageing

Older adults complain more about problems with memory, attention, mental speed, planning and decision making (Ponds et al., 2000). Compared to older adults without memory complaints, older adults with cognitive complaints show higher scores on ratings for depression, anxiety and neuroticism as well as physical health problems (Comijs et al., 2002; Ponds et al., 2000). When investigating subscales of memory tests in more detail, subjective memory impairment is associated only with objective impairment on delayed recall but not with other aspects of memory (Jessen et al., 2007). Subjective memory complaints can, however, predict future objective memory problems (Dufouil et al., 2005; Schmand et al., 1997). Older adults with memory complaints unaccompanied by objective neuropsychological findings show mild brain atrophy similar to older adults diagnosed with mild cognitive impairment (Saykin et al., 2006). Thus, although cognitive complaints may in part be related to depression and physical health problems, they may be indicative of abnormal brain changes, which can be detected only with more specific imaging techniques. Since these complaints are predictive of future objective cognitive deficits, more sensitive neuropsychological tests may be needed to facilitate earlier diagnosis of neurodegenerative processes.

Insomnia

Insomnia patients report more daytime functional impairments than good sleepers (Alapin et al., 2000). In particular, they report suffering from cognitive problems, for example as related to concentration and memory (Roth and Ancoli-Israel, 1999; Shochat et al., 1999). They generally have a tendency to rate their subjective performance as more negative than subjective good sleepers (Broman et al., 1992). Insomnia patients also report more mood disturbances, a lower quality of life (Rombaut et al., 1990; Shochat et al., 1999; Zammit et al., 1999) and more anxiety (Riedel and Lichstein, 2000). They also show dysfunctional sleep-related ideas compared to self-defined good sleepers. In particular, they have stronger beliefs about the negative consequences of sleep problems, feel more hopeless about losing control of their sleep and feel more helpless about the unpredictability of their insomnia. These psychological characteristics are found to be more predictive of subjective sleep complaints than of objective sleep disturbances (Edinger et al., 2000). In conclusion, although insomnia patients complain more about daytime cognitive impairments and mood disturbances, there is also evidence that they tend to misjudge their performance (Bastien et al., 2003; Broman et al., 1992).

Integration: contribution of sleep changes to cognitive ageing?

The tendency of insomniacs to rate their subjective performance as worse suggests that the poor sleep that many elderly people experience may contribute to the age-related increase in complaints about attention, mental speed, planning, decision making and memory. We are not aware of studies that specifically address this association by analysing complaints about performance within a group of elderly people with various degrees of sleep complaints. Subjective sleep problems can, however, be predictive for objective cognitive decline in later life (Jelicic et al., 2002). With subjective cognitive functioning as a predictor of future objective cognitive deficits, it seems worthwhile to investigate the relation between sleep complaints and objective sleep problems as a predictor for future cognitive functioning on more specified cognitive tests. Moreover, the influence of sleep interventions on this development could reduce or stabilize some of its progress.

Objective functioning in everyday life

A second possibility to address cognitive functioning is by inspection of objective reports on functioning in everyday life.

Normal ageing

'Old age has its infirmities', the saying goes. Older age comes with a higher risk for invalidity and metabolic, cardiovascular and neurological diseases. Mobility is reduced, physical strength diminishes and cognitive performance is affected. In older adults, work-related accidents are more often accompanied by hospitalization than in younger employees (Chau et al., 2004). The influence of physical job demands and lifestyle on injury rates is higher for older than for younger employees (Chau et al., 2009). At the same time, the elderly show, of all age groups, the largest variation between individuals in functioning, with many aged functioning well until a very high age. It thus appears of interest to investigate whether poor sleep is also associated with compromised functioning and might thus contribute to this variation.

Insomnia

Insomniacs are three times more likely than non-insomniacs to have serious accidents (Godet-Cayre et al., 2006). Measured over a year, 8% of insomniacs compared to 1% of non-insomniacs have an industrial accident (Leger et al., 2002). Days spent in bed due to illness are about twice as common among insomniacs compared to non-insomniacs, even after correcting for age, gender and chronic disease (Simon and VonKorff, 1997). Work absenteeism in days per year is estimated at 5.4 for insomniacs compared to 2.4 for good sleepers in France (Godet-Cayre et al., 2006). Combining the costs of health care, insomnia-related work absenteeism and productivity losses, a recent Canadian study estimated the average annual costs per insomnia patient at $5.010 a year (Daley et al., 2009). In the United States, direct (e.g. medication, consultations etc.) and indirect costs (e.g. work absenteeism) during months were estimated to be $1253 per person higher for insomniacs than for non-insomniacs among young adults and $1143 per person higher for elderly insomniacs compared to elderly non-insomniacs (Ozminkowski et al., 2007).

Integration: contribution of sleep changes to cognitive ageing?

The increased risk among insomniacs for accidents, illness and absenteeism suggests that the poor sleep that many elderly people experience may contribute to the age-related increase in accidents, illness and absenteeism. Evidence for a causal relationship between poor sleep and an age-related increase in accidents is, however, yet lacking. We are not aware of studies that specifically addressed the association of sleep with everyday life functioning within a group of elderly people with various degrees of sleep complaints.

Neuropsychological task performance

Neuropsychological tests have been developed to obtain a more formal investigation of different domains of cognitive functioning than can be obtained from subjective experience or objective reports on global functioning in everyday life.

Normal ageing

Many studies have unequivocally shown age-related performance decreases in several cognitive domains including mental speed, attention, memory and complex problem solving (Daselaar et al., 2005; Grady, 2008; Van Der Werf et al., 2001; Hooren et al., 2007). Of all cognitive domains that deteriorate with age, the executive functions requiring integrity of the prefrontal cortical circuitry may show the most marked changes. Older adults are less able to regulate behaviour on the basis of plans, abstract concepts, environmental feedback or one's own responses (Daigneault et al., 1992), whereas their performance on memory tasks is relatively less affected (Cabeza et al., 2000; Tisserand et al., 2005). In addition to the marked change in executive functions including working memory, set shifting and inhibition, some newer studies indicate that ageing also markedly affects the integration of cognitive and emotional processes. Baena et al. (2010) recently showed that older adults are less able to recognize and/or interpret affective information for ongoing decision-making purposes in the Iowa Gambling Task. Older adults also showed slower response times when recognizing emotional faces, in particular for angry faces. Generally, however, emotion regulation per se is preserved in normal ageing as opposed to many cognitive functions (Reuter-Lorenz and Lustig, 2005), although amygdala activation is reduced when performing emotional valence tasks (Gunning-Dixon et al., 2003; Mather et al., 2004).

Insomnia

Although patients with chronic insomnia complain about concentration and memory problems and a decreased ability to accomplish daily tasks as a consequence of their sleeping problems, behavioural studies generally failed to present conclusive results for cognitive correlates of this condition (Fulda and Schulz, 2001; Sateia et al., 2000). Orff et al. (2007) did not find performance differences between 32 PI patients and 17 good sleepers on tests for motor speed, attention, verbal fluency, verbal learning and memory. Investigating the more complex Wisconsin Card Sorting Test (WCST), which measures working memory and set shifting functions, Fang et al. (2008) similarly found no performance differences between 18 insomniacs and 21 normal sleepers in the age range of 20–63 years. Szelenberger and Niemcewicz (2000), however, showed that insomniacs need more repetitions than controls before they master the Selective Reminding Test and, moreover, that the number of repetitions required correlated with insomnia severity as measured by the Athens Insomnia Scale. Dividing a large group of insomniacs according to their sleep duration, Fernandez-Mendoza et al. (2010) found that insomniacs with short sleep duration showed deficits in neuropsychological performance on tests measuring set-switching and processing speed, whereas insomniacs with normal sleep duration did not.

Integration: contribution of sleep changes to cognitive ageing?

Age-related cognitive decline thus appears most pronounced in several executive functions that require integrity of the prefrontal cortical circuitry. Since executive function seems unaffected in insomnia, the contribution of the age-related increased risk of insomnia to this decline in executive cognitive functioning is not clear. However, studies on effects of insomnia on executive functions concerned adults with sleep complaints, not elderly insomniacs. We are aware of only a few studies that specifically addressed neuropsychological functioning within a group of elderly people with various degrees of disordered sleep. In one study on 144 home-dwelling elderly people around the age of 70 years, mental speed, memory and executive function showed small to moderate correlations with actigraphically determined 24-h sleep-wake rhythm fragmentation (Oosterman et al., 2009). The fragmentation of sleep and wakefulness towards an ultradian polyphasic rather than the adult circadian monophasic pattern is typical of ageing and age-related dementia and involves structural and functional changes in the suprachiasmatic nucleus, the clock of the brain (Baena et al., 2010; Harper et al., 2008).

Surprisingly, Altena et al. showed that elderly people with a clinical diagnosis of insomnia show better executive functioning than age-matched controls without sleep complaints. Elderly insomniacs generated more words on both a category and a letter fluency task. After sleep therapy, performance on the more complex letter fluency tasks increased even more (Altena et al., 2008a). Because this task requires more prefrontal activation than the category fluency task, sleep therapy may improve prefrontal function. The unexpected better performance in insomniacs than in controls might be related to the previously reported high level of arousal and high standards and perfectionism in insomnia. Integrating the findings of Oosterman et al. (2009) and Altena et al. (2008a), the poor sleep in elderly people comes in different phenotypes, each with specific sleep and cognitive changes. Thus, the phenotype of a fragmented 24-h sleep-wake rhythm – suggestive of inability to sustain extended periods of both sleep and wakefulness – may indeed aggravate the cognitive decline associated with ageing (Oosterman et al., 2009) or Alzheimer's dementia (Carvalho-Bos et al., 2007), and respond favourably to stimulation of the biological clock of the brain (e.g. Dowling et al., 2008; Scherder et al., 1999; Van Someren et al., 1998). On the other hand, elderly people with the phenotype of insomnia – with selective complaints of the inability to fall and stay asleep, but not to stay awake – may have enhanced executive functioning, possibly due to hyperarousal and perfectionism-related effort to reach high standards of performance. Insomniacs with short sleep duration, in fact, showed deficits of neuropsychological performance on tests measuring set-switching and processing speed, whereas insomniacs with normal sleep duration did not (Fernandez-Mendoza et al., 2010). This dissociation indicates that our understanding of the contribution of sleep changes to cognitive ageing requires dissociating not only different cognitive domains but also different phenotypes of disordered sleep.

It should be noted that the majority of standard neuropsychological tests measure neurological deficits. In spite of their sensitivity to measure the effects of total sleep deprivation for one or two nights, these tests may not be sensitive or specific enough to assess subtle changes in cognitive performance that may be associated with chronic insomnia. The next section discusses how computerized assessment of reaction times and responses during task performance allows researchers a better insight into subtle changes in cognitive functioning and how it is affected by age-related changes in sleep.

Computerized psychomotor task performance

Computerized psychomotor tasks have become an indispensable tool in cognitive neuroscience. Excellent control over stimulus properties and precise monitoring of their effect on response choices and their timing have been shown to be extremely valuable in sorting out cognitive processes and how they are affected by ageing and disorders. In contrast to numerous studies on psychomotor task performance in ageing, relatively few studies have used this powerful tool to elucidate how cognitive processing in insomnia may be affected and whether this might contribute to what we refer to as age-related cognitive decline.

Normal ageing

Although older adults rate themselves as more alert and less tired than younger adults, they generally perform slower on a psychomotor task, more so on more complex tasks than on simple tasks (Birren and Fisher, 1995; Rees et al., 1999). Fozard et al. (1994) performed a longitudinal study with large numbers of participants on changes in reaction time and ageing. A general slowing with age was found, more so on a more complex reaction time task (go–no go) than on simpler reaction time tasks (serial reaction time task). Moreover, slowing with age was found to be greater in women than in men. Elderly may set higher criteria for giving a correct response and spend more time on action monitoring, which may further explain increases in reaction time. This last observation may also explain why older adults, though being slower on a vigilance task which required decision making, make fewer errors than younger adults; response time is negatively correlated with the number of errors (Brache et al., 2010). Elderly require additional brain activity to perform complex motor tasks at the same level as young adults do. Motor control also becomes more reliant on the prefrontal cortex and basal ganglia. All can be interpreted as compensatory activation (Seidler et al., 2010). The slower reaction times in elderly, however, worsen less with time awake and circadian modulation than in young adults (Blatter et al., 2006).

Insomnia

Not all studies consistently report quantitative performance deficits in insomnia. The reasons may be multiple, including insensitivity of the applied measure and uncontrolled variance. The best-controlled study is probably the one by Varkevisser and Kerkhof (2005) who obtained quantitative performance on tasks addressing vigilance, working memory and motor control in insomniacs and controls throughout a 26-h constant routine protocol with minimal physical activity and no sleep. Unlike the small effects in less controlled studies, attenuated performance could be clearly demonstrated in insomniacs under these controlled circumstances.

In spite of the large number of studies investigating the effect of sleep on the process of memory consolidation, only one study addressed possible abnormalities in this process in insomnia (Nissen et al., 2006). The approach appears useful; while performance on a mirror tracing task before sleep did not differ between insomniacs and controls, insomniacs showed only half of the overnight improvement that is typical in normal sleepers.

In conclusion, computerized tasks applied under controlled circumstances show affected performance across a number of cognitive domains in insomnia and affected overnight motor learning.

Integration: contribution of sleep changes to cognitive ageing?

Age-related changes in psychomotor performance on computerized tasks are relatively small for simple reaction time tasks and are more pronounced on complex tasks. Under controlled conditions, adult insomniacs may show a somewhat comparable profile of attenuated performance, suggesting that the age-related increased risk of insomnia may contribute to age-related changes in psychomotor performance. However, the mentioned studies on effects of insomnia on psychomotor performance concerned adults with sleep complaints, not elderly insomniacs. A few studies that specifically addressed psychomotor performance within a group of elderly people with various degrees of disordered sleep will allow for a more conclusive statement. Under constant routine conditions keeping subjects in a supine position, psychomotor speed on a sustained attention task was reduced more in elderly insomniacs than in elderly without sleep complaints (Raymann and Van Someren, 2007). Furthermore, the typical decrease in performance with increasing time on task occurred earlier in elderly insomniacs. Under less controlled conditions, Altena et al. (2008b) showed that – compared to elderly controls without sleep complaints – elderly insomnia patients perform faster on a simple vigilance task but slower on a more complex vigilance task and interpreted this interaction effect in terms of the inverted U-shaped association between arousal and performance.

Crenshaw and Edinger (1999) aimed to relate changes in psychomotor performance to brain activity during sleep and showed in elderly insomniacs, but not in elderly controls, a negative correlation of simple reaction times with the power in the sleep–EEG slow wave frequency band. In conclusion, the increased prevalence of insomnia in old age may contribute to the age-related attenuated performance on reaction time tasks that appears to be most pronounced on more complex tasks. A comparison between different studies suggests that psychomotor performance deficits surface more pronounced in conditions in which participants are kept in a supine position (Raymann and Van Someren, 2007; Varkevisser and Kerkhof, 2005) which promotes sleepiness, possibly mediated by a reduction in sympathetic outflow and the resulting increase in skin blood flow and skin temperature (Van Someren, 2004).

Structural magnetic resonance imaging

MRI is a technique based on the magnetization properties of hydrogen nuclei. Because different amounts of these nuclei are present in different brain tissues, a very detailed image of the different brain structures can be generated. Ideally, investigations of changes in brain structure in ageing and insomnia could facilitate our understanding of the underlying mechanisms of age-related and insomnia-related changes in cognitive performance.

Normal ageing

Several structural brain alterations take place with increasing age. Global cortical volume decreases, with an anterior–posterior gradient: frontal and parietal regions show greater rates of decline than temporal and occipital regions (Thambisetty et al., 2010).

Grey matter changes take place in frontal regions such as the lateral frontal and cingulate regions, the lateral and orbital frontal regions (Tisserand et al., 2002) and the inferior frontal and insular regions; the inferior parietal cortex also shows higher rates of volume decrease than other regions (Resnick et al., 2003). In a 20-year longitudinal study of 48 post-menopausal women, the degree of grey matter loss in the right hippocampus and right orbitofrontal cortex was predicted by higher perceived stress (Gianaros et al., 2007).

White matter changes are more widespread and less confined to one region; still, there is a clear topography in age-related changes in white matter signal intensity with the most pronounced decreases in superior and medial frontal regions, the cingulum and medial and lateral temporal regions (Salat et al., 2009). In a diffusion tensor imaging study, O'Sullivan et al. (2001) showed that particularly in the frontal regions of the brain, white matter tract integrity is reduced and mean diffusivity is higher for older compared to younger adults. Mean diffusivity correlates with executive function as measured by the Trailmaking Test. Voineskos et al. (2010) showed that white matter integrity decline is related to cognitive decline. In particular, the inferior longitudinal fasciculus (ILF) is related to visuomotor dexterity, the inferior occipitofrontal fasciculus to visuospatial construction and the posterior fibres (i.e. splenium) of the corpus callosum to memory and executive function.

Insomnia

In a pilot study investigating structural brain differences in middle-aged insomnia patients in preselected prefrontal and temporal regions, Riemann et al. (2007) showed that they had a lower hippocampal volume than controls without sleep complaints. Patients and controls with a current or lifetime psychiatric disorder were excluded from this study. A reduced hippocampal volume could not be confirmed, however, in a considerably larger group of 20 slightly younger male insomnia patients compared to 15 controls (Winkelman et al., 2010). In patients suffering from post-traumatic stress disorder, insomnia severity is associated with a decreased volume of the CA3/dentate gyrus hippocampal subfield (Neylan et al., 2010).

Integration: contribution of sleep changes to cognitive ageing?

Hall et al. demonstrated a positive relation of hippocampus grey matter volume with reported sleep duration in 50 older women without sleep complaints (Baena et al., 2010). In our own unpublished data on 138 home-dwelling elderly people around, medial temporal lobe atrophy showed a moderate correlation with actigraphically determined 24-h sleep-wake rhythm fragmentation. In the only study to date using a whole-brain analysis in elderly clinically diagnosed insomniacs and controls, Altena et al. (2010) did not confirm hippocampal volume differences, but reported insomnia patients to have a lower grey matter density in the orbitofrontal cortex and precuneus.

The orbitofrontal grey matter density reduction reported by Altena et al. showed a strong negative relation with insomnia severity. The affected middle subregion of the orbitofrontal cortex, on the border of area 13l and 12/47, is a prime candidate for the neuronal coding of the subjective experience of pleasure and comfort (Kringelbach, 2005; Kringelbach and Berridge, 2009) such as thermal comfort judgements (Dunn et al., 2010; Rolls et al., 2008), which are compromised in insomniacs (Raymann and Van Someren, 2008). The important function of the orbitofrontal cortex in emotion regulation and reward processing (Kringelbach and Rolls, 2004) and its connections with the amygdala may also be related to the disturbances in emotion regulation which characterize insomniacs (Baglioni et al., 2010; Kales et al., 1987; Lombardo et al., 2008; Morin et al., 2003; Pavlova et al., 2001; Shaver et al., 2002). In summary, structural imaging studies suggest that different symptom clusters that may all be experienced as 'poor sleep', may be differentially associated with age-related localized reductions in brain volume. First, age-related volume reductions of the hippocampus and medial temporal lobe may worsen in association with a fragmented 24-h sleep-wake rhythm, with stress, for example from poor sleep. The volume reduction might be involved in the reported negative association of disturbed sleep and performance on memory tasks (Backhaus et al., 2006; Oosterman et al., 2009; Szelenberger and Niemcewicz, 2000). Second, elderly with a lower orbitofrontal volume may be the ones that are more prone to perceive stress and insomnia as more severe and possibly the ones that have the most compromised abilities to evaluate thermal comfort, which is indeed affected with ageing (Van Someren et al., 2002). Third, a single study found elderly insomniacs to have a lower grey matter volume in the precuneus. Further research is needed to evaluate this insomnia-associated structural change in a key part of the so-called default mode network (DMN). This brain network is active in the absence of task demands, during restful waking and sleep (Fukunaga et al., 2006) Insomnia patients show a decreased ability to disengage from external information processing at sleep onset (Bastien et al., 2003). The findings of reduced grey matter density in part of this network (Altena et al., 2010) may be related to an insufficiency for insomniacs to enter this resting state. If so, this insomnia feature may contribute to the reported age-related changes in this network, notably the smaller and slower deactivations of the DMN when performing a task (Sambataro et al., 2010).

Some inconsistency in the findings on structural imaging studies should be noted. We suggest these to be due to subtle differences in the profiles of objective sleep and sleep-wake rhythms and subjective sleep complaints, once more indicating that our understanding of the contribution of sleep changes to cognitive ageing requires dissociating not only different cognitive domains and corresponding brain networks but also different phenotypes of disordered sleep.

Functional magnetic resonance imaging

Functional MRI (fMRI) is based on the principle that a local increase in mass neuronal activity leads to a subsequent increase in local blood flow. This in turn causes a decrease in the concentration of deoxygenated haemoglobin in the microvasculature surrounding the activated region (Malonek and Grinvald, 1996). This change leads to an increase in the blood oxygenation level-dependent (BOLD) signal (D'Esposito et al., 2003; Kwong et al., 1992; Ogawa et al., 1990, 1992).

Normal ageing

Changes in the BOLD signal as a function of normal ageing in fMRI tasks are found in various regions including the medial temporal lobe (Daselaar et al., 2003, 2006), but are particularly prominent in prefrontal regions. Findings suggest both an attenuated activation in some regions and a compensatory increased activation in other, mostly prefrontal, regions (Davis et al., 2008). Aged subjects may thus show both hypo-activation in task-related prefrontal areas and hyper-activation in non-task-related areas, reflecting attempts at compensation (Cabeza et al., 1997; Grady et al., 2005, 2006). In a meta-analysis, Rajah and D'Esposito (2005) showed that with age a differentiation of cortical function occurs in the bilateral ventral prefrontal cortex. Deficits in function occur in the right dorsal and anterior prefrontal cortex. As a result of these changes, functional compensation in left dorsal and anterior prefrontal cortex may occur. Such compensatory mechanisms indicate the use of less effective cognitive strategies (Burgmans et al., 2010). fMRI studies comparing younger and older participants showed that elderly have a decreased signal-to-noise ratio when performing a simple motor reaction time task (D'Esposito et al., 1999). When performing a finger-tapping task, a decrease with age of both the signal amplitude and the number of activated voxels is found (Hesselmann et al., 2001).

Insomnia

To date, only one published study used fMRI to investigate changes in insomnia. Altena et al. (2008a) showed that when insomnia patients perform letter and category fluency tasks in fMRI, they show less activation in task-related prefrontal regions (inferior frontal gyrus, medial prefrontal cortex) compared to controls without sleep complaints. Sleep therapy, but not waitlist control, results in partial recovery of this hypo-activation. In spite of the initial hypo-activation, insomnia patients generate more words on both fluency tasks than controls do. After sleep therapy, but not after waitlist control, the number of words generated on the most complex task, the letter fluency task, increases even more. The high performance level on word production deserves further attention and might be related to the high levels of arousal and a tendency for perfectionism that are characteristic of many insomniacs (Bonnet and Arand, 1997; Lundh et al., 1994; Pavlova et al., 2001; Vincent and Walker, 2000).

Integration: contribution of sleep changes to cognitive ageing?

Combining the reported age-related and insomnia-related changes in brain function found with fMRI, it can be tentatively suggested that poor sleep may contribute to the age-related decline in task-induced prefrontal activation. The partial reversibility of this effect with short-term non-pharmacological sleep therapy is striking. It may inspire more research into the reversibility of hypofrontality at high age by promoting sound sleep. Data are too limited to make statements about the involvement of poor sleep in compensatory activation processes. The absence of compensatory activation in the only fMRI insomnia study may indicate that different subjects activate different brain regions as such, so that no mean group effect is found. Further subtyping of insomnia might be of help to map possibly compensatory brain processes.

Electroencephalography (EEG)

Both sleep stages and characteristics of wakefulness can be studied using EEG. Using this technique, electrodes are placed on the scalp with which the electrical activity produced by mass neuronal activity can be measured.

Normal ageing

The wake EEG of older people performing a word recognition task shows less frontal midline theta power than in younger adults. The attenuated midline theta power can be seen also during a wake resting state, although it may be less evident (Cummins and Finnigan, 2007). Studying brain connectivity patterns by applying causality analysis of multichannel EEG with partial directed coherence in different age groups, Zhu et al. (2010) conclude there is loss of connectivity in cortical interactive networks with ageing, particularly in the left frontal and central brain areas.

During sleep, the EEG shows typical age-related changes. Nocturnal sleep is more shallow, as indicated by an increased number of brief arousals and a marked decrease in the power in the 0.5–4 Hz frequency band, usually referred to as slow wave activity (Bliwise, 1993).

The pronounced difference in daytime versus nocturnal EEG profiles also becomes smaller with age. Power spectral density of sleep EEG shows that day–night differences in the lower alpha and spindle frequency range are smaller in older people (Munch et al., 2005). Age is also associated with a higher prevalence of daytime naps (Buysse et al., 1991, 1992). Munch et al. (2005) showed that during a 40 h nap protocol, more sleep occurs at normal waking time in older than in younger adults. Older adults also show a reduced circadian modulation in REM sleep.

Insomnia

When measuring wake resting state EEG, insomniacs show less alpha power than normal controls (Lamarche and Ogilvie, 1997; Staner et al., 2003). Szelenberger et al. measured high-density EEG during the Continuous Attention Test (CAT), a visual recognition task, and quantified brain activation using low-resolution brain electromagnetic tomography (LORETA) (Szelenberger and Niemcewicz, 2001). They found that compared to controls, insomnia patients showed less event-related current density in orbitofrontal, medial prefrontal, anterior cingulate, premotor and parietal cortex, but increased activation in the left dorsolateral prefrontal cortex. Notably, as also reported in an fMRI study (Altena et al., 2008a), differences in brain activation occurred in the absence of compromised performance.

At sleep onset, insomniacs show elevated beta power (high-frequency EEG activity) and decreased delta power (low-frequency EEG activity) compared to normal sleeping controls (Lamarche and Ogilvie, 1997; Staner et al., 2003). Particularly in PI patients, in comparison to good sleepers and 'secondary' insomnia patients, high-frequency EEG activity increases across NREM cycles, with its highest rate of occurrence during stage 1 and REM sleep (Perlis et al., 2001). It may be that an accelerated EEG profile is representative of only a specific subtype of insomnia, and it is tempting to suggest specific treatment options aimed at increasing slow oscillations and suppressing faster frequencies (Raymann et al., 2008; Van Someren, 2004). Several studies, but certainly not all, describe prolonged sleep latency, increased wake time after sleep onset and reduced sleep efficiency in insomnia. Subjective complaints typically diverge from objective findings. Reductions in slow wave sleep and REM sleep are found in only a minority of studies (Benca et al., 1992; Hudson et al., 1992; Reite et al., 1995).

Integration: contribution of sleep changes to cognitive ageing?

As described above for imaging studies, the effect of age on prefrontal EEG activation and brain connectivity patterns during wakefulness is in part also found in adult insomniacs, suggesting a possible contribution of poor sleep to the age-related changes. Also, the sleep EEGs of elderly and insomniacs show similar deviations from young adults without sleep complaints, notably the increased beta power at sleep onset and increase in high-frequency EEG activity in NREM sleep.

Event-related potentials

EEG constitutes one of the most used non-invasive methods to investigate the temporal dynamics of neural processes; resting state background EEG itself, however, is limited in providing insights into information processes since the recording tends to reflect the brain's global electrical activity. A more powerful approach is the study of modulation of brain activity in response to a particular stimulus. By presenting series of stimuli, EEG signals are averaged together after aligning these signals with the onset of the stimulus or response. This averaging procedure cancels out noise and activities unrelated to the event of interest. This results in ERP, a series of peaks and troughs in the average brain activity that are related to specific parts of the information processing (Naatanen and Picton, 1987). Modulations in polarity, latency and scalp distributions of these components can be used to evaluate group differences on different aspects of information processes. Because the temporal resolution is in the range of milliseconds, ERP permit the determination of the sequence of activity of fast cognitive processes in real time. During wakefulness, early evoked components between 50 and 100 ms reflect sensory-related processing whereas later evoked components are related not only to attention and arousal but also to complex cognitive processing. During sleep, later evoked components between 300 and 900 ms are thought to reflect synchronized activity related to cortical and thalamo-cortical mechanisms (see for a review Colrain and Campbell, 2007). A highly selective overview of the most reported ERP components in ageing and insomnia is given below.

Normal ageing

Studies investigating healthy ageing have covered processes such as perception, executive functions, memory and emotion. Early components, associated with processes such as arousal (N1) and inhibition of attentional processes (P2), show increase in P2 amplitude with age (e.g. Crowley et al., 2002; Crowley and Colrain, 2004; Garcia-Larrea et al., 1992). The higher order processing P300 component typically shows a shift in activation from posterior to anterior areas as a function of age, implying that age alters activations from different brain areas at different rates (e.g. Fjell and Walhovd, 2001; Polich, 2007).

Brain potentials can also be studied during sleep using auditory stimuli. Compared to young adults, elderly people showed a decreased N1 amplitude, an augmented and delayed P2 component, a long lasting late positivity (LLP) and smaller N350 and N550 components (e.g. Crowley et al., 2002; Crowley and Colrain, 2004). These changes were associated with a reduced density of K-complexes.

Taken together, research into age-related changes in ERPs show mixed results; as in fMRI studies, this has led to the view that reduced activity of a component could reflect impaired activation of the neuronal processes that would be most optimal for the information process under consideration, while increased activity may reflect compensatory mechanisms (for a review, see Grady, 2008).

Insomnia

Primary (psychophysiological) insomnia has been associated with hyperarousal both in the psychological and in the physiological sense (Edinger et al., 2001; Perlis et al., 2001). This may interfere with processes necessary to block the sensory and information processing system, thus contributing to impaired sleep onset and sleep maintenance. ERP studies investigating the underlying mechanisms of PI found several neurophysiological alterations in auditory oddball tasks and sensory gating tasks, but results are inconsistent and interpretations equivocal. The early component P50, related to sensory gating, is maintained during sleep but attenuated during wake, supporting the notion that poor sleepers have deficient sensory blocking (Milner et al., 2009).

The mid-latency components such as P1, N1, P2 and N2 also showed to be affected in insomnia, depending on time of measurement and stimulus type. The results are somewhat inconsistent with components reported to be enhanced in amplitude (Bastien et al., 2008; Regestein et al., 1993; Turcotte and Bastien, 2009; Yang and Lo, 2007), show no effects (Sforza and Haba-Rubio, 2006) or, for the later N350 component, are diminished (Bastien et al., 2008; Hairston et al., 2010; Harsh et al., 1994; Turcotte and Bastien, 2009; Yang and Lo, 2007). The N350 has therefore been associated with the sensory gating mechanism (e.g. Harsh et al., 1994) necessary to inhibit cortical arousal (Bastien et al., 2008; Colrain and Campbell, 2007). It has moreover been suggested to be involved with K-complexes, vertex sharp waves and the normal process of sleep initiation (Campbell et al., 1992; Colrain and Campbell, 2007). In addition, the gating of the P450 component, which is observed only during sleep, is less strong in insomnia patients (Hairston et al., 2010) and is thought to be analogous to the N350, a subcomponent of the K-complex (Bastuji and Garcia-Larrea, 1999; Bastuji et al., 1995).

Findings on the P300 are equivocal. The P300 amplitude was found to be smaller in awake insomnia patients (Hairston et al., 2010), to be larger in awake insomnia patients after a poor night of sleep (Devoto et al., 2003, 2005) or to not differ from the P300 of controls (Sforza and Haba-Rubio, 2006).

In summary, most components appeared to be sensitive to the changing levels of arousal in insomnia; the early components show mixed results, whereas the later components, the N350 and P450, seem to be consistently smaller in insomnia patients compared to good sleepers, both during sleep and wake.

Integration: contribution of sleep changes to cognitive ageing?

Most studies have shown age-related cognitive decline and its effect on particularly executive functioning, although compensatory mechanisms are facilitated to achieve optimal performance. In insomnia studies with young subjects, the presence of hyperarousal is seen as one of the causes underlying this disorder. Although ERP studies on the effects of insomnia on executive functioning in elderly insomniacs are limited, the influence of sleep changes on cognitive ageing is thought to affect components such as the N1 and P300 which are influenced by arousal fluctuations. Elevated arousal during sleep may result in more 'age-related' changes in the N350 and P450 in poorly sleeping compared to well-sleeping elderly.

Positron emission tomography

With PET, a radioactively labelled ligand is injected into the blood, after which its regional density in the brain can be measured. For example, labelled glucose can be used to study regional metabolic activity in the brain.

Normal ageing

In a PET study by Cabeza et al. (2000), younger adults show recruitment of right prefrontal cortex during the encoding of a verbal memory task. High-performing older adults show bilateral activation of these prefrontal regions. The bilateral prefrontal activation in high-performing older adults is suggestive of the necessity for compensatory prefrontal activation to be able to perform the task well. The recruitment of additional brain regions next to regions expected to be activated by a given task is regarded as a compensatory process in the brain, and found in many conditions and diseases (Drummond et al., 2000; Feigin et al., 2006; Staffen et al., 2002). A similar finding of prefrontal compensatory mechanisms in ageing was found by Grady et al. (1994). When performing a face- and location-matching task, older adults showed less activation in occipital but more in prefrontal regions. Reuter-Lorenz et al. (2000) used PET to investigate older and younger participants performing both a verbal and a spatial working memory task. Although lateralization for each task (left prefrontal regions for verbal, right prefrontal regions for the spatial task) was very clear in younger participants, older participants showed bilateral activation for both tasks, which is again interpreted as compensatory mechanisms coming into play. Reduced activation in brain regions normally critical for task performance (the dorsolateral prefrontal cortex in the WCST and the inferolateral temporal cortex in Raven's Progressive Matrices (RPM)) was found in elderly compared to younger subjects in a study by D'Esposito et al. (1999). Increased activation was found in brain regions not normally involved in these tasks: the hippocampal region during the WCST and the mesial polar frontal prefrontal cortex during both WCST and RPM.

In summary, PET studies show a decrease in task-related activation with ageing, accompanied by compensatory activation in non-task-related regions, in particular in the prefrontal cortex. If a task shows unilateral activation in younger adults, a more bilateral activation is observed in older adults.

Insomnia

During wakefulness, insomniacs show a lower metabolic rate in the prefrontal cortex than controls without sleep complaints do (Nofzinger et al., 2004). During the transition from wake to sleep, insomnia patients show a relative lack of inactivation of the hypothalamus, thalamus, insular cortex, hippocampus and amygdala and of the anterior cingulate and medial prefrontal cortex. These findings are difficult to reconcile with a single photon emission computed tomography (SPECT) study demonstrating that insomniacs have a global hypoperfusion during initial stages of NREM sleep (Smith et al., 2002) which reversed after successful behavioural therapy, in particular in the basal ganglia (Smith et al., 2005). Additional studies should resolve this discrepancy which may not only be due to the difference in sleep stages measured and neuroimaging techniques applied but could also be due to variance in subtypes of insomnia, which have not been clearly defined yet.

Integration: contribution of sleep changes to cognitive ageing?

Because the only known PET study in insomnia was performed during resting state and not during task performance, no conclusion can be reached on a possible contribution of poor sleep to age-related changes. In normal ageing, the same pattern of reduced task-related activation and prefrontal compensatory mechanisms emerges that was found in other functional imaging studies. It would be interesting to investigate whether insomnia, like ageing, is associated with the bilateral compensatory activation in tasks that normally induce unilateral activation only. With the one unilateral task applied thus far in fMRI, verbal fluency, no such patterns were found for insomniacs (Altena et al., 2008a). As mentioned above though, group analyses are insensitive if compensatory activation regionally differs between individuals. Unaffected performance on most neuropsychological tasks (see 'Neuropsychological task performance' section) suggests that some compensatory processes yet to be defined are effective in insomnia.

Transcranial magnetic stimulation

With TMS, electric currents are induced in the brain through electromagnetic induction, using a rapidly changing magnetic field in predefined brain regions, which makes it possible to study functions and interconnections of the brain (Chen, 2000). It allows to investigate the excitability of the cerebral cortex, by measuring facilitation and inhibition (Kobayashi and Pascual-Leone, 2003).

Normal ageing

TMS studies in elderly people have shown that in particular short- and long-interval intracortical inhibitions are increased in older compared to younger adults. Under resting conditions, there is less intracortical facilitation in this age group. The authors interpret this as a suggestion for increased GABA-mediated intracortical inhibition with age (McGinley et al., 2010).

Insomnia

Van Der Werf et al. evaluated intracortical inhibition and facilitation using double pulse TMS in elderly insomniacs (Van Der Werf et al., 2010). Both after a single and a double pulse, the physiological motor response was higher for insomniacs than for controls, suggestive once more of hyperarousability. The intracortical facilitation effect after double pulse stimulation is lower for the insomniacs, however, possibly due to the already higher baseline (single pulse) response. Group differences were not altered after sleep therapy. This attenuation appears specific to insomnia and has not been reported in previous experimental sleep deprivation studies.

Integration: contribution of sleep changes to cognitive ageing?

The results reported by Van Der Werf et al. (2010) are consistent with the notion of hyperarousal. The fact that the exaggerated response does not normalize after sleep therapy suggests that hyperarousal may not normalize completely at all levels of brain functionality, and may in part be a trait. Such a trait might lead to an increased risk of developing insomnia. Preliminary findings show that insomnia patients have reduced brain levels of the inhibitory and sleep-promoting neurotransmitter GABA, which could be related to this increased motor response. Reduced levels of GABA can lead to increased levels of glutamate, which may in turn increase CRH. CRH plays an important role in arousal and promotes wakefulness. An important but complex role of CRH in the onset and maintenance of insomnia has been suggested. The increasing risk of insomnia in old age may contribute to the age-related decrease in intracortical facilitation.

Concluding remarks

This chapter evaluated whether the sleep complaints that are so typical in older people might contribute to what is generally referred to as 'age-related cognitive decline'. Only a limited number of studies specifically address this question by comparing cognition and brain functional and structural indices in elderly insomniacs versus elderly without sleep complaints. A possible involvement of poor sleep was, therefore, also pursued by comparing changes that have been found to be associated with ageing and insomnia.

Ageing affects many brain functions, of which those related to prefrontal processing are most prominent. Older adults need more effort and make more mistakes on executive tasks (Daselaar et al., 2005; Grady, 2008; Van Der Werf et al., 2001) and are slower on computerized psychomotor tasks, more so with more complex tasks (Blatter et al., 2006). Brain imaging shows attenuated activation in task-related regions and compensatory mechanisms effective in particularly prefrontal regions (Burgmans et al., 2010; Cabeza et al., 1997; Davis et al., 2008; D'Esposito et al., 1999; Grady et al., 2005, 2006). Tasks that require unilateral prefrontal activation in younger adults require bilateral prefrontal activation in older adults (Reuter-Lorenz et al., 2000).

The compromised, insomnia-like sleep of many elderly is likely to contribute to 'age-related' changes. With respect to psychomotor task performance, poor sleep was shown to reversibly contribute to the preferential slowing on more complex tasks that is typical of ageing (Altena et al., 2008a). With respect to functional imaging, the prefrontal hypoactivation that is typical of ageing is also present in insomnia, both during rest (Nofzinger et al., 2004) and during task performance (Altena et al., 2008a). Disturbed sleep may contribute to ERP changes seen in ageing due to its association with increased arousal; perhaps in line with this, TMS studies show that loss of intracortical facilitation occurs both in ageing and in insomnia, indicating that disturbed sleep may be a shared mechanism. Another emerging observation is that changes in brain activation patterns do not necessarily translate into compromised task performance because of compensatory activation. The hyperarousal characteristic of insomnia may be interpreted within the compensatory framework because in some tasks it will help compensate deficits and result in normal performance. Too few studies on insomnia have addressed other ways of compensation, that is by activation of other brain areas, as has consistently been found in ageing studies. Even if this compensation occurs, it may go unnoticed in group analyses if individuals are not homogeneous with respect to the brain areas they activate for compensation.

Further subtyping of insomnia is called for (Van Someren et al., 2009). For example, there is a striking difference in neuropsychological performance between insomniacs with and without short sleep duration (Fernandez-Mendoza et al., 2010). Fernandez-Mendoza et al. suggest that the hypercortisolemia typical only for insomniacs with a short sleep duration could be involved in executive deficits. The contribution of poor sleep to cognitive ageing, and its underlying mechanisms, may surface more readily if future studies would include adult and elderly subjects with and without hypercortisolemia and with and without sleep complaints. Subtyping according to daytime behaviour may be fruitful as well; while some poorly sleeping elderly are hyperaroused and are active throughout the day, others may have a fragmented activity rhythm due to intrusions of daytime naps that in turn contribute to a less consolidated sleep during the night. Since insomnia in the elderly can, at least partly and in some cases, be treated using nonpharmacological means, we suggest that age-related changes in brain function may be counteracted when sleep problems can be treated appropriately.

To conclude, it can be stated that the poor sleep that many elderly are confronted with contributes to what we are used to call 'age-related' cognitive decline. For a better understanding of mechanisms involved, it seems essential to be aware of, and quantify, the different profiles of compromised sleep.

References

Alapin, I., Fichten, C. S., Libman, E., Creti, L., Bailes, S., & Wright, J. (2000). How is good and poor sleep in older adults and college students related to daytime sleepiness, fatigue, and ability to concentrate? *Journal of Psychosomatic Research*, *49*, 381–390.

Altena, E., Van Der Werf, Y. D., Sanz-Arigita, E. J., Voorn, T. A., Rombouts, S. A., & Kuijer, J. P., et al., (2008a). Prefrontal hypoactivation and recovery in insomnia. *Sleep*, *31*, 1271–1276.

Altena, E., Van Der Werf, Y. D., Strijers, R. L., & Van Someren, E. J. (2008b). Sleep loss affects vigilance: Effects of chronic insomnia and sleep therapy. *Journal of Sleep Research*, *17*, 335–343.

Altena, E., Vrenken, H., Van Der Werf, Y. D., van den Heuvel, O. A., & Van Someren, E. J. (2010). Reduced orbitofrontal and parietal gray matter in chronic insomnia: A voxel-based morphometric study. *Biological Psychiatry*, *67*, 182–185.

American Academy of Sleep, M. (2000). *International classification of sleep disorders, Revised: Diagnostic and coding manual.* American Academy of Sleep Medicine, Rochester.

Backhaus, J., Junghanns, K., Born, J., Hohaus, K., Faasch, F., & Hohagen, F. (2006). Impaired declarative memory consolidation during sleep in patients with primary insomnia: Influence of sleep architecture and nocturnal cortisol release. *Biological Psychiatry*, *60*, 1324–1330.

Baena, E., Allen, P. A., Kaut, K. P., & Hall, R. J. (2010). On age differences in prefrontal function: The importance of emotional/cognitive integration. *Neuropsychologia*, *48*, 319–333.

Baglioni, C., Spiegelhalder, K., Lombardo, C., & Riemann, D. (2010). Sleep and emotions: A focus on insomnia. *Sleep Medicine Reviews*, *14*, 227–238.

Basta, M., Chrousos, G. P., Vela-Bueno, A., & Vgontzas, A. N. (2007). Chronic insomnia and stress system. *Sleep Medicine Clinics*, *2*, 279–291.

Bastien, C. H., Fortier-Brochu, E., Rioux, I., LeBlanc, M., Daley, M., & Morin, C. M. (2003). Cognitive performance and sleep quality in the elderly suffering from chronic insomnia. Relationship between objective and subjective measures. *Journal of Psychosomatic Research*, *54*, 39–49.

Bastien, C. H., St-Jean, G., Morin, C. M., Turcotte, I., & Carrier, J. (2008). Chronic psychophysiological insomnia:

Hyperarousal and/or inhibition deficits? An ERPs investigation. *Sleep*, *31*, 887–898.

Bastuji, H., & Garcia-Larrea, L. (1999). Evoked potentials as a tool for the investigation of human sleep. *Sleep Medicine Reviews*, *3*, 23–45.

Bastuji, H., Garcia-Larrea, L., Franc, C., & Mauguiere, F. (1995). Brain processing of stimulus deviance during slow-wave and paradoxical sleep: A study of human auditory evoked responses using the oddball paradigm. *Journal of Clinical Neurophysiology*, *12*, 155–167.

Beaulieu-Bonneau, S., LeBlanc, M., Merette, C., Dauvilliers, Y., & Morin, C. M. (2007). Family history of insomnia in a population-based sample. *Sleep*, *30*, 1739–1745.

Benca, R. M., Obermeyer, W. H., Thisted, R. A., & Gillin, J. C. (1992). Sleep and psychiatric disorders. A meta-analysis. *Archives of General Psychiatry*, *49*, 651–668 discussion 669–670.

Birren, J. E., & Fisher, L. M. (1995). Aging and speed of behavior: Possible consequences for psychological functioning. *Annual Review of Psychology*, *46*, 329–353.

Bixler, E., Vgontzas, A., Lin, H., & Vela-Bueno, A. (2007). Menopause and hormone replacement therapy: Effects on objective sleep patterns. *Sleep*, *30*, A258–A259.

Blatter, K., Graw, P., Munch, M., Knoblauch, V., Wirz-Justice, A., & Cajochen, C. (2006). Gender and age differences in psychomotor vigilance performance under differential sleep pressure conditions. *Behavioural Brain Research*, *168*, 312–317.

Bliwise, D. L. (1993). Sleep in normal aging and dementia. *Sleep*, *16*, 40–81.

Bonnet, M. H., & Arand, D. L. (1995). 24-Hour metabolic rate in insomniacs and matched normal sleepers. *Sleep*, *18*, 581–588.

Bonnet, M. H., & Arand, D. L. (1997). Hyperarousal and insomnia. *Sleep Medicine Reviews*, *1*, 97–108.

Bonnet, M. H., & Arand, D. L. (2003). Insomnia, metabolic rate and sleep restoration. *Journal of Internal Medicine*, *254*, 23–31.

Boomsma, DI., van Someren, E. J., Beem, A. L., de Geus, E. J., & Willemsen, G. (2008). Sleep during a regular week night: A twin-sibling study. *Twin Research and Human Genetics*, *11*, 538–545.

Brache, K., Scialfa, C., & Hudson, C. (2010). Aging and vigilance: Who has the inhibition deficit? *Experimental Aging Research*, *36*, 140–152.

Broman, J. -E., Lundh, L. G., Aleman, K., & Hetta, J. (1992). Subjective and objective performance in patients with persistent insomnia. *Cognitive Behavior Therapy*, *21*, 115–126.

Burgmans, S., van Boxtel, M. P., Vuurman, E. F., Evers, E. A., & Jolles, J. (2010). Increased neural activation during picture encoding and retrieval in 60-year-olds compared to 20-year-olds. *Neuropsychologia*, *48*, 2188–2197.

Buysse, D. J. (2008). Chronic insomnia. *American Journal of Psychiatry*, *165*, 678–686.

Buysse, D. J., Ancoli-Israel, S., Edinger, J. D., Lichstein, K. L., & Morin, C. M. (2006). Recommendations for a standard research assessment of insomnia. *Sleep*, *29*, 1155–1173.

Buysse, D. J., Browman, K. E., Monk, T. H., Reynolds 3rd, C. F., Fasiczka, A. L., & Kupfer, D. J. (1992). Napping and 24-hour sleep/wake patterns in healthy elderly and young adults. *Journal of the American Geriatrics Society*, *40*, 779–786.

Buysse, D. J., Reynolds 3rd, C. F., Monk, T. H., Hoch, C. C., Yeager, A. L., & Kupfer, D. J. (1991). Quantification of subjective sleep quality in healthy elderly men and women using the Pittsburgh Sleep Quality Index (PSQI). *Sleep*, *14*, 331–338.

Cabeza, R., Anderson, N. D., Houle, S., Mangels, J. A., & Nyberg, L. (2000). Age-related differences in neural activity during item and temporal-order memory retrieval: A positron emission tomography study. *Journal of Cognitive Neuroscience*, *12*, 197–206.

Cabeza, R., Grady, C. L., Nyberg, L., McIntosh, A. R., Tulving, E., & Kapur, S., et al., (1997). Age-related differences in neural activity during memory encoding and retrieval: A positron emission tomography study. *Journal of Neuroscience*, *17*, 391–400.

Campbell, K. B., Bell, I., & Bastien, C. H. (1992). Evoked potential measures of information processing during natural sleep. In: Broughton, R. J., Ogilvie, R. D. (Eds.), *Sleep, arousal, and performance*. Birkhauser, Boston, pp. 88–116.

Carvalho-Bos, S. S., Riemersma-van der Lek, R. F., Waterhouse, J., Reilly, T., & Van Someren, E. J. (2007). Strong association of the rest-activity rhythm with well-being in demented elderly women. *American Journal of Geriatric Psychiatry*, *15*, 92–100.

Chang, P. P., Ford, D. E., Mead, L. A., Cooper-Patrick, L., & Klag, M. J. (1997). Insomnia in young men and subsequent depression. The Johns Hopkins Precursors Study. *American Journal of Epidemiology*, *146*, 105–114.

Chau, N., Bhattacherjee, A., & Kunar, B. M. (2009). Relationship between job, lifestyle, age and occupational injuries. *Occupational Medicine*, *59*, 114–119.

Chau, N., Gauchard, G. C., Siegfried, C., Benamghar, L., Dangelzer, J. L., & Francais, M., et al., (2004). Relationships of job, age, and life conditions with the causes and severity of occupational injuries in construction workers. *International Archives of Occupational and Environmental Health*, *77*, 60–66.

Chen, R. (2000). Studies of human motor physiology with transcranial magnetic stimulation. *Muscle and Nerve*, *9*, S26–S32.

Chesson Jr., A., Hartse, K., Anderson, W. M., Davila, D., Johnson, S., & Littner, M., et al., (2000). Practice parameters for the evaluation of chronic insomnia. An American Academy of Sleep Medicine report. Standards of Practice Committee of the American Academy of Sleep Medicine. *Sleep*, *23*, 237–241.

Colrain, I. M., & Campbell, K. B. (2007). The use of evoked potentials in sleep research. *Sleep Medicine Reviews*, *11*, 277–293.

Comijs, H. C., Deeg, D. J., Dik, M. G., Twisk, J. W., & Jonker, C. (2002). Memory complaints; the association with psycho-affective and health problems and the role of personality characteristics. A 6-year follow-up study. *Journal of Affective Disorders*, *72*, 157–165.

Crenshaw, M. C., & Edinger, J. D. (1999). Slow-wave sleep and waking cognitive performance among older adults with and without insomnia complaints. *Physiology & Behavior*, *66*, 485–492.

Crowley, K. E., & Colrain, I. M. (2004). A review of the evidence for P2 being an independent component process: Age, sleep and modality. *Clinical Neurophysiology*, *115*, 732–744.

Crowley, K., Trinder, J., & Colrain, I. M. (2002). An examination of evoked K-complex amplitude and frequency of occurrence in the elderly. *Journal of Sleep Research*, *11*, 129–140.

Cummins, T. D., & Finnigan, S. (2007). Theta power is reduced in healthy cognitive aging. *International Journal of Psychophysiology*, *66*, 10–17.

Daigneault, S., Braun, C. M. J., & Whitaker, H. A. (1992). Early effects of normal aging on perseverative and non-perseverative prefrontal measures. *Developmental Neuropsychology*, *8*, 99–114.

Daley, M., Morin, C. M., LeBlanc, M., Gregoire, J. P., & Savard, J. (2009). The economic burden of insomnia: Direct and indirect costs for individuals with insomnia syndrome, insomnia symptoms, and good sleepers. *Sleep*, *32*, 55–64.

Daselaar, S. M., Fleck, M. S., Dobbins, I. G., Madden, D. J., & Cabeza, R. (2006). Effects of healthy aging on hippocampal and rhinal memory functions: An event-related fMRI study. *Cerebral Cortex*, *16*, 1771–1782.

Daselaar, S. M., Veltman, D. J., Rombouts, S. A., Raaijmakers, J. G., & Jonker, C. (2003). Deep processing activates the medial temporal lobe in young but not in old adults. *Neurobiology of Aging*, *24*, 1005–1011.

Daselaar, S. M., Veltman, D. J., Rombouts, S. A., Raaijmakers, J. G., & Jonker, C. (2005). Aging affects both perceptual and lexical/semantic components of word stem priming: An event-related fMRI study. *Neurobiology of Learning and Memory*, *83*, 251–262.

Davis, S. W., Dennis, N. A., Daselaar, S. M., Fleck, M. S., & Cabeza, R. (2008). Que PASA? The posterior-anterior shift in aging. *Cerebral Cortex*, *18*, 1201–1209.

der Werf, S. Y., Kaptein, K. I., de Jonge, P., Spijker, J., de Graaf, R., & Korf, J. (2006). Major depressive episodes and random mood. *Archives of General Psychiatry*, *63*, 509–518.

D'Esposito, M., Deouell, L. Y., & Gazzaley, A. (2003). Alterations in the BOLD fMRI signal with ageing and disease: A challenge for neuroimaging. *Nature Reviews Neuroscience*, *4*, 863–872.

D'Esposito, M., Zarahn, E., Aguirre, G. K., & Rypma, B. (1999). The effect of normal aging on the coupling of neural activity to the bold hemodynamic response. *Neuroimage*, *10*, 6–14.

Devoto, A., Manganelli, S., Lucidi, F., Lombardo, C., Russo, P. M., & Violani, C. (2005). Quality of sleep and P300 amplitude in primary insomnia: A preliminary study. *Sleep*, *28*, 859–863.

Devoto, A., Violani, C., Lucidi, F., & Lombardo, C. (2003). P300 amplitude in subjects with primary insomnia is modulated by their sleep quality. *Journal of Psychosomatic Research*, *54*, 3–10.

Dowling, G. A., Burr, R. L., Van Someren, E. J. W., Hubbard, E. M., Luxenberg, J. S., & Mastick, J., et al., (2008). Melatonin and bright light treatment for rest-activity disruption in institutionalized patients with Alzheimer's disease. *Journal of the American Geriatrics Society*, *56*, 239–246.

Drummond, S. P., Brown, G. G., Gillin, J. C., Stricker, J. L., Wong, E. C., & Buxton, R. B. (2000). Altered brain response to verbal learning following sleep deprivation. *Nature*, *403*, 655–657.

Dufouil, C., Fuhrer, R., & Alperovitch, A. (2005). Subjective cognitive complaints and cognitive decline: Consequence or predictor? The epidemiology of vascular aging study. *Journal of the American Geriatrics Society*, *53*, 616–621.

Dunn, B.J., Conover, K., Plourde, G., Munro, D., Kilgour, R., & Shizgal, P. (2010). Hedonic valuation during thermal alliesthesia. *Abstracts of the 16th Annual Meeting of the Organization for Human Brain Mapping*.

Edinger, J. D., Fins, A. I., Glenn, D. M., Sullivan Jr., R. J., Bastian, L. A., & Marsh, G. R., et al., (2000). Insomnia and the eye of the beholder: Are there clinical markers of objective sleep disturbances among adults with and without insomnia complaints? *Journal of Consulting and Clinical Psychology*, *68*, 586–593.

Edinger, J. D., Glenn, D. M., Bastian, L. A., Marsh, G. R., Daile, D., & Hope, T. V., et al., (2001). Sleep in the laboratory and sleep at home II: Comparisons of middle-aged insomnia sufferers and normal sleepers. *Sleep*, *24*, 761–770.

Fang, S. C., Huang, C. J., Yang, T. T., & Tsai, P. S. (2008). Heart rate variability and daytime functioning in insomniacs and normal sleepers: Preliminary results. *Journal of Psychosomatic Research*, *65*, 23–30.

Feigin, A., Ghilardi, M. F., Huang, C., Ma, Y., Carbon, M., & Guttman, M., et al., (2006). Preclinical Huntington's disease: Compensatory brain responses during learning. *Annals of Neurology*, *59*, 53–59.

Fernandez-Mendoza, J., Calhoun, S., Bixler, E. O., Pejovic, S., Karataraki, M., & Liao, D., et al., (2010). Insomnia with objective short sleep duration is associated with deficits in neuropsychological performance: A general population study. *Sleep*, *33*, 459–465.

Fjell, A. M., & Walhovd, K. B. (2001). P300 and neuropsychological tests as measures of aging: Scalp topography and cognitive changes. *Brain Topography*, *14*, 25–40.

Foley, D. J., Monjan, A. A., Brown, S. L., Simonsick, E. M., Wallace, R. B., & Blazer, D. G. (1995). Sleep complaints among elderly persons: An epidemiologic study of three communities. *Sleep*, *18*, 425–432.

Ford, D. E., & Kamerow, D. B. (1989). Epidemiologic study of sleep disturbances and psychiatric disorders. An opportunity for prevention? *Journal of the American Medical Association*, *262*, 1479–1484.

Fozard, J. L., Vercryssen, M., Reynolds, S. L., Hancock, P. A., & Quilter, R. E. (1994). Age differences and changes in reaction time: The Baltimore Longitudinal Study of Aging. *Journal of Gerontology*, *49*, P179–189.

Fukunaga, M., Horovitz, S. G., van Gelderen, P., de Zwart, J. A., Jansma, J. M., & Ikonomidou, V. N., et al., (2006). Large-amplitude, spatially correlated fluctuations in BOLD fMRI signals during extended rest and early sleep stages. *Magnetic Resonance Imaging*, *24*, 979–992.

Fulda, S., & Schulz, H. (2001). Cognitive dysfunction in sleep disorders. *Sleep Medicine Reviews*, *5*, 423–445.

Garcia-Larrea, L., Lukaszewicz, A. C., & Mauguiere, F. (1992). Revisiting the oddball paradigm. Non-target vs. neutral stimuli and the evaluation of ERP attentional effects. *Neuropsychologia*, *30*, 723–741.

Gianaros, P. J., Jennings, J. R., Sheu, L. K., Greer, P. J., Kuller, L. H., & Matthews, K. A. (2007). Prospective reports of chronic life stress predict decreased grey matter volume in the hippocampus. *Neuroimage*, *35*, 795–803.

Godet-Cayre, V., Pelletier-Fleury, N., Le Vaillant, M., Dinet, J., Massuel, M. A., & Leger, D. (2006). Insomnia and absenteeism at work. Who pays the cost? *Sleep*, *29*, 179–184.

Grady, C. L. (2008). Cognitive neuroscience of aging. *Annals of the New York Academy of Sciences*, *1124*, 127–144.

Grady, C. L., Maisog, J. M., Horwitz, B., Ungerleider, L. G., Mentis, M. J., & Salerno, J. A., et al., (1994). Age-related changes in cortical blood flow activation during visual processing of faces and location. *Journal of Neuroscience*, *14*, 1450–1462.

Grady, C. L., McIntosh, A. R., & Craik, F. I. (2005). Task-related activity in prefrontal cortex and its relation to recognition memory performance in young and old adults. *Neuropsychologia*, *43*, 1466–1481.

Grady, C. L., Springer, M. V., Hongwanishkul, D., McIntosh, A. R., & Winocur, G. (2006). Age-related changes in brain activity across the adult lifespan. *Journal of Cognitive Neuroscience*, *18*, 227–241.

Gunning-Dixon, F. M., Gur, R. C., Perkins, A. C., Schroeder, L., Turner, T., & Turetsky, B. I., et al., (2003). Age-related differences in brain activation during emotional face processing. *Neurobiology of Aging*, *24*, 285–295.

Hairston, I. S., Talbot, L. S., Eidelman, P., Gruber, J., & Harvey, A. G. (2010). Sensory gating in primary insomnia. *European Journal of Neuroscience*, *31*, 2112–2121.

Harper, D. G., Stopa, E. G., Kuo-Leblanc, V., McKee, A. C., Asayama, K., & Volicer, L., et al., (2008). Dorsomedial SCN neuronal subpopulations subserve different functions in human dementia. *Brain*, *131*, 1609–1617.

Harsh, J., Voss, U., Hull, J., Schrepfer, S., & Badia, P. (1994). ERP and behavioral changes during the wake/sleep transition. *Psychophysiology*, *31*, 244–252.

Hesselmann, V., Zaro Weber, O., Wedekind, C., Krings, T., Schulte, O., & Kugel, H., et al., (2001). Age related signal decrease in functional magnetic resonance imaging during motor stimulation in humans. *Neuroscience Letters*, *308*, 141–144.

Hooren, S. A., Valentijn, A. M., Bosma, H., Ponds, R. W., van Boxtel, M. P., & Jolles, J. (2007). Cognitive functioning in healthy older adults aged 64–81: A cohort study into the effects of age, sex, and education. *Neuropsychology, Development, and Cognition B: Aging Neuropsychology and Cognition*, *14*, 40–54.

Hudson, J. I., Pope, H. G., Sullivan, L. E., Waternaux, C. M., Keck, P. E., & Broughton, R. J. (1992). Good sleep, bad sleep: A meta-analysis of polysomnographic measures in insomnia, depression, and narcolepsy. *Biological Psychiatry*, *32*, 958–975.

Jelicic, M., Bosma, H., Ponds, R. W., Van Boxtel, M. P., Houx, P. J., & Jolles, J. (2002). Subjective sleep problems in later life as predictors of cognitive decline. Report from the Maastricht Ageing Study (MAAS). *International Journal of Geriatric Psychiatry*, *17*, 73–77.

Jessen, F., Wiese, B., Cvetanovska, G., Fuchs, A., Kaduszkiewicz, H., & Kolsch, H., et al., (2007). Patterns of subjective memory impairment in the elderly: Association with memory performance. *Psychological Medicine*, *37*, 1753–1762.

Kales, A., Caldwell, A. B., Soldatos, C. R., Bixler, E. O., & Kales, J. D. (1983). Biopsychobehavioral correlates of insomnia. II. Pattern specificity and consistency with the Minnesota Multiphasic Personality Inventory. *Psychosomatic Medicine*, *45*, 341–356.

Kales, A., Soldatos, C. R., & Kales, J. D. (1987). Sleep disorders: Insomnia, sleepwalking, night terrors, nightmares, and enuresis. *Annals of Internal Medicine*, *106*, 582–592.

Kaptein, K. I., De Jonge, P., Korf, J., Spijker, J., De Graaf, R., & van der Werf, S. Y. (2007). Random-mood interpretation of determinants for major depression. *Psychological Medicine*, *37*, 1261–1271.

Kato, M., Phillips, B. G., Sigurdsson, G., Narkiewicz, K., Pesek, C. A., & Somers, V. K. (2000). Effects of sleep deprivation on neural circulatory control. *Hypertension*, *35*, 1173–1175.

Kobayashi, M., & Pascual-Leone, A. (2003). Transcranial magnetic stimulation in neurology. *Lancet Neurology*, *2*, 145–156.

Kringelbach, M. L. (2005). The human orbitofrontal cortex: Linking reward to hedonic experience. *Nature Reviews Neuroscience*, *6*, 691–702.

Kringelbach, M. L., & Berridge, K. C. (2009). Towards a functional neuroanatomy of pleasure and happiness. *Trends in Cognitive Sciences*, *13*, 479–487.

Kringelbach, M. L., & Rolls, E. T. (2004). The functional neuroanatomy of the human orbitofrontal cortex: Evidence from neuroimaging and neuropsychology. *Progress in Neurobiology*, *72*, 341–372.

Kwong, K. K., Belliveau, J. W., Chesler, D. A., Goldberg, I. E., Weisskoff, R. M., & Poncelet, B. P., et al., (1992). Dynamic magnetic resonance imaging of human brain activity during primary sensory stimulation. *Proceedings of the National Academy of Sciences of the United States of America*, *89*, 5675–5679.

Lamarche, C. H., & Ogilvie, R. D. (1997). Electrophysiological changes during the sleep onset period of psychophysiological insomniacs, psychiatric insomniacs, and normal sleepers. *Sleep*, *20*, 724–733.

Landis, C. A., Savage, M. V., Lentz, M. J., & Brengelmann, G. L. (1998). Sleep deprivation alters body temperature dynamics to mild cooling and heating not sweating threshold in women. *Sleep*, *21*, 101–108.

Leger, D., Guilleminault, C., Bader, G., Levy, E., & Paillard, M. (2002). Medical and socio-professional impact of insomnia. *Sleep*, *25*, 625–629.

Lichstein, K. L., Durrence, H. H., Taylor, D. J., Bush, A. J., & Riedel, B. W. (2003). Quantitative criteria for insomnia. *Behavioral Research and Therapy*, *41*, 427–445.

Lombardo, C., Baglioni, C., Devoto, A., Lucidi, F., & Violani, C. (2008). Sympathetic arousal and arousability predicts subsequent sleep quality. *International Journal of Psychophysiology*, *69*, 224–1224.

Lugaresi, E., Zucconi, M., & Bixler, E. O. (1987). Epidemiology of sleep disorders. *Psychiatric Annals*, *17*, 446–450.

Lundh, L., Broman, J., Hetta, J., & Saboonchi, F. (1994). Perfectionism and insomnia. *Scandinavian Journal of Behaviour Therapy*, *23*, 3–18.

Malonek, D., & Grinvald, A. (1996). Interactions between electrical activity and cortical microcirculation revealed by imaging spectroscopy: Implications for functional brain mapping. *Science*, *272*, 551–554.

Mather, M., Canli, T., English, T., Whitfield, S., Wais, P., & Ochsner, K., et al., (2004). Amygdala responses to emotionally valenced stimuli in older and younger adults. *Psychological Science*, *15*, 259–263.

McGinley, M., Hoffman, R. L., Russ, D. W., Thomas, J. S., & Clark, B. C. (2010). Older adults exhibit more intracortical inhibition and less intracortical facilitation than young adults. *Experimental Gerontology*

Milner, C. E., Cuthbert, B. P., Kertesz, R. S., & Cote, K. A. (2009). Sensory gating impairments in poor sleepers during presleep wakefulness. *Neuroreport*, *20*, 331–336.

Morin, C. M., Rodrigue, S., & Ivers, H. (2003). Role of stress, arousal, and coping skills in primary insomnia. *Psychosomatic Medicine*, *65*, 259–267.

Morphy, H., Dunn, K. M., Lewis, M., Boardman, H. F., & Croft, P. R. (2007). Epidemiology of insomnia: A longitudinal study in a UK population. *Sleep*, *30*, 274–280.

Muenter, N. K., Watenpaugh, D. E., Wasmund, W. L., Wasmund, S. L., Maxwell, S. A., & Smith, M. L. (2000). Effect of sleep restriction on orthostatic cardiovascular control in humans. *Journal of Applied Physiology*, *88*, 966–972.

Munch, M., Knoblauch, V., Blatter, K., Schroder, C., Schnitzler, C., & Krauchi, K., et al., (2005). Age-related attenuation of the evening circadian arousal signal in humans. *Neurobiology of Aging*, *26*, 1307–1319.

Naatanen, R., & Picton, T. (1987). The N1 wave of the human electric and magnetic response to sound: A review and an analysis of the component structure. *Psychophysiology*, *24*, 375–425.

National Institutes of Health State of the Science Conference Statement. (2005). Manifestations and Management of Chronic Insomnia in Adults June 13–15, 2005. *Sleep*, *28*, 1049–1057.

Neylan, T. C., Mueller, S. G., Wang, Z., Metzler, T. J., Lenoci, M., & Truran, D., et al., (2010). Insomnia severity is associated with a decreased volume of the CA3/dentate gyrus hippocampal subfield. *Biological Psychiatry*, *68*, 494–496.

Nissen, C., Kloepfer, C., Nofzinger, E. A., Feige, B., Voderholzer, U., & Riemann, D. (2006). Impaired sleep-related memory consolidation in primary insomnia – A pilot study. *Sleep*, *29*, 1068–1073.

Nofzinger, E. A., Buysse, D. J., Germain, A., Price, J. C., Miewald, J. M., & Kupfer, D. J. (2004). Functional neuroimaging evidence for hyperarousal in insomnia. *American Journal of Psychiatry*, *161*, 2126–2128.

Ogawa, S., Lee, T. M., Kay, A. R., & Tank, D. W. (1990). Brain magnetic resonance imaging with contrast dependent on blood oxygenation. *Proceedings of the National Academy of Sciences of the United States of America*, *87*, 9868–9872.

Ogawa, S., Tank, D. W., Menon, R., Ellermann, J. M., Kim, S. G., & Merkle, H., et al., (1992). Intrinsic signal changes accompanying sensory stimulation: Functional brain mapping with magnetic resonance imaging. *Proceedings of the National Academy of Sciences of the United States of America*, *89*, 5951–5955.

Oosterman, J. M., van Someren, E. J., Vogels, R. L., Van Harten, B., & Scherder, E. J. (2009). Fragmentation of the rest-activity rhythm correlates with age-related cognitive deficits. *Journal of Sleep Research*, *18*, 129–135.

Orff, H. J., Drummond, S. P., Nowakowski, S., & Perils, M. L. (2007). Discrepancy between subjective symptomatology and objective neuropsychological performance in insomnia. *Sleep*, *30*, 1205–1211.

O'Sullivan, M., Jones, D. K., Summers, P. E., Morris, R. G., Williams, S. C., & Markus, H. S. (2001). Evidence for cortical "disconnection" as a mechanism of age-related cognitive decline. *Neurology*, *57*, 632–638.

Ozminkowski, R. J., Wang, S., & Walsh, J. K. (2007). The direct and indirect costs of untreated insomnia in adults in the United States. *Sleep*, *30*, 263–273.

Pallesen, S., Nordhus, I. H., Kvale, G., Havik, O. E., Nielsen, G. H., & Johnsen, B. H., et al., (2002). Psychological characteristics of elderly insomniacs. *Scandinavian Journal of Psychology*, *43*, 425–432.

Pavlova, M., Berg, O., Gleason, R., Walker, F., Roberts, S., & Regestein, Q. (2001). Self-reported hyperarousal traits among insomnia patients. *Journal of Psychosomatic Research*, *51*, 435–441.

Perlis, M. L., Kehr, E. L., Smith, M. T., Andrews, P. J., Orff, H., & Giles, D. E. (2001). Temporal and stagewise distribution of high frequency EEG activity in patients with primary and secondary insomnia and in good sleeper controls. *Journal of Sleep Research*, *10*, 93–104.

Polich, J. (2007). Updating P300: An integrative theory of P3a and P3b. *Clinical Neurophysiology*, *118*, 2128–2148.

Ponds, R. W., Van Boxtel, M. P., & Jolles, J. (2000). Age-related changes in subjective cognitive functioning. *Educational Gerontology*, *26*, 67–81.

Rajah, M. N., & D'Esposito, M. (2005). Region-specific changes in prefrontal function with age: A review of PET and fMRI studies on working and episodic memory. *Brain*, *128*, 1964–1983.

Raymann, R. J., & Van Someren, E. J. (2007). Time-on-task impairment of psychomotor vigilance is affected by mild skin warming and changes with aging and insomnia. *Sleep*, *30*, 96–103.

Raymann, R. J., & Van Someren, E. J. (2008). Diminished capability to recognize the optimal temperature for sleep initiation may contribute to poor sleep in elderly people. *Sleep*, *31*, 1301–1309.

Raymann, R. J. E. M., Swaab, D. F., & Van Someren, E. J. W. (2008). Skin deep: Cutaneous temperature determines sleep depth. *Brain*, *131*, 500–513.

Rees, K., Allen, D., & Lader, M. (1999). The influences of age and caffeine on psychomotor and cognitive function. *Psychopharmacology*, *145*, 181–188.

Regestein, Q. R., Dambrosia, J., Hallett, M., Murawski, B., & Paine, M. (1993). Daytime alertness in patients with primary insomnia. *American Journal of Psychiatry*, *150*, 1529–1534.

Reite, M., Buysse, D., Reynolds, C., & Mendelson, W. (1995). The use of polysomnography in the evaluation of insomnia. *Sleep*, *18*, 58–70.

Resnick, S. M., Pham, D. L., Kraut, M. A., Zonderman, A. B., & Davatzikos, C. (2003). Longitudinal magnetic resonance imaging studies of older adults: A shrinking brain. *Journal of Neuroscience*, *23*, 3295–3301.

Reuter-Lorenz, P. A., & Lustig, C. (2005). Brain aging: Reorganizing discoveries about the aging mind. *Current Opinion in Neurobiology*, *15*, 245–251.

Reuter-Lorenz, P. A., Jonides, J., Smith, E. E., Hartley, A., Miller, A., & Marshuetz, C., et al., (2000). Age differences in the frontal lateralization of verbal and spatial working memory revealed by PET. *Journal of Cognitive Neuroscience*, *12*, 174–187.

Riedel, B. W., & Lichstein, K. L. (2000). Insomnia and daytime functioning. *Sleep Medicine Reviews*, *4*, 277–298.

Riemann, D., Voderholzer, U., Spiegelhalder, K., Hornyak, M., Buysse, D. J., & Nissen, C., et al., (2007). Chronic insomnia and MRI-measured hippocampal volumes: A pilot study. *Sleep*, *30*, 955–958.

Rodenbeck, A., Huether, G., Ruther, E., & Hajak, G. (2002). Interactions between evening and nocturnal cortisol secretion and sleep parameters in patients with severe chronic primary insomnia. *Neuroscience Letters*, *324*, 159–163.

Rolls, E. T., Grabenhorst, F., & Parris, B. A. (2008). Warm pleasant feelings in the brain. *Neuroimage*, *41*, 1504–1513.

Rombaut, N., Maillard, F., Kelly, F., & Hindmarch, I. (1990). The quality of life of insomniacs questionnaire (QOLI). *Medical Science Research*, *18*, 845–847.

Roth, T., & Ancoli-Israel, S. (1999). Daytime consequences and correlates of insomnia in the United States: Results of the 1991 National Sleep Foundation Survey. II. *Sleep*, *22*(Suppl. 2); S354–S358.

Salat, D. H., Lee, S. Y., van der Kouwe, A. J., Greve, D. N., Fischl, B., & Rosas, H. D. (2009). Age-associated alterations in cortical gray and white matter signal intensity and gray to white matter contrast. *Neuroimage*, *48*, 21–28.

Sambataro, F., Murty, V. P., Callicott, J. H., Tan, H. Y., Das, S., & Weinberger, D. R., et al., (2010). Age-related alterations in default mode network: Impact on working memory performance. *Neurobiology of Aging*, *31*, 839–852.

Sateia, M. J. (2009). Update on sleep and psychiatric disorders. *Chest*, *135*, 1370–1379.

Sateia, M. J., Doghramji, K., Hauri, P. J., & Morin, C. M. (2000). Evaluation of chronic insomnia. *Sleep*, *23*, 243–308.

Saykin, A. J., Wishart, H. A., Rabin, L. A., Santulli, R. B., Flashman, L. A., & West, J. D., et al., (2006). Older adults with cognitive complaints show brain atrophy similar to that of amnestic MCI. *Neurology*, *67*, 834–842.

Scherder, E. J. A., Van Someren, E. J. W., & Swaab, D. F (1999). Transcutaneous Electrical Nerve Stimulation (TENS) improves the rest-activity rhythm in midstage Alzheimer's disease. *Behavioural Brain Research*, *101*, 105–107.

Schmand, B., Jonker, C., Geerlings, M. I., & Lindeboom, J. (1997). Subjective memory complaints in the elderly: Depressive symptoms and future dementia. *British Journal of Psychiatry*, *171*, 373–376.

Seidler, R. D., Bernard, J. A., Burutolu, T. B., Fling, B. W., Gordon, M. T., & Gwin, J. T., et al., (2010). Motor control and aging: Links to age-related brain structural, functional, and biochemical effects. *Neuroscience & Biobehavioral Reviews*, *34*, 721–733.

Sforza, E., & Haba-Rubio, J. (2006). Event-related potentials in patients with insomnia and sleep-related breathing disorders: Evening-to-morning changes. *Sleep*, *29*, 805–813.

Shaver, J. L., Johnston, S. K., Lentz, M. J., & Landis, C. A. (2002). Stress exposure, psychological distress, and physiological stress activation in midlife women with insomnia. *Psychosomatic Medicine*, *64*, 793–802.

Shochat, T., Umphress, J., Israel, A. G., & Ancoli-Israel, S. (1999). Insomnia in primary care patients. *Sleep*, *22*(Suppl. 2); S359–S365.

Simon, G. E., & VonKorff, M. (1997). Prevalence, burden, and treatment of insomnia in primary care. *American Journal of Psychiatry*, *154*, 1417–1423.

Smith, M. T., Perlis, M. L., Chengazi, V. U., Pennington, J., Soeffing, J., & Ryan, J. M., et al., (2002). Neuroimaging of NREM sleep in primary insomnia: A Tc-99-HMPAO single photon emission computed tomography study. *Sleep*, *25*, 325–335.

Smith, M. T., Perlis, M. L., Chengazi, V. U., Soeffing, J., & McCann, U. (2005). NREM sleep cerebral blood flow before and after behavior therapy for chronic primary insomnia: Preliminary single photon emission computed tomography (SPECT) data. *Sleep Medicine*, *6*, 93–94.

Spielman, A. J. (1986). Assessment of insomnia. *Clinical Psychology Review*, *6*, 11–25.

Staffen, W., Mair, A., Zauner, H., Unterrainer, J., Niederhofer, H., & Kutzelnigg, A., et al., (2002). Cognitive function and fMRI in patients with multiple sclerosis: Evidence for compensatory cortical activation during an attention task. *Brain*, *125*, 1275–1282.

Staner, L., Cornette, F., Maurice, D., Viardot, G., Le Bon, O., & Haba, J., et al., (2003). Sleep microstructure around sleep onset differentiates major depressive insomnia from primary insomnia. *Journal of Sleep Research*, *12*, 319–330.

Stepanski, E. J., & Rybarczyk, B. (2006). Emerging research on the treatment and etiology of secondary or comorbid insomnia. *Sleep Medicine Reviews*, *10*, 7–18.

Stepanski, E. J., Zorick, F., Roehrs, T., Young, D., & Roth, T. (1988). Daytime alertness in patients with chronic insomnia compared with asymptomatic control subjects. *Sleep*, *11*, 54–60.

Szelenberger, W., & Niemcewicz, S. (2000). Severity of insomnia correlates with cognitive impairment. *Acta Neurobiologiae Experimentalis*, *60*, 373.

Szelenberger, W., & Niemcewicz, S. (2001). Event-related current density in primary insomnia. *Acta Neurobiologiae Experimentalis*, *61*, 299–308.

Thambisetty, M., Wan, J., Carass, A., An, Y., Prince, J. L., & Resnick, S. M. (2010). Longitudinal changes in cortical thickness associated with normal aging. *Neuroimage*

Tisserand, D. J., McIntosh, A. R., van der Veen, F. M., Backes, W. H., & Jolles, J. (2005). Age-related reorganization of encoding networks directly influences subsequent recognition memory. *Brain Research. Cognitive Brain Research*, *25*, 8–18.

Tisserand, D. J., Pruessner, J. C., Sanz Arigita, E. J., van Boxtel, M. P., Evans, A. C., & Jolles, J., et al., (2002). Regional frontal cortical volumes decrease differentially in aging: An MRI study to compare volumetric approaches and voxel-based morphometry. *Neuroimage*, *17*, 657–669.

Turcotte, I., & Bastien, C. H. (2009). Is quality of sleep related to the N1 and P2 ERPs in chronic psychophysiological insomnia sufferers? *International Journal of Psychophysio- logy*, *72*, 314–322.

Van Der Werf, Y. D., Altena, E., Van Dijk, K. D., Strijers, R. L., Rijke, W. D., & Stam, C. J., et al., (2010). Is disturbed intracortical excitability a stable trait of chronic insomnia? A study using transcranial magnetic stimulation before and after multimodal sleep therapy. *Biological Psychiatry*. doi: 10.1016/j.biopsych.2010.06.028

Van Der Werf, Y. D., Tisserand, D. J., Visser, P. J., Hofman, P. A., Vuurman, E., & Uylings, H. B., et al., (2001). Thalamic volume predicts performance on tests of cognitive speed and decreases in healthy aging. A magnetic resonance imaging-based volumetric analysis. *Cognitive Brain Research*, *11*, 377–385.

Van Someren, E. J. (2000). Circadian and sleep disturbances in the elderly. *Experimental Gerontology*, *35*, 1229–1237.

Van Someren, E. J. W. (2004). Sleep propensity is modulated by circadian and behavior-induced changes in cutaneous temperature. *Journal of Thermal Biology*, *29*, 437–444.

Van Someren, E. J. W., Pollmächer, T., Leger, D., Espie, C., Bassetti, C., & Riemann, D. (2009). The European insomnia network. *Frontiers in Neuroscience*, *3*, 436.

Van Someren, E. J. W., Raymann, R. J. E. M., Scherder, E. J. A., Daanen, H. A. M., & Swaab, D. F. (2002). Circadian and age-related modulation of thermoreception and temperature regulation: Mechanisms and functional implications. *Aging Research Reviews*, *1*, 721–778.

Van Someren, E. J. W., Scherder, E. J. A., & Swaab, D. F. (1998). Transcutaneous electrical nerve stimulation (TENS) improves circadian rhythm disturbances in Alzheimer's disease. *Alzheimer Disease and Associated Disorders*, *12*, 114–118.

Varkevisser, M., & Kerkhof, G. A. (2005). Chronic insomnia and performance in a 24-h constant routine study. *Journal of Sleep Research*, *14*, 49–59.

Vgontzas, A. N., Bixler, E. O., Lin, H. M., Prolo, P., Mastorakos, G., & Vela-Bueno, A., et al., (2001). Chronic insomnia is associated with nyctohemeral activation of the hypothalamic-pituitary-adrenal axis: Clinical implications. *Journal of Clinical Endocrinology & Metabolism*, *86*, 3787–3794.

Vgontzas, A. N., Zoumakis, M., Papanicolaou, D. A., Bixler, E. O., Prolo, P., & Lin, H. M., et al., (2002). Chronic insomnia is associated with a shift of interleukin-6 and tumor necrosis factor secretion from nighttime to daytime. *Metabolism: Clinical & Experimental*, *51*, 887–892.

Vincent, N. K., & Walker, J. R. (2000). Perfectionism and chronic insomnia. *Journal of Psychosomatic Research*, *49*, 349–354.

Voineskos, A. N., Rajji, T. K., Lobaugh, N. J., Miranda, D., Shenton, M. E., & Kennedy, J. L., et al., (2010). Age-related decline in white matter tract integrity and cognitive performance: A DTI tractography and structural equation modeling study. *Neurobiology of Aging*. doi: 10.1016/j.neurobiolaging.2010.02.009.

Winkelman, J. W., Benson, K. L., Buxton, O. M., Lyoo, I. K., Yoon, S., & O'Connor, S., et al., (2010). Lack of hippocampal volume differences in primary insomnia and good sleeper controls: An MRI volumetric study at 3 Tesla. *Sleep Medicine*, *11*, 576–582.

Yang, C. M., & Lo, H. S. (2007). ERP evidence of enhanced excitatory and reduced inhibitory processes of auditory stimuli during sleep in patients with primary insomnia. *Sleep*, *30*, 585–592.

Zammit, G. K., Weiner, J., Damato, N., Sillup, G. P., & McMillan, C. A. (1999). Quality of life in people with insomnia. *Sleep*, *22*(Suppl. 2); S379–S385.

Zhang, B., & Wing, Y. K. (2006). Sex differences in insomnia: A meta-analysis. *Sleep*, *29*, 85–93.

Zhu, C., Guo, X., Jin, Z., Sun, J., Qiu, Y., & Zhu, Y., et al., (2010). Influences of brain development and ageing on cortical interactive networks. *Clinical Neurophysiology*. doi: 10.1016/j.clinph.2010.06.016.

Index

D

E

F

G

H

I

J

K

L

M

N

O

P

Q

R

S

T

V

W

Volume 149: Cortical Function: A View from the Thalamus, by V.A. Casagrande, R.W. Guillery and S.M. Sherman (Eds.) – 2005, ISBN 0-444-51679-4.
Volume 150: The Boundaries of Consciousness: Neurobiology and Neuropathology, by Steven Laureys (Ed.) – 2005, ISBN 0-444-51851-7.
Volume 151: Neuroanatomy of the Oculomotor System, by J.A. Büttner-Ennever (Ed.) – 2006, ISBN 0-444-51696-4.
Volume 152: Autonomic Dysfunction after Spinal Cord Injury, by L.C. Weaver and C. Polosa (Eds.) – 2006, ISBN 0-444-51925-4.
Volume 153: Hypothalamic Integration of Energy Metabolism, by A. Kalsbeek, E. Fliers, M.A. Hofman, D.F. Swaab, E.J.W. Van Someren and R.M. Buijs (Eds.) – 2006, ISBN 978-0-444-52261-0.
Volume 154: Visual Perception, Part 1, Fundamentals of Vision: Low and Mid-Level Processes in Perception, by S. Martinez-Conde, S.L. Macknik, L.M. Martinez, J.M. Alonso and P.U. Tse (Eds.) – 2006, ISBN 978-0-444-52966-4.
Volume 155: Visual Perception, Part 2, Fundamentals of Awareness, Multi-Sensory Integration and High-Order Perception, by S. Martinez-Conde, S.L. Macknik, L.M. Martinez, J.M. Alonso and P.U. Tse (Eds.) – 2006, ISBN 978-0-444-51927-6.
Volume 156: Understanding Emotions, by S. Anders, G. Ende, M. Junghofer, J. Kissler and D. Wildgruber (Eds.) – 2006, ISBN 978-0-444-52182-8.
Volume 157: Reprogramming of the Brain, by A.R. Møller (Ed.) – 2006, ISBN 978-0-444-51602-2.
Volume 158: Functional Genomics and Proteomics in the Clinical Neurosciences, by S.E. Hemby and S. Bahn (Eds.) – 2006, ISBN 978-0-444-51853-8.
Volume 159: Event-Related Dynamics of Brain Oscillations, by C. Neuper and W. Klimesch (Eds.) – 2006, ISBN 978-0-444-52183-5.
Volume 160: GABA and the Basal Ganglia: From Molecules to Systems, by J.M. Tepper, E.D. Abercrombie and J.P. Bolam (Eds.) – 2007, ISBN 978-0-444-52184-2.
Volume 161: Neurotrauma: New Insights into Pathology and Treatment, by J.T. Weber and A.I.R. Maas (Eds.) – 2007, ISBN 978-0-444-53017-2.
Volume 162: Neurobiology of Hyperthermia, by H.S. Sharma (Ed.) – 2007, ISBN 978-0-444-51926-9.
Volume 163: The Dentate Gyrus: A Comprehensive Guide to Structure, Function, and Clinical Implications, by H.E. Scharfman (Ed.) – 2007, ISBN 978-0-444-53015-8.
Volume 164: From Action to Cognition, by C. von Hofsten and K. Rosander (Eds.) – 2007, ISBN 978-0-444-53016-5.
Volume 165: Computational Neuroscience: Theoretical Insights into Brain Function, by P. Cisek, T. Drew and J.F. Kalaska (Eds.) – 2007, ISBN 978-0-444-52823-0.
Volume 166: Tinnitus: Pathophysiology and Treatment, by B. Langguth, G. Hajak, T. Kleinjung, A. Cacace and A.R. Møller (Eds.) – 2007, ISBN 978-0-444-53167-4.
Volume 167: Stress Hormones and Post Traumatic Stress Disorder: Basic Studies and Clinical Perspectives, by E.R. de Kloet, M.S. Oitzl and E. Vermetten (Eds.) – 2008, ISBN 978-0-444-53140-7.
Volume 168: Models of Brain and Mind: Physical, Computational and Psychological Approaches, by R. Banerjee and B.K. Chakrabarti (Eds.) – 2008, ISBN 978-0-444-53050-9.
Volume 169: Essence of Memory, by W.S. Sossin, J.-C. Lacaille, V.F. Castellucci and S. Belleville (Eds.) – 2008, ISBN 978-0-444-53164-3.
Volume 170: Advances in Vasopressin and Oxytocin – From Genes to Behaviour to Disease, by I.D. Neumann and R. Landgraf (Eds.) – 2008, ISBN 978-0-444-53201-5.
Volume 171: Using Eye Movements as an Experimental Probe of Brain Function—A Symposium in Honor of Jean Büttner-Ennever, by Christopher Kennard and R. John Leigh (Eds.) – 2008, ISBN 978-0-444-53163-6.
Volume 172: Serotonin–Dopamine Interaction: Experimental Evidence and Therapeutic Relevance, by Giuseppe Di Giovanni, Vincenzo Di Matteo and Ennio Esposito (Eds.) – 2008, ISBN 978-0-444-53235-0.
Volume 173: Glaucoma: An Open Window to Neurodegeneration and Neuroprotection, by Carlo Nucci, Neville N. Osborne, Giacinto Bagetta and Luciano Cerulli (Eds.) – 2008, ISBN 978-0-444-53256-5.
Volume 174: Mind and Motion: The Bidirectional Link Between Thought and Action, by Markus Raab, Joseph G. Johnson and Hauke R. Heekeren (Eds.) – 2009, 978-0-444-53356-2.
Volume 175: Neurotherapy: Progress in Restorative Neuroscience and Neurology — Proceedings of the 25th International Summer School of Brain Research, held at the Royal Netherlands Academy of Arts and Sciences, Amsterdam, The Netherlands, August 25–28, 2008, by J. Verhaagen, E.M. Hol, I. Huitinga, J. Wijnholds, A.A. Bergen, G.J. Boer and D.F. Swaab (Eds.) – 2009, ISBN 978-0-12-374511-8.
Volume 176: Attention, by Narayanan Srinivasan (Ed.) – 2009, ISBN 978-0-444-53426-2.
Volume 177: Coma Science: Clinical and Ethical Implications, by Steven Laureys, Nicholas D. Schiff and Adrian M. Owen (Eds.) – 2009, ISBN 978-0-444-53432-3.

Volume 178: Cultural Neuroscience: Cultural Influences On Brain Function, by Joan Y. Chiao (Ed.) – 2009, ISBN 978-0-444-53361-6.
Volume 179: Genetic models of schizophrenia, by Akira Sawa (Ed.) – 2009, ISBN 978-0-444-53430-9.
Volume 180: Nanoneuroscience and Nanoneuropharmacology, by Hari Shanker Sharma (Ed.) – 2009, ISBN 978-0-444-53431-6.
Volume 181: Neuroendocrinology: The Normal Neuroendocrine System, by Luciano Martini, George P. Chrousos, Fernand Labrie, Karel Pacak and Donald W. Pfaff (Eds.) – 2010, ISBN 978-0-444-53617-4.
Volume 182: Neuroendocrinology: Pathological Situations and Diseases, by Luciano Martini, George P. Chrousos, Fernand Labrie, Karel Pacak and Donald W. Pfaff (Eds.) – 2010, ISBN 978-0-444-53616-7.
Volume 183: Recent Advances in Parkinson's Disease: Basic Research, by Anders Björklund and M. Angela Cenci (Eds.) – 2010, ISBN 978-0-444-53614-3.
Volume 184: Progress in Brain Research: Recent Advances in Parkinson's Disease: Translational and Clinical Research, by Anders Björklund and M. Angela Cenci (Eds.) – 2010, ISBN 978-0-444-53702-7.